Puberty

Philip Kumanov • Ashok Agarwal
Editors

Puberty

Physiology and Abnormalities

Springer

Editors
Philip Kumanov
Medical University of Sofia
Sofia, Bulgaria

Ashok Agarwal
American Center for Reproductive Medicine
Cleveland Clinic Foundation
Cleveland, OH, USA

ISBN 978-3-319-32120-2 ISBN 978-3-319-32122-6 (eBook)
DOI 10.1007/978-3-319-32122-6

Library of Congress Control Number: 2016948364

Printed on acid-free paper

This Springer imprint is published by Springer Nature
The registered company is Springer International Publishing AG Switzerland

Preface

'T was strange that one so young should thus concern
His brain about the action of the sky;
If you think 't was philosophy that this did,
I can't help thinking puberty assisted.

Lord Byron "*Don Juan*"
Canto the First, XCIII

The exact neuroendocrinological mechanisms that bring childhood to an end still remain unclear, and the subsequent period of puberty represents a sequence of profound hormonal, physical, and psychical changes. The social relationships of maturing individuals are likewise altered. The transition from girl to woman and from boy to man, respectively, is a time of raised concerns: Both parents and children constantly worry about growth and sexual maturation advancing normally. Some diseases, hidden to this point, become apparent. As a complex process of profound changes, puberty is one of the most vulnerable periods of life. No one has represented so skillfully the drama of those who are no longer children but not yet mature, overshadowed by the dark uncertainty of the future, as the Norwegian artist Edvard Munch in his masterpiece, *Puberty*.

With that in mind, the need for a comprehensive textbook on the growth and development of children, as well as on the most important abnormalities and deviations of puberty, is more than imperative. The responsibility of the medical community to growing children is substantial, as this period of transformation from childhood to maturity is crucial for lifelong health. An insufficient or inadequate approach to the mental or physical stability of adolescents may have serious consequences afterwards. The problem has escalated in the last few decades given the aging population and lower worldwide birth rates. Normal reproduction would be impossible without a healthy puberty.

This book is mainly clinically oriented but extends to also cover corresponding theoretical aspects. It will be useful for pediatricians, endocrinologists, gynecologists, andrologists, urologists, family practitioners, child psychologists, and public health specialists—all those who are challenged in their everyday practice with the problems of puberty. The chapters are prepared by internationally reputed experts, whose contributions are thankfully acknowledged.

Throughout the book, the reader should keep in mind that the second most remarkable phenomenon, after birth of normal child, is its transition to a healthy mature person.

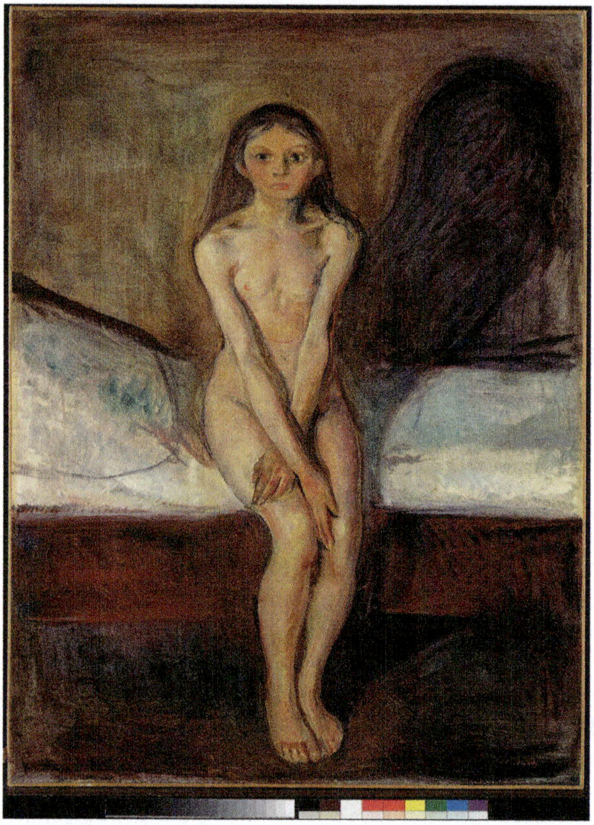

Edvard Munch "Puberty"

The National Museum of Art, Architecture and Design, Oslo

[Reprinted with kind permission from National Museum of Art, Architecture and Design]

Sofia, Bulgaria
Cleveland, United States
July 2016

Philip Kumanov, MD, PhD, DMedSci
Ashok Agarwal, PhD

Contents

1 **Maturation and Physiology of Hypothalamic Regulation of the Gonadal Axis** 1
Yoshihisa Uenoyama, Naoko Inoue, Nahoko Ieda, Vutha Pheng, Kei-ichiro Maeda, and Hiroko Tsukamura

2 **Genetics of Puberty** 13
Shehla Tabassum and Salman Kirmani

3 **Hormonal Changes in Childhood and Puberty** 23
Rodolfo A. Rey, Stella M. Campo, María Gabriela Ropelato, and Ignacio Bergadá

4 **Physical Changes During Pubertal Transition** 39
Ralitsa Robeva and Philip Kumanov

5 **Growth in Childhood and Puberty** 65
Michael Hermanussen

6 **Bone Development in Children and Adolescents** 77
Mihail A. Boyanov

7 **Body Weight and Puberty** 95
Analia Tomova

8 **The Environmental Factors and Epigenetics of Gametogenesis in Puberty** 109
Sezgin Gunes and Mehmet Alper Arslan

9 **Timing of Puberty and Secular Trend in Human Maturation** 121
Anastasios Papadimitriou

10 **Precocious Puberty** 137
Juliane Léger and Jean-Claude Carel

11 **Constitutional Delayed Puberty** 155
Peter A. Lee and Christopher P. Houk

12 Pubertal Dysfunction: A Disorder of GnRH Pulsatility 169
Lauren C. Passby, Kavitha Rozario, and Jyothis T. George

13 Pubertal Gynecomastia 183
Philip Kumanov

14 Pubertal Acne 197
Devinder Mohan Thappa and Munisamy Malathi

15 Adolescent Varicocele 211
Ahmad Majzoub and Edmund Sabanegh Jr.

16 Polycystic Ovary Syndrome in Adolescent Girls 229
Sajal Gupta, Elizabeth Pandithurai, and Ashok Agarwal

17 Growth Hormone and Steroid Assays' Problems in Childhood and Puberty 247
Dobrin A. Svinarov

18 Psychosocial Development of Adolescents With and Without Deviations 263
Yolanda N. Evans

19 Substance Use in Adolescence 273
Candice E. Van Skike, Shannon L. Zandy, and Douglas B. Matthews

Index 287

Contributors

Ashok Agarwal, PhD, HCLD (ABB), ELD (ACE) American Center for Reproductive Medicine, Cleveland Clinic, Cleveland, OH, USA

Mehmet Alper Arslan, PhD Department of Medical Biology, Faculty of Medicine, Health Sciences Institute, Samsun, Turkey

Department of Multidisciplinary Molecular Medicine, Health Sciences Institute, Ondokuz Mayis University, Samsun, Turkey

Ignacio Bergadá, MD Centro de Investigaciones Endocirnológicas "Dr. César Bergadá" (CEDIE), CONICET-FEI-División de Endocirnología, Hospital de Niños Ricardo Gutiérrez, Buenos Aires, Argentina

Mihail A. Boyanov, PhD, DMSc Department of Internal Medicine, Clinic of Endocrinology and Metabolism, University Hospital Alexandrovska, Medical University Sofia, Sofia, Bulgaria

Stella M. Campo, MSc, PhD Centro de Investigaciones Endocirnológicas "Dr. César Bergadá" (CEDIE), CONICET-FEI-División de Endocirnología, Hospital de Niños Ricardo Gutiérrez, Buenos Aires, Argentina

Jean-Claude Carel, MD Department of Paediatric, Endocrinology and Diabetology, INSERM UMR 1141, DHU PROTECT, Reference Center for Rare Endocrine Growth Diseases, Denis Diderot Paris 7 University, Hôpital Robert Debré, Paris, France

Yolanda N. Evans, MD, MPH Department of Pediatrics, Seattle Children's Hospital/University of Washington, Seattle, WA, USA

Jyothis T. George, PhD, FRCP Royal Berkshire Hospital, Reading, UK

Boehringer Ingelheim, Bracknell, UK

Sezgin Gunes, PhD Department of Medical Biology, Faculty of Medicine, Ondokuz Mayis University, Samsun, Turkey

Department of Multidisciplinary Molecular Medicine, Health Sciences Institute, Ondokuz Mayis University, Samsun, Turkey

Sajal Gupta, MD Andrology Center, Cleveland Clinic, Cleveland, OH, USA

Michael Hermanussen, PhD, MD Aschauhof 3, Altenhof, Germany

Christopher P. Houk, MD Department of Pediatrics, Georgia Regents University, Augusta, GA, USA

Nahoko Ieda, PhD Graduate School of Bioagricultural Sciences, Nagoya University, Nagoya, Aichi, Japan

Naoko Inoue, PhD Graduate School of Bioagricultural Sciences, Nagoya University, Nagoya, Aichi, Japan

Salman Kirmani, MBBS, FABP, FABMG Departments of Paediatrics and Child Health, Aga Khan University Hospital, Karachi, Sindh, Pakistan

Philip Kumanov, MD, PhD, DMedSci Clinical Center of Endocrinology, Medical Faculty, Medical University of Sofia, Sofia, Bulgaria

Peter A. Lee, MD, PhD Department of Pediatrics, Hershey Medical Center, Penn State College of Medicine, Hershey, PA, USA

Juliane Léger, MD Department of Paediatric Endocrinology and Diabetology, INSERM UMR 1141, DHU PROTECT, Reference Center for Rare Endocrine Growth Diseases, Denis Diderot Paris 7 University, Hopital Robert Debre, Paris, France

Kei-ichiro Maeda, DVM, PhD Graduate School of Agricultural and Life Sciences, The University of Tokyo, Tokyo, Japan

Ahmad Majzoub, MD Department of Urology, Glickman Urological and Kidney Institute/Cleveland Clinic Foundation, Cleveland, OH, USA

Munisamy Malathi, MD, DNB Department of Dermatology and Sexually Transmitted Diseases, Jawaharlal Institute of Postgraduate Medical Education and Research (JIPMER), Puducherry, Pondicherry, India

Douglas B. Matthews, PhD Department of Psychology, University of Wisconsin-Eau Claire, Eau Claire, WI, USA

Elizabeth Pandithurai, MBBS Department of Urology, Cleveland Clinic, Cleveland, OH, USA

Anastasios Papadimitriou, MD Third Department of Pediatrics, 'Attikon' University Hospital, Athens, Greece

Lauren C. Passby, BA (Hons) (Oxon) Medical Sciences Division, University of Oxford, John Radcliffe Hospital, Oxford, Oxfordshire, UK

Vutha Pheng Asian Satellite Campus-Cambodia, Nagoya University, Phnom Penh, Cambodia

Rodolfo A. Rey, MD, PhD Centro de Investigaciones Endocirnológicas "Dr. César Bergadá" (CEDIE), CONICET-FEI-División de Endocirnología, Hospital de Niños Ricardo Gutiérrez, Buenos Aires, Argentina

Ralitsa Robeva, MD, PhD Clinical Center of Endocrinology, Medical Faculty, Medical University of Sofia, Sofia, Bulgaria

María Gabriela Ropelato, MSc, PhD Centro de Investigaciones Endocirnológicas, CONICET-FEI-División de Endocirnología, Hospital de Niños Ricardo Gutiérrez, Buenos Aires, Argentina

Kavitha Rozario, MBBS, MRCPCH Department of Paediatric Endocrinology, Oxford University Hospitals NHS Foundation Trust, Oxford, UK

Edmund Sabanegh Jr., MD Department of Urology, Glickman Urological and Kidney Institute, Cleveland Clinic Foundation, Cleveland, OH, USA

Candice E. Van Skike, PhD Department of Pharmaceutical Sciences, University of Kentucky, Lexington, KY, USA

Dobrin A. Svinarov, MD, PhD, Dr Med Sc Department of Therapeutic Drug Management and Clinical Pharmacology, Alexander Hospital, Medical University of Sofia, Sofia, Bulgaria

Shehla Tabassum, MBBS, FCPS Department of Diabetes, Endocrinology and Metabolism, Aga Khan University, Karachi, Pakistan

Devinder Mohan Thappa, MD, DHA, FAMS, FIMSA Department of Dermatology and Sexually Transmitted Diseases, Jawaharlal Institute of Postgraduate Medical Education and Research (JIPMER), Puducherry, Pondicherry, India

Analia Tomova, MD, PhD Clinical Center of Endocrinology, Medical Faculty, Medical University of Sofia, Sofia, Bulgaria

Hiroko Tsukamura, PhD Graduate School of Bioagricultural Sciences, Nagoya University, Nagoya, Aichi, Japan

Yoshihisa Uenoyama, PhD Graduate School of Bioagricultural Sciences, Nagoya University, Nagoya, Aichi, Japan

Shannon L. Zandy, PharmD Department of Pharmacy, The University of Texas at Austin, Austin, TX, USA

Abbreviations

BMD	Bone mineral density
BMI	Body mass index
BPA	Bisphenol A
CALIPER	Canadian Laboratory Initiative on Pediatric Reference Interval Database
CB1Rs	Cannabinoid-1 receptors
CBG	Cortisol binding globulin
CDGP	Constitutional delay of growth and puberty
CDP	Constitutional delayed puberty
CGIs	CpG islands
CYP19A1	Cytochrome P 450 19 A1
DBCP	Dibromochloropropane
DDT	Dichlorodiphenyltrichloroethane
DHEA	Dehydroepiandrosterone
DHEAS	DHEA-sulfate
DNMTs	DNA methyltransferases
e-cigarette	Electronic cigarette
EDC	Endocrine disrupting chemicals
endo-siRNAs	Endogenous sinus
FSH	Follicle stimulating hormone
GALP	Galanin-like peptide
GC-MS	Gas chromatography-mass spectrometry
GH	Growth hormone
GHBP	Growth hormone binding protein
GHD	GH deficiency
GHRH	GH-releasing hormone
GnRH	Gonadotropin-releasing hormone
GNRH	Gonadotropin-releasing hormone
GNRHR	Gonadotropin-releasing hormone receptor
H	Histone
HDM	Histone demethylases

HPC	Hypothalamic-pituitary-gonadal
HTM	Methyltransferases
IA(s)	Immunoassay(s)
ID-MS	Isotope dilution MS
IGF	Insulin-like growth factor
IGFBP	IGF-binding protein
IGF-I	Insulin-like growth factor-I
IHH	Idiopathic hypogonadotopic hypogonadism
IS	International standard
K	Lysine
KISS-1	Kisspeptin 1
LC-MS	Liquid chromatography coupled to mass spectrometry
LC-MS/MS	Liquid chromatography coupled to tandem mass spectrometry
LH	Luteinizing hormone
miRNAs	MicroRNAs
MS	Mass spectrometry
nAChR	Nicotinic acetylcholine receptor
NHANES	National Health and Nutrition Examination Survey
NIBSC	National Institute of Biological Standards and Control
NPY	Neuropeptide Y
PCBs	Polychlorinated biphenyls
POP	Persistent organic pollutants
QC	Quality control
RISC	RNA-induced silencing complex
SHBG	Sex hormone binding globulin
THC	Δ9-Tetrahydrocannabinol
TPs	Transition proteins
UTR	Untranslated region

Chapter 1
Maturation and Physiology of Hypothalamic Regulation of the Gonadal Axis

Yoshihisa Uenoyama, Naoko Inoue, Nahoko Ieda, Vutha Pheng, Kei-ichiro Maeda, and Hiroko Tsukamura

Introduction

It is well accepted that the hypothalamus plays a pinnacle role in the hierarchical control of the gonadal axis through the anterior lobe of the pituitary gland in mammals. The concept of hypothalamic regulation of the gonadal axis dates back to the late 1940s, when Geoffrey Harris and colleagues [1] predicted the presence of neurohumoral substances, which control the pituitary gland. By this time, two gonadotropins, i.e., follicle-stimulating hormone (FSH) and luteinizing hormone (LH), had already been isolated from the pituitary gland [2]. Intensive studies have been performed to isolate the predicted substance(s) controlling FSH and/or LH release. In the early 1970s, a decapeptide, which stimulates both FSH and LH release [3], was isolated from porcine and ovine hypothalami by two groups, led by Andrew Schally [4] and Roger Guillemin [5], respectively. The discovery of the gonadotropin-releasing hormone (GnRH) facilitated the studies on the involvement of hypothalamic neurotransmitters and neuropeptides in GnRH/gonadotropin release system during the last three decades of the twentieth century. It has become increasingly clear that the activity of GnRH neurons is under a complex influence of afferent inputs, which mediates the feedback action of gonadal steroids, timing of sexual

Y. Uenoyama (✉) • N. Inoue • N. Ieda • H. Tsukamura
Graduate School of Bioagricultural Sciences, Nagoya University,
Chikusa-ku, Furo-cho, Nagoya, Aichi 464-8601, Japan
e-mail: uenoyama@nagoya-u.jp; ninoue@agr.nagoya-u.ac.jp;
ieda@agr.nagoya-u.ac.jp; htsukamura@nagoya-u.jp

V. Pheng
Asian Satellite Campus-Cambodia, Nagoya University, Phnom Penh, Cambodia
e-mail: vutha1@yahoo.com

K.-i. Maeda
Graduate School of Agricultural and Life Sciences, The University of Tokyo,
Tokyo 113-8657, Japan
e-mail: akeimaed@mail.ecc.u-tokyo.ac.jp

P. Kumanov, A. Agarwal (eds.), *Puberty*, DOI 10.1007/978-3-319-32122-6_1

maturation at puberty, drives estrous/menstrual cycles, and arrests gonadal activity under the adversity such as lactation, malnutrition, and diseases [6–11].

At the turn of the twenty-first century, discoveries via inactivating mutations of novel neuropeptide signaling, i.e., kisspeptin-GPR54 signaling, in humans suffering the hypogonadotropic hypogonadism, provided a breakthrough in our understanding of the hypothalamic mechanism controlling GnRH/gonadotropin release at the onset of puberty. This review focuses on our current understanding of how the hypothalamus regulates pubertal maturation of gonadal axis in mammals via GnRH/gonadotropin release.

Tonic GnRH/Gonadotropin Release Controls Pubertal Maturation of Gonadal Activity

There are two modes of GnRH/gonadotropin release in mammals. Males exhibit only tonic GnRH/gonadotropin release, whereas females exhibit both tonic and surge-mode GnRH/gonadotropin release. The tonic GnRH/gonadotropin release is characterized by its pulsatile nature, which was originally detected by a combination of frequent blood sampling and radioimmunoassay for LH in primates [12], and controls follicular development and maintenance of corpus luteum in females, and spermatogenesis in males, along with the steroidogenesis in both sexes. The surge-mode GnRH/gonadotropin release is observed at the mid-menstrual cycle in primates [13, 14] and the end of the follicular phase in other animals [15, 16] to trigger ovulation and the corpus luteum formation.

Sexual maturation at the puberty onset seems to be timed by an increase in tonic GnRH/gonadotropin release in several mammals examined to date [17–21]. Experimentally, a pioneer study by Ernst Knobil and colleagues demonstrated that intermittent GnRH stimulation to the pituitary at a physiological frequency observed in adulthood induced puberty onset in immature female rhesus monkeys and that its withdrawal reverted to the immature state [22]. This finding strongly suggests that an increase in tonic GnRH/gonadotropin release is the first step in the pubertal onset. Knobil and colleagues also established a method for electrophysiological recording of multiple unit neuronal activity (MUA) that is synchronized with LH pulses [23] and suggested that the neuronal activity recorded in the mediobasal hypothalamus could be derived from the so-called GnRH pulse generator. The periodic increase in electrical activity, called MUA volleys, is considered as a manifestation of GnRH release and seems to be suppressed in prepubertal animals. The onset of puberty, therefore, is considered to be dependent on the activation of the GnRH pulse generator.

KNDy Neurons as a Master Regulator of Tonic GnRH/Gonadotropin Release

An intrinsic source of the GnRH pulse generator had been deemed as a great enigma of the GnRH/gonadotropin-releasing system before the discovery of kisspeptin (first named metastin [24]). To date, the most plausible interpretation is that kisspeptin neurons localized in the hypothalamic arcuate nucleus (ARC) (also known as KNDy neurons as described below) serve as a master regulator of tonic GnRH/gonadotropin release in mammals. A critical role of kisspeptin in puberty onset has emerged from clinical studies for familial hypogonadotropic hypogonadism, characterized by pubertal failure due to gonadotropin deficiency. Two years after the deorphanization of GPR54 as a receptor for kisspeptin in 2001 [24, 25], two studies demonstrated that inactivating mutations of *GPR54* gene caused pubertal failure in humans [26, 27]. Subsequently, the phenotype of humans with inactivating mutations of the *GPR54* gene was recapitulated in humans bearing inactivating mutations of the *KISS1* gene (coding kisspeptin) [28] and in rodent models carrying targeted mutations of *Kiss1* or *Gpr54* loci [27, 29–33]. In particular, *Kiss1* knockout rats showed a severe hypogonadotropic hypogonadal phenotype, suggesting an indispensable role of kisspeptin in pubertal maturation of gonadal axis in both sexes [33]. Because *Gpr54* gene expression in GnRH neurons is evident in rodents [29, 34], kisspeptin is thought to directly control GnRH release and thus gonadotropin release. Indeed, increasing evidence indicates that kisspeptin stimulates gonadotropin release via GnRH neurons in several mammals [34–36].

Clinical studies for hypogonadotropic hypogonadism also demonstrated a critical role of neurokinin B (NKB), a member of tachykinin family, in hypothalamic regulation of puberty onset. Inactivating mutations of *TAC3* (coding NKB) or its cognate *TACR3* (coding tachykinin NK3 receptor) gene were found in humans suffering from the hypogonadotropic hypogonadism [37–40]. It should be noted that kisspeptin, NKB, and an endogenous opioid, dynorphin A, are co-localized in a cohort of ARC neurons in mammalian species [41–43], and thus the cohort of neurons has now become known as the KNDy neurons for the names of three neuropeptides, such as kisspeptin, NKB, and dynorphin A. Our previous studies demonstrated that the neuronal activity accompanied with LH pulses is successfully detected in the area near the cluster of KNDy neurons in goats [43, 44], suggesting that KNDy neurons are an intrinsic source of the GnRH pulse generator. Based on the results currently available [43–45], we envision that NKB and dynorphin A regulate the intermittent discharge of KNDy neurons in an autocrine and/or paracrine manner, resulting in pulsatile GnRH/gonadotropin release. Indeed, our recent study indicates the involvement of NKB and dynorphin A in pubertal maturation of GnRH/gonadotropin release [46], i.e., chronic administration of tachykinin NK3 receptor agonist or kappa-opioid receptor antagonist facilitated puberty onset along with the induction of tonic LH release in female rats. This result suggests that a lack of NKB signaling and relatively high dynorphin A tone may play a key role in suppression of the intermittent discharge of KNDy neurons, which drive pulsatile GnRH/gonadotropin release. In other words, it is likely that an increase in NKB stimulation and/or decrease in the inhibitory tone of dynorphin A (#1 in Fig. 1.1) drives intermittent discharge of KNDy neurons and hence GnRH/gonadotropin release (#2 in Fig. 1.1), resulting in puberty onset along with follicular development in the ovary (#3 in Fig. 1.1). Double-labeled immunoelectron microscopic studies indicate that an action site of kisspeptin seems GnRH neuronal terminals in the median eminence, where kisspeptin exerts stimulatory influence on GnRH neurons via volume transmission [47, 48]. Direct evidence for pubertal increase in kisspeptin release was proposed

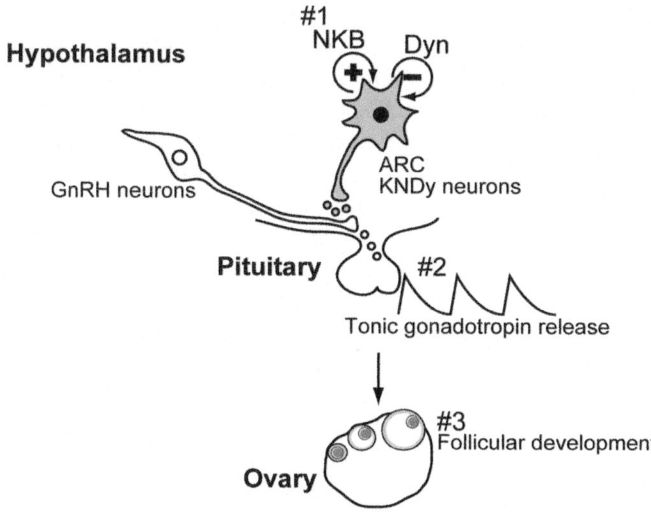

Fig. 1.1 Schematic illustration showing the possible hypothalamic mechanism regulating pubertal increase in GnRH/gonadotropin release in female mammals. KNDy neurons localized in the hypothalamic arcuate nucleus (ARC) play a key role in pubertal increase in GnRH/gonadotropin release in mammals. At the onset of puberty, an increase in neurokinin B stimulation and/or decrease in the inhibitory tone of dynorphin A (#1) may drive the intermittent discharge of KNDy neurons in an autocrine/paracrine manner. Kisspeptin stimulates tonic GnRH release at the median eminence and thus gonadotropin secretion (#2), which times puberty onset along with the follicular development in females (#3)

from a previous study, in which Keen et al. [49] showed a pubertal increase in both kisspeptin and GnRH release and coordinated release of pulsatile kisspeptin and GnRH at the median eminence in rhesus monkeys.

Estrogen-Dependent and Estrogen-Independent Prepubertal Restraint of GnRH/Gonadotropin-Releasing System

The GnRH/gonadotropin-releasing system seems to be already matured before the onset of puberty. Indeed, ARC *Kiss1* gene expression and pulsatile LH release immediately increased after ovariectomy in prepubertal rats [50, 51]. Estrogen replacement restores the prepubertal restraint of the ARC *Kiss1* gene expression and LH pulses in female rats [50, 51], suggesting that the prepubertal suppression of the tonic GnRH/gonadotropin-releasing system is dependent on a circulating estrogen derived from the immature ovaries. A possible mechanism involved in the prepubertal restraint of tonic GnRH/gonadotropin-releasing system is illustrated in Fig. 1.2. Based on the results currently available [50, 51], we envisage that estrogen derived from the immature ovaries (#1 in Fig. 1.2) may play a key role in prepubertal suppression of ARC *Kiss1* gene expression (#2 in Fig. 1.2), resulting

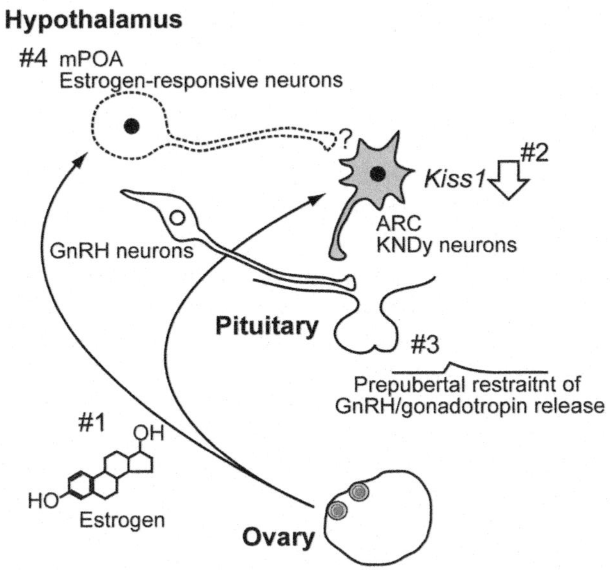

Fig. 1.2 Schematic illustration showing a possible mechanism regulating the pubertal restraint of the GnRH/gonadotropin release system in female mammals. During the prepubertal period, estrogen derived from the immature gonads (#1) strongly suppresses ARC *Kiss1* gene expression in KNDy neurons (#2) and hence GnRH/gonadotropin release (#3). Estrogen may exert an inhibitory influence on ARC *Kiss1* gene expression via direct or indirect pathways (#1). Estrogen-responsive neurons in the medial preoptic area (mPOA) may exert an inhibitory influence on GnRH/gonadotropin release via suppression of ARC *Kiss1* gene expression (#4)

in a restraint of tonic GnRH/gonadotropin release during the prepubertal period (#3 in Fig. 1.2). Since kisspeptin neuron-specific estrogen receptor α (ERα) knockout mice show precocious puberty onset along with a higher ARC *Kiss1* gene expression than wild-type mice [52], estrogen-dependent prepubertal restraint of *Kiss1* gene expression and LH pulses would be directly mediated by ERα in ARC KNDy neurons. Similarly, in males, the prepubertal suppression of the tonic GnRH/gonadotropin-releasing system seems dependent on a circulating testosterone derived from the immature testes, because castration increases plasma LH levels in prepubertal male rats [53].

In addition to the direct inhibitory effect on ARC *Kiss1* gene expression, estrogen may indirectly inhibit *Kiss1* gene expression and/or GnRH/gonadotropin-releasing system during the prepubertal period. Our recent study showed that site-specific micro-implants of estradiol in the medial preoptic area (mPOA) or ARC restored suppression of LH pulses in prepubertal ovariectomized rats [50]. This suggests that estrogen-responsive neurons, at least, in the mPOA and ARC, are involved in the estrogen-dependent prepubertal restraint of GnRH/gonadotropin-releasing system in female rats. Given the critical role of kisspeptin and NKB in pubertal maturation in humans and rodents, KNDy neurons could be a first candidate for the estrogen-responsive neurons in the ARC. Additionally, estrogen-responsive neurons in the mPOA may exert an inhibitory influence on ARC *Kiss1* gene expression (#4 in Fig. 1.2).

The inhibitory influence of estrogen on ARC *Kiss1* gene expression and GnRH/gonadotropin release appears to decrease during the pubertal transition, resulting in upregulation of ARC *Kiss1* gene expression and GnRH/gonadotropin release [51]. This scenario is consistent with the classical gonadostat hypothesis [54] that changes in hypothalamic sensitivity to negative feedback action of estrogen are associated with pubertal maturation of the GnRH/gonadotropin-releasing system in rodents. We envisage that pubertal decrease in the responsiveness to estrogen in ARC KNDy neurons plays a role in pubertal increase in *Kiss1* gene expression. It is unlikely that changes in responsiveness to estrogen negative feedback action during the pubertal transition are simply caused by a change in the expression of ERα, because our previous study showed that the number of ERα-expressing cells and *Esr1* gene (encoding ERα) expression in the POA and ARC was comparable between pre- and postpubertal periods in female rats [50]. Further studies are warranted to address this issue.

It should be noted that the central mechanism controlling the prepubertal restraint of GnRH/gonadotropin-releasing system in primates appears to differ from other species such as rodents and sheep [10, 11]. In monkeys, gonadectomy induces an increase in gonadotropin release during the neonatal period and after the onset of puberty, but not during the prepubertal period [11]. This indicates that both steroid-dependent and steroid-independent pathways are responsible for restraint of GnRH/gonadotropin-releasing system. Terasawa and Fernandez [10] suggest that the steroid-independent inhibition may be due to the abundant synaptogenesis in primate brain than other species and that the decrease in the number of synapse to the adult levels could lead to pubertal increase in GnRH/gonadotropin release via removal of inhibitory inputs in primates. The characteristic steroid-independent restraint period of GnRH/gonadotropin-releasing system in primates is called the juvenile period [55]. In humans, the juvenile hiatus in GnRH/gonadotropin secretion is seen between the ages of 4–9 years [55], even in girls suffering from Turner syndrome with gonadal dysgenesis [56] and boys with testicular defects [57], both which exhibit elevated plasma gonadotropin levels in infantile and peripubertal period.

Cues Relieving Prepubertal Restraint of GnRH/Gonadotropin-Releasing System

It is well demonstrated that the timing of puberty onset is dependent on body weight rather than chronological age [58]. Epidemiologic studies showed that age of menarche in girls declined from 17 years old in the nineteenth century to 13 years old in the twentieth century in developed countries [58]. This secular trend can be understood in terms of the faster somatic growth in humans in the twentieth century [58].

Thus, nutritional cues are likely to contribute to the regulation of pubertal maturation of GnRH/gonadotropin-releasing system. Energy storage in the body fat has been considered to be a possible determinant for the onset of puberty for a long time [59, 60]. Leptin, the first hormone discovered from fat tissue [61, 62], was then considered as a signal that relays the attainment of energy storage to the brain, because leptin-deficient mice do not show puberty and exogenous leptin restores fertility [63]. In fact, the leptin receptor is expressed in several hypothalamic and extra-hypothalamic nuclei including ARC [64]. Recently, KNDy neurons were found to express leptin receptors [65]. Mice with a leptin deficiency showed decreased ARC *Kiss1* gene expression [65], suggesting that leptin seems to be a nutritional cue relieving the prepubertal restraint of GnRH/gonadotropin-releasing system. Leptin, however, could be a prerequisite of normal puberty, because the increase in leptin secretion is not necessarily synchronized with the onset of puberty [58].

In addition to nutrition, the photoperiod tightly regulates the timing of puberty onset in seasonal breeders such as sheep and Syrian hamsters. Foster et al. [18] clearly showed that the onset of puberty is postponed to the next breeding season in lambs, which achieved critical body size in late winter. Earlier studies showed that *Kiss1* gene expression is higher in the breeding season than in the nonbreeding season in sheep and Syrian hamsters [66, 67]. Taken together, KNDy neurons may integrate multiple external cues, such as nutrition or photoperiod, to control pubertal maturation of the GnRH/gonadotropin-releasing system.

Conclusions and Unanswered Questions

Studies during the last few decades have provided a new framework for the understanding of pubertal maturation of hypothalamic regulation of gonadal axis in mammals. It is now well accepted that KNDy neurons are responsible for the regulation of pubertal increase and GnRH/gonadotropin release in mammals. But, there are still some important unanswered questions. Little is known about the cellular and molecular mechanisms controlling the prepubertal restraint of and pubertal increase in kisspeptin biosynthesis, which is tightly controlled by steroid-dependent and steroid-independent mechanism. In particular, mechanisms underlying the relationship between nutritional statuses and relieving the prepubertal restraint of kisspeptin biosynthesis are still unanswered questions. Further studies, therefore, are needed to fully elucidate the pubertal maturation of hypothalamic mechanism regulating gonadal axis in mammals.

Acknowledgments We wish to thank Dr Nicola Skoulding for editorial assistance. The present study was supported in part by a grant from the Science and Technology Research Promotion Program for Agriculture, Forestry, Fisheries, and Food Industry, Grants-in-Aid 26252046 (to HT), 24380157 (to KM), from the Japan Society for the Promotion of Science, and from the Ito Foundation (to YU).

References

1. Harris GW. Neural control of the pituitary gland. Physiol Rev. 1948;28:139–79.
2. Fevold H, Hisaw F, Leonard S. The gonad stimulating and the luteinizing hormones of the anterior lobe of the hypophysis. Am J Physiol. 1931;97:291–301.
3. Schally AV. Aspects of hypothalamic regulation of the pituitary gland. Science. 1978;202:18–28.
4. Schally AV, Arimura A, Kastin AJ, Matsuo H, Baba Y, Redding TW, Nair RM, Debeljuk L, White WF. Gonadotropin-releasing hormone: one polypeptide regulates secretion of luteinizing and follicle-stimulating hormones. Science. 1971;173:1036–8.
5. Amoss M, Burgus R, Blackwell R, Vale W, Fellows R, Guillemin R. Purification, amino acid composition and N-terminus of the hypothalamic luteinizing hormone releasing factor (LRF) of ovine origin. Biochem Biophys Res Commun. 1971;44:205–10.
6. Maeda K, Tsukamura H. Neuroendocrine mechanism mediating fasting-induced suppression of luteinizing hormone secretion in female rats. Acta Neurobiol Exp. 1996;56:787–96.
7. Herbison AE. Multimodal influence of estrogen upon gonadotropin-releasing hormone neurons. Endocr Rev. 1998;19:302–30.
8. Cunningham MJ, Clifton DK, Steiner RA. Leptin's actions on the reproductive axis: perspectives and mechanisms. Biol Reprod. 1999;60:216–22.
9. Ojeda SR, Prevot V, Heger S, Lomniczi A, Dziedzic B, Mungenast A. The neurobiology of female puberty. Horm Res. 2003;60 Suppl 3:15–20.
10. Terasawa E, Fernandez DL. Neurobiological mechanisms of the onset of puberty in primates. Endocr Rev. 2001;22:111–51.
11. Plant TM, Barker-Gibb ML. Neurobiological mechanisms of puberty in higher primates. Hum Reprod Update. 2004;10:67–77.
12. Dierschke DJ, Bhattacharya AN, Atkinson LE, Knobil E. Circhoral oscillations of plasma LH levels in the ovariectomized rhesus monkey. Endocrinology. 1970;87:850–3.
13. Neill JD, Johansson ED, Datta JK, Knobil E. Relationship between the plasma levels of luteinizing hormone and progesterone during the normal menstrual cycle. J Clin Endocrinol Metab. 1967;27:1167–73.
14. Monroe SE, Atkinson LE, Knobil E. Patterns of circulating luteinizing hormone and their relation to plasma progesterone levels during the menstrual cycle of the Rhesus monkey. Endocrinology. 1970;87:453–5.
15. Legan SJ, Karsch FJ. A daily signal for the LH surge in the rat. Endocrinology. 1975;96: 57–62.
16. Moenter SM, Caraty A, Locatelli A, Karsch FJ. Pattern of gonadotropin-releasing hormone (GnRH) secretion leading up to ovulation in the ewe: existence of a preovulatory GnRH surge. Endocrinology. 1991;129:1175–82.
17. Andrews WW, Ojeda SR. A detailed analysis of the serum luteinizing hormone secretory profile in conscious, free-moving female rats during the time of puberty. Endocrinology. 1981;109:2032–9.
18. Foster DL, Yellon SM, Olster DH. Internal and external determinants of the timing of puberty in the female. J Reprod Fertil. 1985;75:327–44.
19. Foster DL, Ebling FJP, Vannerson LA, Wood RI, Fenner DE. Regulation of puberty in the lamb: internal and external cues. In: Imura H, Shizume K, Yoshida S, editors. Progress in endocrinology. Amsterdam: Elsevier; 1988. p. 861–6.
20. Watanabe G, Terasawa E. In vivo release of luteinizing hormone releasing hormone increases with puberty in the female rhesus monkey. Endocrinology. 1989;125:92–9.
21. Sisk CL, Richardson HN, Chappell PE, Levine JE. In vivo gonadotropin-releasing hormone secretion in female rats during peripubertal development and on proestrus. Endocrinology. 2001;142:2929–36.
22. Wildt L, Marshall G, Knobil E. Experimental induction of puberty in the infantile female rhesus monkey. Science. 1980;207:1373–5.

23. Wilson RC, Kesner JS, Kaufman JM, Uemura T, Akema T, Knobil E. Central electrophysiologic correlates of pulsatile luteinizing hormone secretion in the rhesus monkey. Neuroendocrinology. 1984;39:256–60.
24. Ohtaki T, Shintani Y, Honda S, Matsumoto H, Hori A, Kanehashi K, Terao Y, Kumano S, Takatsu Y, Masuda Y, Ishibashi Y, Watanabe T, Asada M, Yamada T, Suenaga M, Kitada C, Usuki S, Kurokawa T, Onda H, Nishimura O, Fujino M. Metastasis suppressor gene KiSS-1 encodes peptide ligand of a G-protein-coupled receptor. Nature. 2001;411:613–7.
25. Kotani M, Detheux M, Vandenbogaerde A, Communi D, Vanderwinden JM, Le Poul E, Brezillon S, Tyldesley R, Suarez-Huerta N, Vandeput F, Blanpain C, Schiffmann SN, Vassart G, Parmentier M. The metastasis suppressor gene KiSS-1 encodes kisspeptins, the natural ligands of the orphan G protein-coupled receptor GPR54. J Biol Chem. 2001;276:34631–6.
26. de Roux N, Genin E, Carel JC, Matsuda F, Chaussain JL, Milgrom E. Hypogonadotropic hypogonadism due to loss of function of the KiSS1-derived peptide receptor GPR54. Proc Natl Acad Sci U S A. 2003;100:10972–6.
27. Seminara SB, Messager S, Chatzidaki EE, Thresher RR, Acierno Jr JS, Shagoury JK, Bo-Abbas Y, Kuohung W, Schwinof KM, Hendrick AG, Zahn D, Dixon J, Kaiser UB, Slaugenhaupt SA, Gusella JF, O'Rahilly S, Carlton MB, Crowley Jr WF, Aparicio SA, Colledge WH. The GPR54 gene as a regulator of puberty. N Engl J Med. 2003;349:1614–27.
28. Topaloglu AK, Tello JA, Kotan LD, Ozbek MN, Yilmaz MB, Erdogan S, Gurbuz F, Temiz F, Millar RP, Yuksel B. Inactivating *KISS1* mutation and hypogonadotropic hypogonadism. N Engl J Med. 2012;366:629–35.
29. Messager S, Chatzidaki EE, Ma D, Hendrick AG, Zahn D, Dixon J, Thresher RR, Malinge I, Lomet D, Carlton MB, Colledge WH, Caraty A, Aparicio SA. Kisspeptin directly stimulates gonadotropin-releasing hormone release via G protein-coupled receptor 54. Proc Natl Acad Sci U S A. 2005;102:1761–6.
30. d'Anglemont de Tassigny X, Fagg LA, Dixon JP, Day K, Leitch HG, Hendrick AG, Zahn D, Franceschini I, Caraty A, Carlton MB, Aparicio SA, Colledge WH: Hypogonadotropic hypogonadism in mice lacking a functional Kiss1 gene. Proc Natl Acad Sci USA. 2007; 104:10714–9.
31. Lapatto R, Pallais JC, Zhang D, Chan YM, Mahan A, Cerrato F, Le WW, Hoffman GE, Seminara SB. *Kiss1−/−* mice exhibit more variable hypogonadism than *Gpr54−/−* mice. Endocrinology. 2007;148:4927–36.
32. Chan YM, Broder-Fingert S, Wong KM, Seminara SB. Kisspeptin/Gpr54-independent gonadotrophin-releasing hormone activity in *Kiss1* and *Gpr54* mutant mice. J Neuroendocrinol. 2009;21:1015–23.
33. Uenoyama Y, Nakamura S, Hayakawa Y, Ikegami K, Watanabe Y, Deura C, Minabe S, Tomikawa J, Goto T, Ieda N, Inoue N, Sanbo M, Tamura C, Hirabayashi M, Maeda KI, Tsukamura H. Lack of pulse and surge modes and glutamatergic stimulation of LH release in *Kiss1* knockout rats. J Neuroendocrinol. 2015;27:187–97.
34. Irwig MS, Fraley GS, Smith JT, Acohido BV, Popa SM, Cunningham MJ, Gottsch ML, Clifton DK, Steiner RA. Kisspeptin activation of gonadotropin releasing hormone neurons and regulation of KiSS-1 mRNA in the male rat. Neuroendocrinology. 2004;80:264–72.
35. Matsui H, Takatsu Y, Kumano S, Matsumoto H, Ohtaki T. Peripheral administration of metastin induces marked gonadotropin release and ovulation in the rat. Biochem Biophys Res Commun. 2004;320:383–8.
36. Shahab M, Mastronardi C, Seminara SB, Crowley WF, Ojeda SR, Plant TM. Increased hypothalamic GPR54 signaling: a potential mechanism for initiation of puberty in primates. Proc Natl Acad Sci U S A. 2005;102:2129–34.
37. Topaloglu AK, Reimann F, Guclu M, Yalin AS, Kotan LD, Porter KM, Serin A, Mungan NO, Cook JR, Ozbek MN, Imamoglu S, Akalin NS, Yuksel B, O'Rahilly S, Semple RK. TAC3 and TACR3 mutations in familial hypogonadotropic hypogonadism reveal a key role for Neurokinin B in the central control of reproduction. Nat Genet. 2009;41:354–8.
38. Guran T, Tolhurst G, Bereket A, Rocha N, Porter K, Turan S, Gribble FM, Kotan LD, Akcay T, Atay Z, Canan H, Serin A, O'Rahilly S, Reimann F, Semple RK, Topaloglu AK.

Hypogonadotropic hypogonadism due to a novel missense mutation in the first extracellular loop of the neurokinin B receptor. J Clin Endocrinol Metab. 2009;94:3633–9.
39. Gianetti E, Tusset C, Noel SD, Au MG, Dwyer AA, Hughes VA, Abreu AP, Carroll J, Trarbach E, Silveira LF, Costa EM, de Mendonca BB, de Castro M, Lofrano A, Hall JE, Bolu E, Ozata M, Quinton R, Amory JK, Stewart SE, Arlt W, Cole TR, Crowley WF, Kaiser UB, Latronico AC, Seminara SB. TAC3/TACR3 mutations reveal preferential activation of gonadotropin-releasing hormone release by neurokinin B in neonatal life followed by reversal in adulthood. J Clin Endocrinol Metab. 2010;95:2857–67.
40. Young J, Bouligand J, Francou B, Raffin-Sanson ML, Gaillez S, Jeanpierre M, Grynberg M, Kamenicky P, Chanson P, Brailly-Tabard S, Guiochon-Mantel A. TAC3 and TACR3 defects cause hypothalamic congenital hypogonadotropic hypogonadism in humans. J Clin Endocrinol Metab. 2010;95:2287–95.
41. Goodman RL, Lehman MN, Smith JT, Coolen LM, de Oliveira CV, Jafarzadehshirazi MR, Pereira A, Iqbal J, Caraty A, Ciofi P, Clarke IJ. Kisspeptin neurons in the arcuate nucleus of the ewe express both dynorphin A and neurokinin B. Endocrinology. 2007;148:5752–60.
42. Navarro VM, Gottsch ML, Chavkin C, Okamura H, Clifton DK, Steiner RA. Regulation of gonadotropin-releasing hormone secretion by kisspeptin/dynorphin/neurokinin B neurons in the arcuate nucleus of the mouse. J Neurosci. 2009;29:11859–66.
43. Wakabayashi Y, Nakada T, Murata K, Ohkura S, Mogi K, Navarro VM, Clifton DK, Mori Y, Tsukamura H, Maeda K, Steiner RA, Okamura H. Neurokinin B and dynorphin A in kisspeptin neurons of the arcuate nucleus participate in generation of periodic oscillation of neural activity driving pulsatile gonadotropin-releasing hormone secretion in the goat. J Neurosci. 2010;30:3124–32.
44. Ohkura S, Takase K, Matsuyama S, Mogi K, Ichimaru T, Wakabayashi Y, Uenoyama Y, Mori Y, Steiner RA, Tsukamura H, Maeda KI, Okamura H. Gonadotrophin-releasing hormone pulse generator activity in the hypothalamus of the goat. J Neuroendocrinol. 2009;21:813–21.
45. Okamura H, Tsukamura H, Ohkura S, Uenoyama Y, Wakabayashi Y, Maeda KI. Kisspeptin and GnRH pulse generation. Adv Exp Med Biol. 2013;784:297–323.
46. Nakahara T, Uenoyama Y, Iwase A, Oishi S, Nakamura S, Minabe S, Watanabe Y, Deura C, Noguchi T, Fujii N, Kikkawa F, Maeda KI, Tsukamura H. Chronic peripheral administration of kappa-opioid receptor antagonist advances puberty onset associated with acceleration of pulsatile luteinizing hormone secretion in female rats. J Reprod Dev. 2013;59:479–84.
47. Uenoyama Y, Inoue N, Pheng V, Homma T, Takase K, Yamada S, Ajiki K, Ichikawa M, Okamura H, Maeda KI, Tsukamura H. Ultrastructural evidence of kisspeptin-gonadotrophin-releasing hormone interaction in the median eminence of female rats: implication of axo-axonal regulation of GnRH release. J Neuroendocrinol. 2011;23:863–70.
48. Matsuyama S, Ohkura S, Mogi K, Wakabayashi Y, Mori Y, Tsukamura H, Maeda K, Ichikawa M, Okamura H. Morphological evidence for direct interaction between kisspeptin and gonadotropin-releasing hormone neurons at the median eminence of the male goat: an immunoelectron microscopic study. Neuroendocrinology. 2011;94:323–32.
49. Keen KL, Wegner FH, Bloom SR, Ghatei MA, Terasawa E. An increase in kisspeptin-54 release occurs with the pubertal increase in luteinizing hormone-releasing hormone-1 release in the stalk-median eminence of female rhesus monkeys in vivo. Endocrinology. 2008;149:4151–7.
50. Uenoyama Y, Tanaka A, Takase K, Yamada S, Pheng V, Inoue N, Maeda KI, Tsukamura H. Central estrogen action sites involved in prepubertal restraint of pulsatile luteinizing hormone release in female rats. J Reprod Dev. 2015;61:351–9.
51. Takase K, Uenoyama Y, Inoue N, Matsui H, Yamada S, Shimizu M, Homma T, Tomikawa J, Kanda S, Matsumoto H, Oka Y, Tsukamura H, Maeda KI. Possible role of oestrogen in pubertal increase of *Kiss1*/kisspeptin expression in discrete hypothalamic areas of female rats. J Neuroendocrinol. 2009;21:527–37.
52. Mayer C, Acosta-Martinez M, Dubois SL, Wolfe A, Radovick S, Boehm U, Levine JE. Timing and completion of puberty in female mice depend on estrogen receptor alpha-signaling in kisspeptin neurons. Proc Natl Acad Sci U S A. 2010;107:22693–8.

53. Negro-Vilar A, Ojeda SR, McCann SM. Evidence for changes in sensitivity to testosterone negative feedback on gonadotropin release during sexual development in the male rat. Endocrinology. 1973;93:729–35.
54. Ramirez DV, McCann SM. Comparison of the regulation of luteinizing hormone (LH) secretion in immature and adult rats. Endocrinology. 1963;72:452–64.
55. Grumbach MM. The neuroendocrinology of human puberty revisited. Horm Res. 2002;57 Suppl 2:2–14.
56. Chrysis D, Spiliotis BE, Stene M, Cacciari E, Davenport ML. Gonadotropin secretion in girls with turner syndrome measured by an ultrasensitive immunochemiluminometric assay. Horm Res. 2006;65:261–6.
57. Dunkel L, Siimes MA, Bremner WJ. Reduced inhibin and elevated gonadotropin levels in early pubertal boys with testicular defects. Pediatr Res. 1993;33:514–8.
58. Foster DL, Nagatani S. Physiological perspectives on leptin as a regulator of reproduction: role in timing puberty. Biol Reprod. 1999;60:205–15.
59. Chehab FF. Leptin as a regulator of adipose mass and reproduction. Trends Pharmacol Sci. 2000;21:309–14.
60. Frisch RE. Body fat, puberty and fertility. Biol Rev Camb Philos Soc. 1984;59:161–88.
61. Zhang Y, Proenca R, Maffei M, Barone M, Leopold L, Friedman JM. Positional cloning of the mouse obese gene and its human homologue. Nature. 1994;372:425–32.
62. Halaas JL, Gajiwala KS, Maffei M, Cohen SL, Chait BT, Rabinowitz D, Lallone RL, Burley SK, Friedman JM. Weight-reducing effects of the plasma protein encoded by the obese gene. Science. 1995;269:543–6.
63. Chehab FF, Lim ME, Lu R. Correction of the sterility defect in homozygous obese female mice by treatment with the human recombinant leptin. Nat Genet. 1996;12:318–20.
64. Elmquist JK, Bjorbaek C, Ahima RS, Flier JS, Saper CB. Distributions of leptin receptor mRNA isoforms in the rat brain. J Comp Neurol. 1998;395:535–47.
65. Smith JT, Acohido BV, Clifton DK, Steiner RA. KiSS-1 neurones are direct targets for leptin in the ob/ob mouse. J Neuroendocrinol. 2006;18:298–303.
66. Smith JT, Clay CM, Caraty A, Clarke IJ. KiSS-1 messenger ribonucleic acid expression in the hypothalamus of the ewe is regulated by sex steroids and season. Endocrinology. 2007;148:1150–7.
67. Revel FG, Ansel L, Klosen P, Saboureau M, Pevet P, Mikkelsen JD, Simonneaux V. Kisspeptin: a key link to seasonal breeding. Rev Endocr Metab Disord. 2007;8:57–65.

Chapter 2
Genetics of Puberty

Shehla Tabassum and Salman Kirmani

Puberty is defined as the physical transition from sexual immaturity to being sexually mature. Adolescence is sometimes considered a synonymous term, but implies more of a psychosocial maturation that comes with puberty. The mean age for the onset of first signs of puberty among girls is around 10.5 years of age (range, 8–13 years), while among boys, it is around 11.5 years (range, 9–14 years) [1–4]. Some variability occurs between individuals with regard to the timing and sequence of pubertal maturation. However, most of boys and girls follow a predictable course through pubertal maturation.

Pubertal onset in both girls and boys appears to be occurring earlier all over the world as compared to that reported in the literature previously [5–7]. Several factors like increased BMI and fat mass have been implicated in causing this earlier pubertal onset, but substantial evidence is still lacking in this regard. Also, pubertal timing varies significantly between different ethnic groups. Genetics seem to play an important role in causing these racial/ethnic differences [8].

Gonadotropin-releasing hormone (GnRH) is the master hormone of the reproductive endocrine system, largely controlling the secretion of luteinizing hormone (LH) and follicle-stimulating hormone (FSH) from pituitary gonadotrope cells. An increase in the pulsatile secretion of GnRH from the hypothalamus is considered to be a critical hormonal event in puberty. FSH and LH then evoke steroidogenesis and gametogenesis from the gonads, culminating in secondary sexual features' development and fertility. There are multiple other factors involved in

S. Tabassum
Department of Diabetes, Endocrinology and Metabolism, Aga Khan University,
Faculty Office Building, Stadium Road, Karachi 74800, Pakistan
e-mail: dr_shehla@hotmail.com

S. Kirmani (✉)
Departments of Paediatrics and Child Health, Aga Khan University Hospital, P.O Box 3500,
Stadium Road, Karachi 74800, Sindh, Pakistan
e-mail: salman.kirmani@aku.edu

P. Kumanov, A. Agarwal (eds.), *Puberty*, DOI 10.1007/978-3-319-32122-6_2

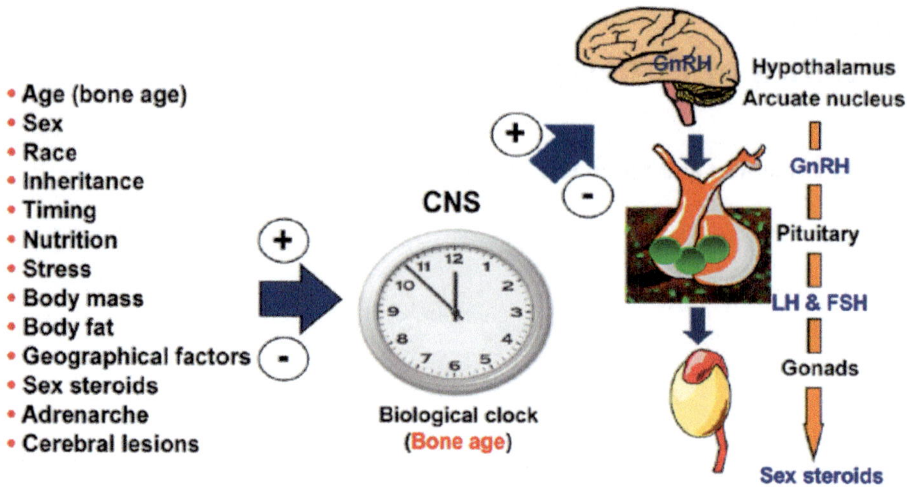

Fig. 2.1 Multiple factors implicated in pubertal onset. *CNS* central nervous system, *GnRH* gonadotropin-releasing hormone, *LH* luteinizing hormone, *FSH* follicle-stimulating hormone (Reprinted from Martos-Moreno GA, Chowen JA, Argente J. Metabolic signals in human puberty: Effects of over and Undernutrition. Molecular and Cellular Endocrinology 2010; 324(1–2): 70–81. With permission from Elsevier.)

the initiation of puberty as well, and the complex interactions between genetic and environmental factors controlling this process are just beginning to be understood (Fig. 2.1).

Regulation of Puberty

Puberty is a mysterious phenomenon, and not all is known to answer the various complicated steps occurring in this process. Several mechanisms have been implicated in the onset of puberty. The process seems to undergo neuropeptide, genetic, metabolic, and environmental regulation.

Neuropeptide Regulation of Puberty

A sustained increase in pulsatile release of gonadotrophin-releasing hormone (GnRH) from the hypothalamus is an essential, final event that defines the initiation of puberty. This depends on coordinated changes in transsynaptic and glial–neuronal communication, consisting of activating neuronal and glial excitatory inputs to the GnRH neuronal network and the loss of transsynaptic inhibitory tone.

The prevalent excitatory systems stimulating GnRH secretion involve a neuronal component and a glial component. The neuronal component consists of excitatory amino acids such as glutamate and peptides such as kisspeptin and neurokinin B. The glial component uses growth factors such as TGF-β, EGF, IGF-1,and bFGF and small molecules for cell–cell signaling such as SynCAM1 and RPTPβ.

KiSS1, located on chromosome 1q32.1, encodes the peptide kisspeptin, which acts via its receptor, encoded by the gene KISS1R (also known as GPR54) located on 19p13.3. It is thought that KISS1 signaling through KISS1R in the hypothalamus at the end of the juvenile phase of development may contribute to the pubertal resurgence of pulsatile GnRH release. The three key features of the kisspeptin–Gpr54–GnRH neuron axis leading up to puberty are (i) the expression of adult-like levels of Gpr54 mRNA in GnRH neurons well in advance of puberty, (ii) a modest increase in the electrical response of GnRH neurons to Gpr54 activation across postnatal development, and (iii) the "sudden" appearance of kisspeptin fibers surrounding GnRH neuron cell bodies/proximal dendrites just prior to puberty onset. Another important pathway in the initiation of puberty may be TAC3 signaling. TAC3 is located on chromosome 12q13.3, and the gene that encodes its receptor TACR3 on chromosome 4q24 and loss-of-function mutation in these genes have been associated with hypogonadotropic hypogonadism [9].

GABAergic and opiatergic neurons provide transsynaptic inhibitory control to the system, but GABA neurons also exert direct excitatory effects on GnRH neurons. New evidence suggests that additional peptides inhibit GnRH neuronal activity. The discovery of such gonadotropin-inhibitory factors, examples of which include the RF amide peptides, RFRP1 and RFRP3 (encoded by the QFRP gene on chromosome 9q34.12), has further clarified the role of genes that inhibit the GnRH axis until the appropriate signals to initiate puberty come into play [10].

Other pathways, especially in the appetite control center of the hypothalamus, have also been shown to influence pubertal onset. Neuropeptide Y (NPY) and agouti-related peptide (AgRP) are orexigenic peptides that have been found to influence the production of pro-opiomelanocortin (POMC), another neuropeptide which affects normal pubertal onset [11].

Genetic Factors Regulating Puberty

Genetic factors have been established to account for 50–75 % of the variability in timing of normal pubertal onset. Several genetic loci have been identified which are associated with age of pubertal onset. The genetic mechanisms that provide encompassing coordination to this cellular network are not clearly known. The timing of puberty varies greatly among healthy individuals in the general population and is influenced by both genetic and environmental factors [8]. The high correlation of the onset of puberty seen within racial/ethnic groups, within families, and between monozygotic compared to dizygotic twins all provides evidence for genetic regulation of pubertal timing. These data suggest that 50–80 % of the variation in pubertal timing is determined by genetic factors. Environmental and physiologic effects also influence the timing of puberty, and there is evidence supporting secular trends in the timing of puberty. It is possible that gene by environment interactions plays an important role in regulating the timing of puberty.

Table 2.1 Genes implicated in the disorders of delayed puberty

Gene	Protein	Function	Disease
KiSS1	Kisspeptin	GnRH secretion	NHH
GPR54 (KiSS1R)	Kisspeptin receptor	GnRH secretion stimulation	NHH
GNRH1	Gonadotropin-releasing hormone	GnRH synthesis	NHH
GNRHR	GnRH receptor	GnRH signaling	NHH
TAC3	Neurokinin B	Unknown	NHH
TACR3	Neurokinin B receptor	Unknown	NHH
FGF8	Fibroblast growth factor 8	Migration of GnRH neurons	KS/NHH
FGFR1	Receptor for FGF8 protein	Migration of GnRH neurons	KS/NHH
PROK2	Prokineticin	Migration of GnRH neurons	KS/NHH
PROKR2	Prokineticin receptor	Migration of GnRH neurons	KS/NHH
CHD7	Chromodomain helicase DNA-binding protein 7	Development of GnRH neurons	CHARGE syndrome, KS/NHH
NELF	Nasal embryonic LHRH factor	Migration of GnRH neurons	KS
KAL1	Anosmin-1	Migration of GnRH neurons	KS
LEP	Leptin	GnRH secretion	Obesity and HH
LEPR	Leptin receptor	GnRH secretion	Obesity and HH
PC1	Prohormone convertase	Cleavage of POMC	Obesity and HH
HESX1	Pituitary transcription factor	Pituitary development	Hypopituitarism
LHX3	Pituitary transcription factor	Pituitary development	Hypopituitarism
PROP1	Pituitary transcription factor	Pituitary development	Hypopituitarism

GnRH gonadotropin-releasing hormone, *NHH* normosmic hypogonadotropic hypogonadism, *HH* hypogonadotropic hypogonadism, *KS* Kallmann syndrome, *POMC* pro-opiomelanocortin

It is tempting to consider that a single gene may be responsible for the initiation of puberty, since mutations in genes such as GNRHR, GPR54, TAC3, TACR3, and KiSS1 result in pubertal failure [12] (Table 2.1). Functional studies have failed to demonstrate that any one of these single genes plays a commanding role in synchronizing the neuronal and glial networks involved in the initiation of puberty. This has led to the current concept of genetic networks regulating the neuroendocrine control of puberty initiation [13]. This network is envisioned to be a host of functionally related genes hierarchically arranged. The highest level of control in this network is likely provided by transcriptional regulators that, by directing expression of key subordinate genes, impose an integrative level of coordination to the neuronal and glial subsets involved in initiating the pubertal process.

The use of new techniques of genetic analysis coupled to systems biology strategies should provide not only the experimental bases supporting this concept but also unveil the existence of crucial components of network control not yet identified. The question of whether the first step in the initiation of puberty is a loss of central restraint, or the activation of stimulatory inputs to GNRH neurons still remains unanswered. It may very well be that transcriptional repression and activation of key

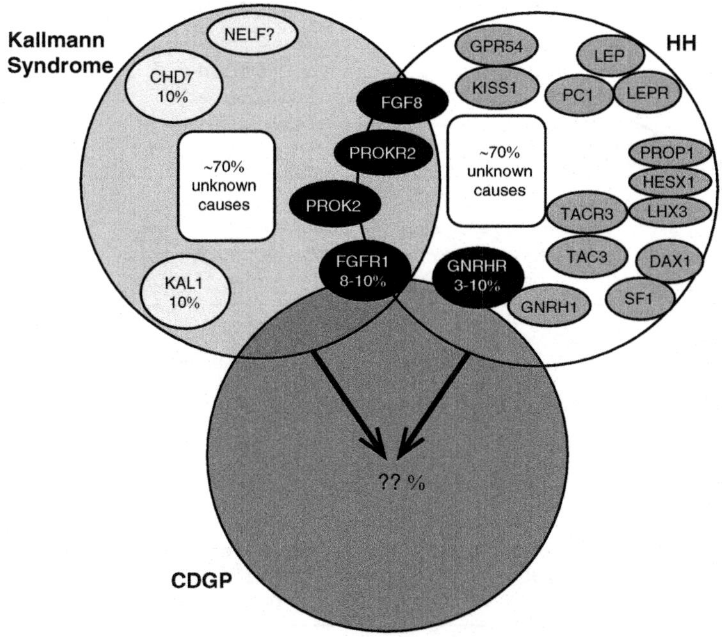

Fig. 2.2 Different genes involved in disorders of delayed puberty. *HH* hypogonadotropic hypogonadism, *CDGP* constitutional delay of growth and development (Reprinted from Gajdos ZKZ, Henderson KD, Hirschhorn JN, Palmert MR. Genetic determinants of pubertal timing in the general population. Molecular and Cellular Endocrinology 2010; 324(1–2):21–29. With permission from Elsevier.)

genes occur simultaneously to orchestrate this complex process. One recent advance in this direction is the identification of the polymorphisms with age at menarche in the leptin and leptin receptor genes in humans [14, 15]. In addition, we are learning more about various transcription factors such as thyroid transcription factor 1 (TTF1) and a transcription factor encoded by the gene C14ORF4 located on chromosome 14q24.3 which modulate gonadotropin-releasing hormone (GnRH) expression [16] (Figs. 2.2 and 2.3).

Metabolic Control of Puberty

Both growth and reproduction consume high levels of energy, requiring suitable energy stores to face these physiological functions. The state of body energy reserves is a key determinant for the onset of puberty. During the last two decades, our knowledge concerning how peptides produced in the digestive tract (in charge of energy intake) and in adipose tissue (in charge of energy storage) provide information regarding metabolic status to the CNS has increased dramatically. Moreover, these peptides have been shown to play an important role in modulating the

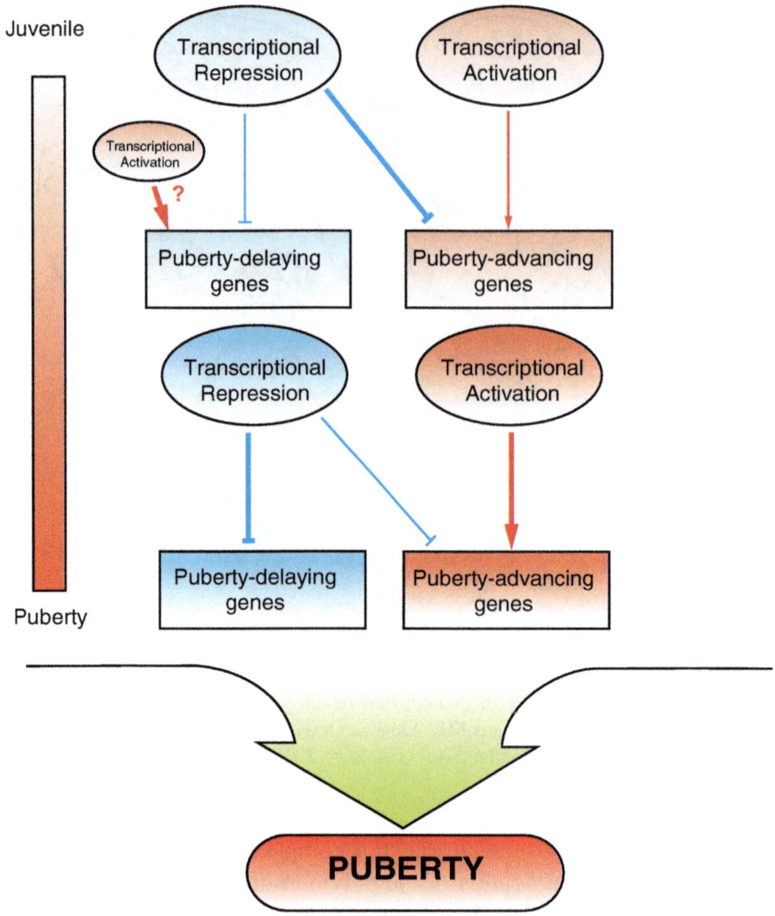

Fig. 2.3 Transcriptional regulation of the initiation of puberty (Reprinted from Ojeda SR, Dubay C, Lomniczi A, Kaidar G, Matagne V, Sandau US, Dissen GA. Gene networks and the neuroendocrine regulation of puberty. Molecular and Cellular Endocrinology 2010; 324(1–2):3–11. With permission from Elsevier.)

gonadotropic axis with their absence or an imbalance in their secretion being able to disturb pubertal onset or progression [11].

Leptin is an adipocyte-derived hormone and its synthesis is directly related to the amount of body fat. Thus, it is involved in the control of energy homeostasis and modulates several neuroendocrine systems, including the HPG axis. Animal knockout models have shown that infertility is characteristic of leptin-deficient mice (ob/ob) and that this can be overcome by leptin treatment. Humans that are leptin deficient due to homozygous gene mutations present with hypogonadotropic hypogonadism, with long-term recombinant leptin treatment being able to achieve pulsatile nocturnal gonadotropin secretion in these patients. Humans with leptin receptor deficiency present with different degrees of hypogonadotropic hypogonadism.

Leptin is considered to be the main peripheral signal providing information about the body's energy stores to the hypothalamic circuits in charge of controlling energy homeostasis, thus communicating this information to the HPG axis by means of mechanisms that are far from being fully understood. Leptin appears to play a permissive role in the initiation of puberty and in the maintenance of the reproductive function. The earlier initiation of puberty seen in obese children may also be partly explained by higher leptin levels. The role of other adipokines such as adiponectin and resistin on the HPG axis is currently poorly understood.

Growing evidence suggests that insulin and leptin interact to downregulate arcuate nucleus (ARC) production of orexigenic peptides such as NPY and AgRP and, in collaboration with serotonin, enhance POMC production and release. Thus, insulin could be another peripheral metabolic signal involved in HPG axis functioning.

Ghrelin is a gut-derived hormone, whose function as a growth hormone secretagogue is well described. More recently, it has been shown that ghrelin modulates energy homeostasis by stimulating the expression of the genes encoding NPY and AgRP in the arcuate nucleus of the hypothalamus and by binding to presynaptic terminals of arcuate NPY and POMC neurons, respectively, stimulating and inhibiting their activity and peptide release. This results in a net orexigenic effect, functionally opposite to that produced by leptin. Thus, it is currently thought that ghrelin plays a role in reporting information regarding the fuel availability in the body to the CNS and that there is an inverse relationship between activation of the HPG axis and ghrelin levels. The role of other gut-derived factors such as peptide YY (PYY) is currently being explored.

Environmental Influences on Puberty

Since genetic background explains 50–80 % of variability in the timing of puberty, it is not surprising that the observed environmental effects are rather modest when individual exposures are assessed. The fact that the age of onset of puberty has been declining in the USA since the mid-1990s, with similar trends are being seen more recently in Europe, points toward such rapid changes having environmental rather than genetic causes [17].

Endocrine-disrupting chemicals have thus been implicated as being such environmental factors affecting pubertal onset. Endocrine disrupters can cause pubertal disorders by several mechanisms. They can act as hormone agonists or antagonists or both depending on the dose and background hormone levels, i.e., the same compound can be an agonist when the level of endogenous hormone is very low (childhood), whereas it can be an antagonist when the real hormone is available (adulthood). Multiple chemical exposures have been considered, but definitive studies are lacking. Examples of such chemicals include polychlorinated and polybrominated biphenyls (PCBs and PBBs), phthalates, dioxins, DDT, and lead. Apart from the association of lead and delayed puberty, the evidence is unclear.

Summary

It is now clear that initiation of puberty involves complex neurohormonal stimuli that are regulated by various genetic and environmental factors. Advances in genetic technologies and a systems biology approach will help with diagnosis and treatment of disorders of pubertal development and help us understand environmental influences that perturb the balance of pubertal development.

References

1. Susman EJ, Houts RM, Steinberg L, et al. Longitudinal development of secondary sexual characteristics in girls and boys between ages 9 ½ and 15 ½ years. Arch Pediatr Adolesc Med. 2010;164:166.
2. Biro FM, Lucky AW, Huster GA, Morrison JA. Pubertal staging in boys. J Pediatr. 1995;127:100.
3. Herman-Giddens ME, Steffes J, Harris D, et al. Secondary sexual characteristics in boys: data from the Pediatric Research in Office Settings Network. Pediatrics. 2012;130, e1058.
4. Rosenfield RL, Lipton RB, Drum ML. Thelarche, pubarche, and menarche attainment in children with normal and elevated body mass index. Pediatrics. 2009;123:84.
5. Sørensen K, Aksglaede L, Petersen JH, Juul A. Recent changes in pubertal timing in healthy Danish boys: associations with body mass index. J Clin Endocrinol Metab. 2010;95:263.
6. Sandhu J, Ben-Shlomo Y, Cole TJ, et al. The impact of childhood body mass index on timing of puberty, adult stature and obesity: a follow-up study based on adolescent anthropometry recorded at Christ's Hospital (1936–1964). Int J Obes (Lond). 2006;30:14.
7. Boyne MS, Thame M, Osmond C, et al. Growth, body composition, and the onset of puberty: longitudinal observations in Afro-Caribbean children. J Clin Endocrinol Metab. 2010;95:3194.
8. Gajdos ZKZ, Henderson KD, Hirschhorn JN, Palmert MR. Genetic determinants of pubertal timing in the general population. Mol Cell Endocrinol. 2010;324:21–9.
9. Topaloglu AK, Reimann F, Guclu M, Yalin AS, Kotan LD, Porter KM, Serin A, Mungan NO, Cook JR, Ozbek MN, Imamoglu S, Akalin NS, Yuksel B, O'Rahilly S, Semple RK. TAC3 and TACR3 mutations in familial hypogonadotropic hypogonadism reveal a key role for neurokinin B in the central control of reproduction. Nat Genet. 2009;41:354–8.
10. Jiang Y, Luo L, Gustafson EL, Yadav D, Laverty M, Murgolo N, Vassileva G, Zeng M, Laz TM, Behan J, Qiu P, Wang L, Wang S, Bayne M, Greene J, Monsma Jr F, Zhang FL. Identification and characterization of a novel RF-amide peptide ligand for orphan G-protein-coupled receptor SP9155. J Biol Chem. 2003;278:27652–7.
11. Martos-Moreno GA, Chowen JA, Argente J. Metabolic signals in human puberty: effects of over and undernutrition. Mol Cell Endocrinol. 2010;324:70–81.
12. Silviera LFG, Trarbach EB, Latronico AC. Genetic basis for GnRH dependant pubertal disorders in humans. Mol Cell Endocrinol. 2010;324:30–8.
13. Ojeda SR, Dubay C, Lomniczi A, Kaidar G, Matagne V, Sandau US, Dissen GA. Gene networks and the neuroendocrine regulation of puberty. Mol Cell Endocrinol. 2010;324:3–11.
14. Riestra P, Garcia-Anguita A, Torres-Cantero A, Bayonas MJ, de Oya M, Garces C. Association of the Q223R polymorphism with age at menarche in the leptin receptor gene in humans. Biol Reprod. 2011;84(4):752–5.
15. Rostami S, Kohan L, Mohammadianpanah M. The LEP G-2548A gene polymorphism is associated with age at menarche and breast cancer susceptibility. Gene. 2015;557(2):154–7.

16. Cukier P, Wright H, Rulfs T, Silveira LF, Teles MG, Mendonca BB, Arnhold IJ, Heger S, Latronico AC, Ojeda SR, Brito VN. Molecular and gene network analysis of thyroid transcription factor 1 (TTF1) and enhanced at puberty (EAP1) genes in patients with GnRH-dependent pubertal disorders. Horm Res Paediatr. 2013;80(4):257–66.
17. Toppari J, Juul A. Trends in pubertal timing in humans and environmental modifiers. Mol Cell Endocrinol. 2010;324:39–44.

Chapter 3
Hormonal Changes in Childhood and Puberty

Rodolfo A. Rey, Stella M. Campo, María Gabriela Ropelato, and Ignacio Bergadá

Introduction

The functional ontogeny of the hypothalamic-pituitary-gonadal axis has particular features that distinguish it from most organs and systems characterized by functional differentiation in early fetal life and complete maturation reached by birth or infancy. Conversely, the gonadal axis displays an incomplete development in utero and during early postnatal life, followed by a functional quiescence of part of the axis during childhood and full maturation during puberty. Although this ontogeny seems to reflect exclusively the changes in the activity of the hypothalamic-gonadotrope axis, a careful look into gonadal developmental physiology uncovers local distinctive features that are also involved in the resulting ontogeny of the reproductive system. In this chapter, we will address the latest understanding on the regulation of the gonadal axis in males and females during development. We will particularly focus on the concept that childhood is not a period of complete quiescence of the gonads and on the differences observed in gonadal function between the early postnatal activation period—which many authors call "mini-puberty"—and canonical puberty. Finally, we will briefly discuss the changes observed in other hormonal axes, which are also related to growth and development.

R.A. Rey (✉) • S.M. Campo • M.G. Ropelato • I. Bergadá
Centro de Investigaciones Endocrinológicas "Dr. César Bergadá" (CEDIE), CONICET-FEI-División de Endocirnología, Hospital de Niños Ricardo Gutiérrez, Gallo 1330, Buenos Aires C1425EFD, Argentina
e-mail: rodolforey@cedie.org.ar; scampo@cedie.org.ar; gropelato@cedie.org.ar; ibergada@cedie.org.ar

P. Kumanov, A. Agarwal (eds.), *Puberty*, DOI 10.1007/978-3-319-32122-6_3

Hormonal Changes in the Male Reproductive Axis

Fetal Life

Initial functional differentiation of endocrine testicular cell populations is independent of pituitary gonadotropins (reviewed in ref [1]). Sertoli and germ cells aggregate to form the seminiferous cords during the seventh fetal week, whereas mesenchymal cells differentiate into Leydig cells in the interstitial tissue in the eighth week. Sertoli cells secrete anti-Müllerian hormone (AMH), responsible for the regression of the Müllerian ducts, i.e., the anlagen of the uterus, fallopian tubes, and upper vagina, and Leydig cells secrete androgens and insulin-like factor 3 (INSL3). Androgens drive fetal virilization of the genitalia and, together with INSL3, are required for testis descent to the scrotum.

In the first trimester, the predominant gonadotropin is human chorionic gonadotropin (hCG) secreted by the placenta. The hypothalamic nuclei that secrete gonadotropin-releasing hormone (GnRH) and the pituitary gonadotrope differentiate later: luteinizing hormone (LH) and follicle-stimulating hormone (FSH) are secreted into the bloodstream from the 17th fetal week (reviewed in [2]). Gonadotropin levels decrease in the third trimester [3], probably due to the negative feedback exerted by placental estrogens.

Placental hCG and pituitary LH induce androgen secretion in Leydig cells. Testosterone levels are high, reaching adult levels, between the 10th and 20th fetal weeks, and decrease during the third trimester (reviewed in [2]).

Basal AMH production is independent of gonadotropins throughout life; however, FSH increases testicular AMH secretion by stimulating Sertoli cell multiplication and upregulating AMH expression in each Sertoli cell [4]. FSH also induces inhibin B secretion by Sertoli cells; inhibin B exerts a negative feedback on FSH.

Birth and Infancy

The circulating levels of gonadotropins and testicular hormones are low at birth (Table 3.1) [5–7]. During the first week of life, gonadotropins increase [6]; in the male, LH levels are higher than FSH (Fig. 3.1). The LH surge drives testosterone and INSL3 secretion. Importantly, for testosterone measurement, serum samples must be extracted to avoid interferences that artificially overestimate results in the first 2 weeks of life [6]. Peak levels of LH, testosterone, and INSL3 are reached during the third month [7–9]; thereafter, they decrease to very low or undetectable from approximately 6 months of age until the onset of puberty (Fig. 3.1).

AMH and inhibin B levels also increase progressively through infancy (Table 3.1) [6, 10–12]. In the first months of life, the surge may be linked to FSH-dependent Sertoli cell proliferation [13]. AMH and inhibin B are useful biomarkers of FSH action [14], as seen in neonates with congenital central hypogonadism [15].

Table 3.1 Reproductive axis hormone levels (median and 3rd and 97th percentiles) in boys from birth to puberty (Tanner stages G1 to G5)

Age	Tanner stage	LH (IU/L)	FSH (IU/L)	Testosterone (ng/dL)	(nmol/L)	Inhibin B (pg/mL)	AMH (pmol/L)	(ng/mL)
1–3 days[a]		0.13 (0–1.10)	0.20 (0–3.97)	48 (18–148)	1.66 (0.62–5.13)	217 (62–444)	328 (140–819)	46 (20–115)
7–14 days[a]		3.50 (0.08–9.57)	1.75 (0.33–6.90)	71 (17–325)	2.46 (0.59–11.27)	297 (95–625)	411 (119–877)	58 (17–123)
20–30 days[a]		2.60 (0.51–5.90)	1.40 (0.54–2.50)	113 (43–508)	3.92 (1.49–17.61)	309 (203–540)	588 (324–1197)	82 (45–168)
1–6 months[b]		0.29 (0.10–2.92)	0.50 (0.15–2.19)	193 (18–355)	6.69 (0.62–12.31)	421 (320–640)	697 (421–1470)	98 (59–206)
6 months–1.9 years[b]		0.10 (0.10–0.35)	0.56 (0.30–1.26)	10 (10–10)	0.35 (0.35–0.35)	240 (80–609)	1132 (684–2329)	159 (96–326)
2.0–8.9 years[b]		0.10 (0.10–0.18)	0.75 (0.24–1.70)	10 (10–10)	0.35 (0.35–0.35)	179 (78–389)	684 (236–1831)	96 (33–256)
9–18 years[b]	G1	0.10 (0.10–2.78)	1.70 (0.58–2.54)	10 (10–108)	0.35 (0.35–3.74)	95 (43–282)	714 (257–1371)	100 (36–192)
	G2	0.80 (0.12–2.76)	2.08 (1.20–4.08)	12 (10–182)	0.42 (0.35–6.31)	156 (67–227)	295 (69–1017)	41 (10–142)
	G3	2.43 (0.67–4.65)	2.96 (1.43–7.44)	182 (12–368)	6.31 (0.42–12.76)	201 (91–371)	71 (30–423)	10 (4–59)
	G4	3.03 (1.44–5.03)	3.55 (2.05–7.94)	392 (187–664)	13.59 (6.48–23.02)	154 (115–271)	65 (33–164)	9 (5–23)
	G5	2.90 (1.34–6.31)	2.55 (1.14–6.99)	438 (114–682)	15.19 (3.95–23.65)	174 (110–278)	82 (38–195)	11 (5–27)

[a]Data from [6]
[b]Data from [10]

This postnatal activation of the hypothalamic-pituitary-gonadal axis has been called "mini-puberty" and is reflected in subtle clinical changes in the male: Sertoli cell proliferation results in a minor increase in testicular volume, which can only be detected by ultrasonography (reviewed in [16]), and Leydig cell androgen production has a trophic effect on the genitalia. Interestingly, the high androgen levels observed during fetal life and the postnatal period are not capable of inducing Sertoli cell maturation and full spermatogenesis, as they do during puberty (see below). The lack of androgen effect on the seminiferous cords may be explained by the fact that the androgen receptor is not expressed in Sertoli cells in the first year of life (Fig. 3.1) [17]. Actually, when the axis activation abnormally continues beyond the age of 1 year, persistently elevated testosterone results in signs of seminiferous tubule maturation like those observed during canonical puberty, e.g., AMH downregulation and inhibin B increase [18].

Key Points

- In the first week after birth, serum levels of gonadotropins and testicular hormones are low.
- Testosterone levels in serum samples should be performed after steroid extraction in the first 2 weeks of life.

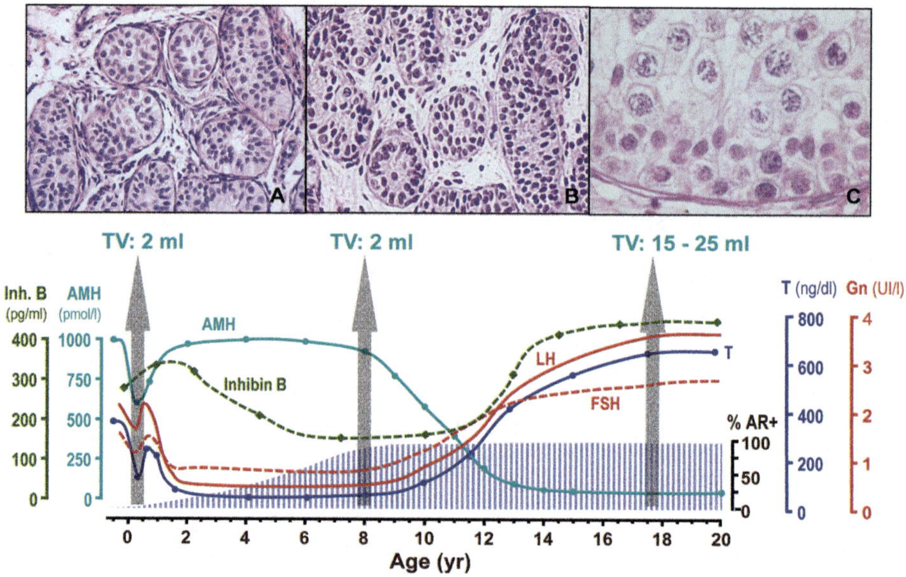

Fig. 3.1 Schematic representation of the ontogeny of pituitary-testicular serum hormone levels from birth to puberty (Tanner stages G1 to G5) and its relationship to androgen receptor (AR) expression in Sertoli cells and testicular histology. At 3 months (**A**), Leydig cells of the interstitial tissue secrete testosterone, but percentage of Sertoli cells positive for AR is extremely low or null; consequently, AMH production is not inhibited by testosterone, and spermatogenesis does not progress into meiosis. At 8 years (**B**), more almost 100 % of Sertoli cells express the AR, but the interstitial tissue does not have mature Leydig cells and testosterone is low; therefore, Sertoli cells remain immature, AMH is high, and no meiosis occurs. At late puberty (**C**), Leydig cells produce high testosterone levels, which provoke the maturation of AR-positive Sertoli cells, reflected in the inhibition of AMH and also in the development of full spermatogenesis. Gn - gonadotropins (Adapted from Rey RA, Musse M, Venara M, Chemes HE. Ontogeny of the androgen receptor expression in the fetal and postnatal testis: its relevance on Sertoli cell maturation and the onset of adult spermatogenesis. Microsc Res Tech 2009; 72: 787–95. With permission from John Wiley & Sons, Inc.)

- Until the age of 3–6 months, basal gonadotropin levels are useful markers of pituitary function, testosterone and INSL3 reflect Leydig cell activity, and AMH and inhibin B are indicative of Sertoli cell function.

Childhood

After the third to sixth months of life in the male, gonadotropins, testosterone, and INSL3 are very low in serum (Fig. 3.1 and Table 3.1). Therefore, the assessment of Leydig cell function during childhood through testosterone or INSL3 determinations requires stimulation with exogenous hCG administration (reviewed in [9]). The decrease in gonadotrope activity during childhood—reflected in low LH and FSH circulating levels—does not seem to be dependent on a negative feedback by testicular factors, since it also occurs in anorchid boys [19].

Classically, childhood has been described as a quiescent period of the gonadal axis, on the basis of low gonadotropin and testosterone serum levels. However, Sertoli cells remain active: they secrete high levels of AMH, a typical marker of the prepubertal testis, and inhibin B (Fig. 3.1). Serum AMH and inhibin B are useful biomarkers to study testicular function during the inadequately called prepubertal "pause" of the reproductive axis.

Key Points

- During childhood, basal serum gonadotropins, testosterone, and INSL3 are very low or undetectable with routine methods in normal boys, so they are not useful markers of the pituitary-Leydig cell axis unless stimulation tests are used.
- Basal serum AMH and inhibin B are high and should be used as primary biomarkers of testicular function.

Puberty

From a clinical standpoint, puberty refers to the period of life spanning 3–5 years characterized by the development of secondary sexual characteristics and the progressive acquisition of the reproductive capacity. In the male, the clinical landmark of pubertal onset is gonadarche, i.e., when testicular volume attains 4 ml (Fig. 3.2). However, it is clear that the physiology of puberty begins somewhat earlier, with a progressive increase in gonadotropin pulse amplitude and frequency (reviewed in [20]). Gonadarche occurs at a mean age of 11.5 years in boys [21]; when it occurs before the age of 9, puberty is considered to be precocious, while it is considered as delayed puberty when gonadarche occurs between 14 and 18 years of age.

At the onset of puberty, the increase in FSH secretion by the gonadotrope induces the proliferation of immature Sertoli cells and boosts testicular volume from 2 to 4 ml, clinically reflected in Tanner stage 2. LH drives the maturation of Leydig cells, which provokes a progressive increase in androgen concentration within the testis resulting in Sertoli cell maturation (reviewed in [22]). Consequently, Sertoli cell proliferation stops, AMH production declines [10, 12], and inhibin B secretion rises [23, 24], as seen in Tanner stages 2–3 (Table 3.1). The increase in serum testosterone levels is a later event, occurring in Tanner stages 3–5 [25], when testicular volume is above 10 ml. Androgens are aromatized to estrogens, and breast development ("gynecomastia") occurs in more than half of normal boys during mid- to late puberty. This physiological event usually reverses spontaneously. Steroid hormones are essential for the occurrence of peak height velocity in Tanner stages 3–4. INSL3 secretion also increases during puberty but becomes gonadotropin independent once adult Leydig cells become fully differentiated (reviewed in [9]).

Germ cells undergo the complete spermatogenic process, leading to sperm production (Fig. 3.1) and to the overt increase in testis volume to 15–25 ml in Tanner stages 4–5 (Fig. 3.2) (reviewed in [22]). FSH and spermatogenesis are essential for inhibin B production, which in turn acts as a negative feedback regulator of pituitary FSH [26]. Therefore, in puberty and adulthood, inhibin B is an extremely informative

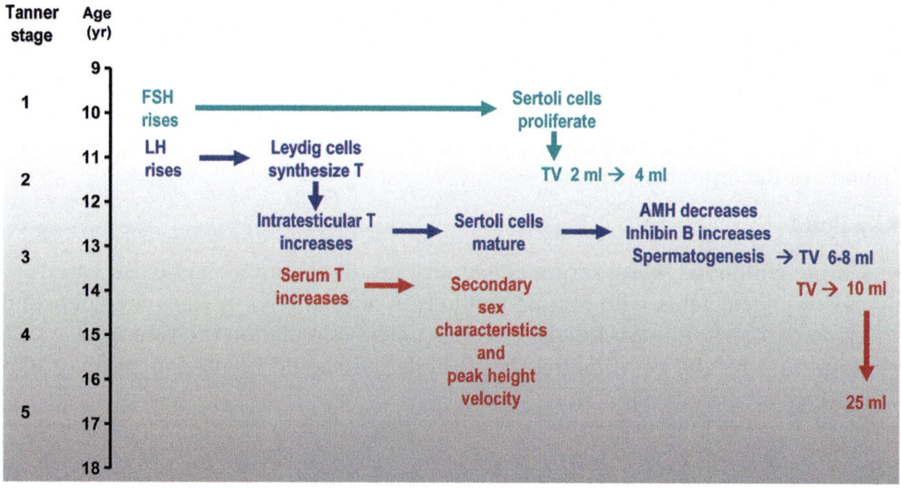

Fig. 3.2 Schematic representation of the pubertal events in the pituitary-testicular axis. The first events are clinically undetectable: when the boy is in Tanner stage 1, gonadotropin levels increase, FSH provokes Sertoli cell proliferation, and LH induces Leydig cell maturation. After some time, the increase in Sertoli cell number is reflected in testicular volume (TV) progression to 4 ml, the clinical milestone of pubertal onset. During Tanner stage 2, intratesticular testosterone concentration increases and provokes Sertoli cell maturation, reflected in downregulation of AMH, increase of inhibin B, and onset of adult spermatogenesis; testicular volume further increases. In Tanner stage 3, the increase in serum testosterone becomes evident, and secondary sex characteristics start developing. During Tanner stages 4 and 5, full testicular volume and secondary sex characteristics are attained

biomarker of testicular function, since it reflects the whole pubertal maturation process, i.e., FSH and testosterone action on Sertoli cells and spermatogenesis.

It is noteworthy that gonadotropin and androgen levels are equally high during fetal life, the postnatal activation (or "mini-puberty"), and puberty, but clinical signs of seminiferous tubule maturation—like AMH downregulation and complete spermatogenesis leading to testis enlargement—only occur during pubertal development. As mentioned before, the ontogeny of the androgen receptor in Sertoli cells seems to be the underlying explanation: in the human, androgen receptor expression appears faintly in few Sertoli cells by the end of the first year. A progressive increase occurs between 2 and 8 years, and by the age of puberty, all Sertoli cells are strongly positive for the androgen receptor (reviewed in [22]).

Key Points

- In the initial steps of puberty, serum LH and FSH increase by pulses.
- Serum AMH decreases and inhibin B increases, reflecting Sertoli cell maturation induced by intratesticular androgens, before serum testosterone increases.
- Serum inhibin B is an excellent biomarker of androgen and FSH action on spermatogenesis.

Hormonal Changes in the Female Reproductive Axis

Fetal Life

The development of the ovary takes longer than that of the testis in fetal life, and it does not occur in the absence of germ cells. Another sexual dimorphism is that oogonia enter meiosis during fetal life, whereas male germ cells only initiate meiosis at puberty. Primary oocytes become surrounded by flattened follicular cells to form primordial follicles, which represent the quiescent follicle ovary reserve. Progressively, flattened cells change to cubic (granulosa) cells, resulting in the formation of primary follicles at around 20 weeks of fetal life. By the 26th week, primary follicles have grown and produce low amounts of AMH [27], which have no effects on Müllerian derivatives because the AMH receptor is no longer expressed. Follicular maturation proceeds to the small antral stage during the last stages of intrauterine life. At this moment, the first meiotic division reaches diplotene stage and becomes arrested until puberty. Estrogen production by the ovary during fetal life is minimal, as compared to high estrogen production by the placenta. Ovarian development up to the seventh month of fetal life occurs independently of fetal gonadotropins [28]. Indeed, follicular development until the small antral stage is mostly gonadotropin independent. During the first half of gestation, female fetuses have higher serum LH and FSH levels than male fetuses. This sex difference has been explained by the absence of a negative feedback. LH and FSH levels decrease toward the end of gestation and are low at term due to high circulating estrogen levels [3].

Birth and Infancy

At birth, gonadotropin levels are low in girls (Table 3.2). Placental hormones are cleared from the newborn circulation during the first postnatal days [5]. By the end of the first week [6], FSH and LH levels start to increase and peak between the first and sixth months [27]. A sexual dimorphism in gonadal inhibin production is evident in the newborn. This dimorphism starts during fetal development, when the inhibin α-subunit is not expressed in the fetal ovaries [29], and is reflected at birth, when inhibins A and B are undetectable in females (Table 3.2). Serum levels of inhibins A and B increase during the first weeks of life [6].

The postnatal gonadotropin surge induces ovarian follicular development and increase of ovarian granulosa cell products, estradiol, inhibin B, and AMH. During the first 2 years, FSH secretion predominates in girls and induces maturation of ovarian follicles; thus, large follicles and measurable estradiol concentrations might be observed [2, 27]. Estradiol levels fluctuate—probably reflecting maturation and atresia of ovarian follicles—and then decrease during the second year of life.

Table 3.2 Reproductive axis hormone levels (median and 3rd and 97th percentiles) in girls from birth to puberty (Tanner stages B1 to B5)

Age	Tanner stage	LH (IU/L)	FSH (IU/L)	E_2 (pg/mL)	Inhibin B[a] (pg/mL)	AMH (pmol/L)	AMH (ng/mL)
2–7 days		0.13 (0.10–1.0)	0.51 (0.19–17.5)	65 (27–94)	Non detectable	6 (ND–25)	0.8 (ND–3.5)
7–30 days		0.45 (0.10–1.8)	6.7 (0.30–20.7)	42 (27–55)	Not available	12 (ND-64)	1.6 (ND–8.9)
1–6 months		0.30 (0.10–0.50)	4.8 (3.5–9.0)	40 (10–60)	48±8.5	15 (4.5–29.5)	2.1 (0.6–4.1)
6 months–2 years		0.17 (0.10–0.30)	3.2 (0.57–7.5)	25 (10–40)	17.5±1.6	8 (3.0–18.9)	1.1 (0.4–2.6)
2–8 years		0.10 (0.10–0.30)	2.2 (0.57–4.6)	10 (10–16)	38.0±8.4	10.9 (1.9–39.2)	1.5 (0.3–5.5)
8–18 years	B1	0.50 (0.10–1.6)	2.8 (0.78–4.8)	25 (10–60)	39±8.3	19.9 (4.7–60.1)	2.8 (0.7–8.4)
	B2	1.2 (0.30–5.3)	4.6 (1.1–7.3)	34 (11–71)	60.6±6.1		
	B3	2.97 (0.41–8.5)	5.4 (2.1–8.6)	42 (20–77)	133.5±14.3		
	B4 and B5[b]	4.97 (1.2–8.7)	5.4 (1.3–10.8)	68 (30–166)	66.9±6.4		

[a]Values are expressed as mean ± SEM
[b]At early follicular phase
ND - non detectable.

Key Points

- At birth, inhibin B and AMH are undetectable in serum. In the first week after birth, gonadotropins and estradiol are low.
- Serum levels of FSH, LH, AMH, and inhibin B increase during the first weeks of life.
- During the first 2 years of age, FSH concentration is higher than LH.
- Serum AMH and inhibin B are useful markers of ovarian function, particularly when highly sensitive estradiol assays are not available.

Childhood

At the end of the 2nd year of life, a gradual dampening of GnRH secretion activity starts in girls, leading to its relative quiescence during childhood because of steroid-independent (predominant) and steroid-dependent inhibitory mechanisms [2]. Consequently, FSH, LH, and estradiol secretion are low (Table 3.2). FSH secretion is predominant (about 10–50 times higher than LH), largely higher than in boys [30, 31]. This gender dimorphism may be due to the lower inhibin B production by the ovary [11]. Serum LH and estradiol levels are hardly detectable in girls, even using ultrasensitive assays [30, 32]. The presence of measurable serum levels of inhibin B and AMH in females during childhood reflects functionally active gonads. However, the absence of inhibin A suggests that the follicles present in the ovary have not reached an advanced stage of antral development. During childhood, serum FSH levels are insufficient to sustain full follicular development, and a large number of small developing follicles become atretic.

Key Points

- FSH concentration is measurable and LH is very low or undetectable LH. FSH response is predominant to stimulation tests with GnRH or with GnRH agonists.
- AMH and inhibin B reflect functionally active gonads and are markers of the ovarian reserve.

Puberty

Like in boys, in girls gonadarche follows a prior increase in the amplitude of GnRH pulses and—consequently—of LH and FSH secretion, taking place initially at night and then, as puberty advances, throughout the day. The clinical onset of puberty or gonadarche in girls is marked by breast development ("thelarche"), which occurs at a mean age of 9.7 years [21]. When thelarche occurs before the age of 8, puberty is considered as precocious.

Progressive increases in LH, FSH, and estradiol serum levels are observed all throughout puberty (Table 3.2). Serum LH concentrations increase 10- to 50-fold as compared to childhood, while FSH concentrations increase two- to threefold. As a result, the serum LH/FSH ratio is approximately 1 at Tanner stages 4 and 5. Also, the onset of puberty is characterized by an increased serum LH response to GnRH or GnRH agonists [33].

From pubertal onset, the "initial recruitment" of primordial follicles to reach the small antral stage—which is gonadotropin independent—is followed by a tonic follicular growth phase stimulated by FSH and finally by a "cyclic recruitment" of the follicle that will be ovulated during each menstrual cycle.

Levels of inhibin B increase through pubertal Tanner stages 2 and 3, possibly reflecting its production by small antral follicles in response to gonadotropin stimulation. Inhibin B levels attained at Tanner stage 3 are higher than those observed in adult women. AMH levels do not change considerably, although the peak seems to be reached peripubertally [34, 35]. It has been proposed that this stage of pubertal development may represent a period of consistently high ovarian follicular activity before the development of the adult menstrual cycle, with ovulation and a luteal phase [36]. The progressive and sustained increment of inhibin B serum levels throughout pubertal development would be the signal that the pituitary gland receives to initiate a full functioning negative feedback mechanism between inhibin and FSH.

Key Points

- Serum LH concentrations rise at puberty to levels 10–50 times higher than prepubertal levels, while FSH concentrations increase 2–3 times during puberty.
- A rise in serum inhibin B levels during puberty may reflect follicle development induced by FSH in early puberty.
- The increment of inhibin B throughout pubertal development initiates full functioning negative feedback between this peptide and FSH.
- AMH reaches its peak levels peripubertally.

Menstrual Cycle

The first menstrual bleeding is known as menarche and occurs between 1.5 and 3 years after thelarche (reviewed in [37]). Gonadotropins, follicular development, and ovarian steroids and inhibins exhibit a well-defined cyclic pattern during menstrual cycles. During the early postmenarcheal years, menstrual cycles can range from 21 to 45 days, and anovulatory cycles are predominant [38]. Regular menstrual cycles are attained 3–5 years post-menarche. The menstrual cycle is divided into a "follicular phase" (first day of bleeding until ovulation) followed by a "luteal phase." As each menstrual cycle begins, FSH concentrations rise over LH concentrations, and consequently, multiple small antral follicles are recruited to begin preovulatory development. By cycle day 8, one follicle becomes selected to ovulate due to its increased responsiveness to FSH and LH, while the remainder follicles become atretic. The dominant follicle reaches more than 10 mm in diameter and increasingly synthesizes estradiol. Later, at the end of follicular phase, it grows up to 20 mm in diameter. This follicle, known as Graafian follicle, produces a sharp increase in serum levels of estradiol that becomes sufficient to produce a positive feedback on pituitary LH secretion. This results in the mid-cycle LH surge, which in turn provokes ovulation [39, 40]. After ovulation, during the luteal phase, the remaining granulosa cells that are not released with the oocyte become luteinized and combine with the newly formed theca lutein cells and surrounding stroma in the ovary to form the corpus luteum, a transient endocrine organ that predominantly secretes progesterone. The high levels of estradiol and progesterone attained at mid-luteal phase slow GnRH pulse frequency [41], which results in a predominance of FSH secretion initiating the next cycle of follicular development.

Serum AMH shows only minimal—clinically irrelevant—variations during the spontaneous menstrual cycle, since it reflects the small follicle ovarian reserve [42]. Inhibin B increases primarily during the follicular phase, while inhibin A predominates in the luteal phase. Inhibin B is produced at early stages of follicular development, whereas inhibin A is preferentially secreted by more differentiated follicular and luteinized cells [43]. The high-molecular-weight precursor of the inhibin α-subunit is present in circulation during the follicular phase as well as during the luteal phase.

Key Points

- Menstrual cycles are irregular and frequently anovulatory in the first 2 years after menarche.
- Gonadotropins, estrogens, and progesterone show a typical cyclic variation.
- AMH barely changes throughout the cycle, whereas inhibin B is higher during the follicular phase and inhibin A during the luteal phase.

Hormonal Changes in Other Axes

The Adrenal Axis

The ontogeny of the adrenal cortex shows major differences between fetal and postnatal steroidogenic activity. During fetal life, the so-called fetal zone of the cortex occupies approximately 80 % of the gland. Steroid synthesis is predominantly represented by pregnenolone, dehydroepiandrosterone (DHEA), and dehydroepiandrosterone sulfate (DHEAS) in the fetal zone. The outer zone is responsible for cortisol production under the influence of fetal adrenocorticotropic hormone (ACTH) from the eighth week and aldosterone. However, the fetal adrenal gland has little 3β-hydroxysteroid dehydrogenase activity. The placenta is rich in this enzyme, catalyzing the conversion of pregnenolone to progesterone, which is used by the fetus in the biosynthesis of aldosterone and cortisol, thus closing the adrenal fetal-placental circuit.

After birth and during the first months of life, a significant regression (approximately 50 %) of the adrenal gland occurs concomitantly with a marked decrease in the production of DHEA. Serum concentrations of cortisol vary widely in neonates with low levels close to the detection limit of the assay [44]. The circadian rhythm of cortisol appears to be installed by the end of the first year of life, although a wide interindividual variability exists [45]. Between the first and fifth years of life, serum concentrations of androstenedione and DHEAS remain very low.

From the age of 5–6 years, adrenarche occurs featuring a progressive increase in the secretion of androstenedione and DHEA. Although they are metabolites with weak androgen activity, in some cases they are responsible for some degrees of clinical manifestation such as body odor, pimples on the face, axillary hair, and/or pubic hair of different magnitude. Usually these manifestations are observed from the age of 7 years in girls and 8 years in boys. The physiological mechanisms of adrenarche have not been well characterized yet, but the potential mechanisms could be ACTH dependent [46].

Basal and ACTH-stimulated levels of DHEA and DHEAS increase throughout puberty, with slightly higher DHEA levels in females in late puberty and higher DHEAS levels in males after puberty. Overall circulating adrenal androgens increase more than tenfold from the onset of adrenarche to peak adult values, around the third decade of life, and thereafter decline progressively. Cortisol secretion and the diurnal rhythm show no changes.

The Growth Axis

Growth hormone (GH)/insulin-like growth factor (IGF) axis is the main responsible for linear growth in humans. The role that each hormone plays in growth varies according to the ontogeny of human growth and development from fetal life to the end of puberty.

Size at birth is the result of multifactorial factors that include environmental, maternal, placental, and fetal factors. Although GH is known to be produced from the end of the first trimester of fetal life and its circulating concentrations reach very high levels by midgestation, the direct action of GH on fetal growth is limited. Probably IGF-I and IGF-II are the most important factors involved in fetal growth regulation. Both increase progressively in fetal circulation until the end of gestation when they drop abruptly. At term the serum concentrations of IGF-I are directly related to birth weight [47]. Circulating insulin-like growth factor-binding protein 3 (IGFBP3) is present in very low concentrations from midgestation suggesting a negligible role comparing to its postnatal role in the maintenance of the binary and ternary complex with IGF-I and the acid labile subunit (ALS). On the contrary, insulin-like growth factor-binding protein 1 (IGFBP1) levels appear to be an indicator of fetal nutrition [47].

Markedly elevated GH values associated to low IGF-I levels are found during the first weeks of life in full-term and preterm neonates. GH secretory pattern is pulsatile governed by neuroendocrine mechanisms [48]. High serum concentrations of GH levels may be due to the lack of negative feedback from low levels of circulating IGF-I and yet to other underdeveloped inhibitory mechanisms [49].

By the end of the first month of life, a progressive maturation of the regulatory mechanisms of GH secretion occurs. Somatostatin and GH-releasing hormone (GHRH), as well as other neuropeptides, lead to the characteristic basal and stimulated serum concentrations of GH during infancy and childhood [50]. GH release occurs over short intervals known as the ultradian rhythms and circadian rhythms that occur during 24 h. Ultradian rhythm of GH is every 20 min with maximum of spontaneous release during the night [51]. Amplitude and frequency of pulsatile GH secretory are regulated and influenced by a variety of different influences such as age, pubertal status and nutrition, and wake-sleep states through complex neural and humoral signals.

Close to pubertal onset, the secretion of growth hormone appears to decrease concomitantly with decreasing growth rate, suggesting a transient decrease in growth hormone secretion that recovers after the onset of puberty. Thereafter, marked changes occur. During puberty there are 1.5 times more amplitude pulses of GH due to higher pulse duration and amplitude, and the integrated GH secretion is 2–2.5 times higher in late puberty [52]. This physiological increment in GH secretion is associated with a significant increase in IGF-I and IGFBP-3 serum concentrations, possibly in response to estrogens.

Insulin and Carbohydrate Metabolism

Insulin sensitivity refers to the ability of insulin to stimulate glucose metabolism, while insulin resistance denotes a situation in which an excess of insulin is required to maintain adequate homeostasis of glucose metabolism. During puberty, there is a physiological transient drop in insulin sensitivity of approximately 30 %. Most of it occurs in Tanner stages 3–4, especially in females. Basal insulin increases throughout puberty. Clearly, there is an inverse relationship between fat mass and insulin sensitivity. The drop in the insulin sensitivity is accompanied by an increase in acute insulin response to glucose and a fall in the disposition index of glucose. Interestingly, IGF-I levels rise and drop in a pattern similar to the rise and fall of insulin across the different stages of puberty, suggesting that the GH/IGF-I axis might also contribute to the physiological insulin resistance of puberty.

References

1. Rey RA, Grinspon RP. Normal male sexual differentiation and aetiology of disorders of sex development. Best Pract Res Clin Endocrinol Metab. 2011;25:221–38.
2. Kuiri-Hänninen T, Sankilampi U, Dunkel L. Activation of the hypothalamic-pituitary-gonadal axis in infancy, minipuberty. Horm Res Paediatr. 2014;82:73–80.
3. Debieve F, Beerlandt S, Hubinont C, Thomas K. Gonadotropins, prolactin, inhibin A, inhibin B, and activin A in human fetal serum from midpregnancy and term pregnancy. J Clin Endocrinol Metab. 2000;85:270–4.
4. Lasala C, Carré-Eusèbe D, Picard JY, Rey R. Subcellular and molecular mechanisms regulating anti-Mullerian hormone gene expression in mammalian and nonmammalian species. DNA Cell Biol. 2004;23:572–85.
5. Corbier P, Dehennin L, Castanier M, Mebazaa A, Edwards DA, Roffi J. Sex differences in serum luteinizing hormone and testosterone in the human neonate during the first few hours after birth. J Clin Endocrinol Metab. 1990;71:1344–8.
6. Bergadá I, Milani C, Bedecarrás P, Andreone L, Ropelato MG, Gottlieb S, et al. Time course of the serum gonadotropin surge, inhibins, and anti-Mullerian hormone in normal newborn males during the first month of life. J Clin Endocrinol Metab. 2006;91:4092–8.
7. Kuiri-Hanninen T, Seuri R, Tyrvainen E, Turpeinen U, Hamalainen E, Stenman UH, et al. Increased activity of the hypothalamic-pituitary-testicular axis in infancy results in increased androgen action in premature boys. J Clin Endocrinol Metab. 2011;96:98–105.
8. Forest MG, Sizonenko PC, Cathiard AM, Bertrand J. Hypophyso-gonadal function in humans during the first year of life. 1. Evidence for testicular activity in early infancy. J Clin Invest. 1974;53:819–28.
9. Bay K, Andersson AM. Human testicular insulin-like factor 3: in relation to development, reproductive hormones and andrological disorders. Int J Androl. 2011;34:97–109.
10. Grinspon RP, Bedecarrás P, Ballerini MG, Iñíguez G, Rocha A, Mantovani Rodrigues Resende EA, et al. Early onset of primary hypogonadism revealed by serum anti-Müllerian hormone determination during infancy and childhood in trisomy 21. Int J Androl. 2011;34:e487–98.
11. Bergadá I, Rojas G, Ropelato MG, Ayuso S, Bergadá C, Campo SM. Sexual dimorphism in circulating monomeric and dimeric inhibins in normal boys and girls from birth to puberty. Clin Endocrinol (Oxf). 1999;51:455–60.
12. Aksglaede L, Sorensen K, Boas M, Mouritsen A, Hagen CP, Jensen RB, et al. Changes in anti-Mullerian hormone (AMH) throughout the life span: a population-based study of 1027 healthy males from birth (cord blood) to the age of 69 years. J Clin Endocrinol Metab. 2010;95:5357–64.
13. Berensztein EB, Sciara MI, Rivarola MA, Belgorosky A. Apoptosis and proliferation of human testicular somatic and germ cells during prepuberty: high rate of testicular growth in newborns mediated by decreased apoptosis. J Clin Endocrinol Metab. 2002;87:5113–8.
14. Valeri C, Schteingart HF, Rey RA. The prepubertal testis: biomarkers and functions. Curr Opin Endocrinol Diabetes Obes. 2013;20:224–33.
15. Bougnères P, François M, Pantalone L, Rodrigue D, Bouvattier C, Demesteere E, et al. Effects of an early postnatal treatment of hypogonadotropic hypogonadism with a continuous subcu-

taneous infusion of recombinant follicle-stimulating hormone and luteinizing hormone. J Clin Endocrinol Metab. 2008;93:2202–5.
16. Rey RA. Mini-puberty and true puberty: differences in testicular function. Ann Endocrinol (Paris). 2014;75:58–63.
17. Chemes HE, Rey RA, Nistal M, Regadera J, Musse M, Gonzalez-Peramato P, Serrano A. Physiological androgen insensitivity of the fetal, neonatal, and early infantile testis is explained by the ontogeny of the androgen receptor expression in Sertoli cells. J Clin Endocrinol Metab. 2008;93:4408–12.
18. Grinspon RP, Andreone L, Bedecarrás P, Ropelato MG, Rey RA, Campo SM, Bergadá I. Male central precocious puberty: serum profile of anti-Mullerian hormone and inhibin B before, during, and after treatment with GnRH analogue. Int J Endocrinol. 2013;2013:823064.
19. Grinspon RP, Ropelato MG, Bedecarrás P, Loreti N, Ballerini MG, Gottlieb S, et al. Gonadotrophin secretion pattern in anorchid boys from birth to pubertal age: pathophysiological aspects and diagnostic usefulness. Clin Endocrinol (Oxf). 2012;76:698–705.
20. Dunkel L, Quinton R. Induction of puberty. Eur J Endocrinol. 2014;170:R229–39.
21. Mouritsen A, Aksglaede L, Soerensen K, Hagen CP, Petersen JH, Main KM, Juul A. The pubertal transition in 179 healthy Danish children: associations between pubarche, adrenarche, gonadarche, and body composition. Eur J Endocrinol. 2013;168:129–36.
22. Rey RA, Musse M, Venara M, Chemes HE. Ontogeny of the androgen receptor expression in the fetal and postnatal testis: its relevance on Sertoli cell maturation and the onset of adult spermatogenesis. Microsc Res Tech. 2009;72:787–95.
23. Trigo RV, Bergadá I, Rey R, Ballerini MG, Bedecarrás P, Bergadá C, et al. Altered serum profile of inhibin B, Pro-alphaC and anti-Mullerian hormone in prepubertal and pubertal boys with varicocele. Clin Endocrinol (Oxf). 2004;60:758–64.
24. Lahlou N, Roger M. Inhibin B in pubertal development and pubertal disorders. Semin Reprod Med. 2004;22:165–75.
25. Pasqualini T, Chemes H, Rivarola MA. Testicular testosterone levels during puberty in cryptorchidism. Clin Endocrinol (Oxf). 1981;15:545–54.
26. Bergadá I, Bergadá C, Campo SM. Role of inhibins in childhood and puberty. J Pediatr Endocrinol Metab. 2001;14:343–53.
27. Kuiri-Hanninen T, Kallio S, Seuri R, Tyrvainen E, Liakka A, Tapanainen J, et al. Postnatal developmental changes in the pituitary-ovarian axis in preterm and term infant girls. J Clin Endocrinol Metab. 2011;96:3432–9.
28. Richards JS, Pangas SA. The ovary: basic biology and clinical implications. J Clin Invest. 2010;120:963–72.
29. Martins da Silva SJ, Bayne RAL, Cambray N, Hartley PS, McNeilly AS, Anderson RA. Expression of activin subunits and receptors in the developing human ovary: activin A promotes germ cell survival and proliferation before primordial follicle formation. Dev Biol. 2004;266:334–45.
30. Apter D, Butzow TL, Laughlin GA, Yen SS. Gonadotropin-releasing hormone pulse generator activity during pubertal transition in girls: pulsatile and diurnal patterns of circulating gonadotropins. J Clin Endocrinol Metab. 1993;76:940–9.
31. Ropelato MG, Escobar ME, Gottlieb S, Bergadá C. Gonadotropin secretion in prepubertal normal and agonadal children evaluated by ultrasensitive time-resolved immunofluorometric assays. Horm Res. 1997;48:164–72.
32. Neely EK, Hintz RL, Wilson DM, Lee PA, Gautier T, Argente J, Stene M. Normal ranges for immunochemiluminometric gonadotropin assays. J Pediatr. 1995;127:40–6.
33. Oerter KE, Uriarte MM, Rose SR, Barnes KM, Cutler Jr GB. Gonadotropin secretory dynamics during puberty in normal girls and boys. J Clin Endocrinol Metab. 1990;71:1251–8.
34. Hagen CP, Aksglaede L, Sorensen K, Mouritsen A, Andersson AM, Petersen JH, et al. Individual serum levels of anti-Mullerian hormone in healthy girls persist through childhood and adolescence: a longitudinal cohort study. Hum Reprod. 2012;27:861–6.
35. Kelsey TW, Wright P, Nelson SM, Anderson RA, Wallace WH. A validated model of serum anti-Mullerian hormone from conception to menopause. PLoS One. 2011;6, e22024.

36. Chada M, Prusa R, Bronsky J, Kotaska K, Sidlova K, Pechova M, Lisa L. Inhibin B, follicle stimulating hormone, luteinizing hormone and testosterone during childhood and puberty in males: changes in serum concentrations in relation to age and stage of puberty. Physiol Res. 2003;52:45–51.
37. Carel JC, Léger J. Precocious puberty. N Engl J Med. 2008;358:2366–77.
38. American Academy of Pediatrics, Committee on Adolescence, American College of Obstetricians and Gynecologists, Committee on Adolescent Health Care, Diaz A, Laufer MR, Breech LL. Menstruation in girls and adolescents: using the menstrual cycle as a vital sign. Pediatrics. 2006;118:2245–50.
39. Karsch FJ, Dierschke DJ, Knobil E. Sexual differentiation of pituitary function: apparent difference between primates and rodents. Science. 1973;179:484–6.
40. Adams JM, Taylor AE, Schoenfeld DA, Crowley Jr WF, Hall JE. The midcycle gonadotropin surge in normal women occurs in the face of an unchanging gonadotropin-releasing hormone pulse frequency. J Clin Endocrinol Metab. 1994;79:858–64.
41. Filicori M, Santoro N, Merriam GR, Crowley Jr WF. Characterization of the physiological pattern of episodic gonadotropin secretion throughout the human menstrual cycle. J Clin Endocrinol Metab. 1986;62:1136–44.
42. Dewailly D, Andersen CY, Balen A, Broekmans F, Dilaver N, Fanchin R, et al. The physiology and clinical utility of anti-Mullerian hormone in women. Hum Reprod Update. 2014;20:370–85.
43. Sehested A, Juul AA, Andersson AM, Petersen JH, Jensen TK, Müller J, Skakkebæk NE. Serum inhibin A and inhibin B in healthy prepubertal, pubertal, and adolescent girls and adult women: relation to age, stage of puberty, menstrual cycle, follicle-stimulating hormone, luteinizing hormone, and estradiol levels. J Clin Endocrinol Metab. 2000;85:1634–40.
44. Ballerini MG, Chiesa A, Scaglia P, Gruneiro-Papendieck L, Heinrich JJ, Ropelato MG. 17alpha-hydroxyprogesterone and cortisol serum levels in neonates and young children: influence of age, gestational age, gender and methodological procedures. J Pediatr Endocrinol Metab. 2010;23:121–32.
45. Knutsson U, Dahlgren J, Marcus C, Rosberg S, Bronnegard M, Stierna P, Albertsson-Wikland K. Circadian cortisol rhythms in healthy boys and girls: relationship with age, growth, body composition, and pubertal development. J Clin Endocrinol Metab. 1997;82:536–40.
46. Auchus RJ. The physiology and biochemistry of adrenarche. Endocr Dev. 2011;20:20–7.
47. Chard T. Insulin-like growth factors and their binding proteins in normal and abnormal human fetal growth. Growth Regul. 1994;4:91–100.
48. Wright NM, Northington FJ, Miller JD, Veldhuis JD, Rogol AD. Elevated growth hormone secretory rate in premature infants: deconvolution analysis of pulsatile growth hormone secretion in the neonate. Pediatr Res. 1992;32:286–90.
49. Giustina A, Veldhuis JD. Pathophysiology of the neuroregulation of growth hormone secretion in experimental animals and the human. Endocr Rev. 1998;19:717–97.
50. Vigneri R, D'Agata R. Growth hormone release during the first year of life in relation to sleep-wake periods. J Clin Endocrinol Metab. 1971;33:561–3.
51. Tannenbaum GS, Ling N. The interrelationship of growth hormone (GH)-releasing factor and somatostatin in generation of the ultradian rhythm of GH secretion. Endocrinology. 1984; 115:1952–7.
52. Veldhuis JD, Roemmich JN, Rogol AD. Gender and sexual maturation-dependent contrasts in the neuroregulation of growth hormone secretion in prepubertal and late adolescent males and females--a general clinical research center-based study. J Clin Endocrinol Metab. 2000;85:2385–94.

Chapter 4
Physical Changes During Pubertal Transition

Ralitsa Robeva and Philip Kumanov

Introduction

Puberty is a period of life during which secondary sex characteristics develop and the gonads reach their endocrine and exocrine maturity. The duration of the pubertal transition is approximately 3–4 years, and at the end of the process, slightly before the body growth ceases, individuals are able to reproduce.

Physical events during puberty reflect the profound endocrine changes in the hypothalamus, pituitary, gonads and adrenal glands. Adolescent reawakening of the hypothalamic–pituitary–gonadal (HPG) axis is preceded by a gender-specific secretion of gonadotropins and sex hormones during foetal life as well as in the postnatal period (minipuberty) [1]. The hormonal peaks during early infancy are followed by a prepubertal HPG quiescence that takes several years. HPG reactivation during adolescence is crucial for the development of puberty, but the underlying mechanisms are not completely understood.

Onset of Puberty: Adrenarche and Gonadarche

The fundaments of pubertal development are two independent but chronologically related processes—*adrenarche* and *gonadarche* [2].

R. Robeva • P. Kumanov (✉)
Clinical Center of Endocrinology, Medical Faculty, Medical University of Sofia,
Zdrave 2 Street, 1431 Sofia, Bulgaria
e-mail: phkumanov@lycos.com

P. Kumanov, A. Agarwal (eds.), *Puberty*, DOI 10.1007/978-3-319-32122-6_4

Adrenarche

Adrenarche is a phenomenon of adrenal zona reticularis activation leading to increased secretion of dehydroepiandrosterone (DHEA) and dehydroepiandrosterone sulphate (DHEAS) [3]. Prepubertally low adrenal androgens begin to rise at around 6–7 years of age and continue to increase in accordance with age and pubertal stages in boys and girls [4]. The development of adrenarche contributes to the appearance of several androgen-dependent phenotypic features after the age of 8–9 years such as occurrence of pubic (*pubarche*) and axillary (*axillarche*) hair, accelerated statural growth, stimulation of apocrine sweat and sebaceous glands associated with adult-type body odour and acne in some children [3, 5, 6]. According to traditional understanding, adrenarche is a process specific for humans and some primates; however, some data describe similar morphological and steroid changes in rat adrenal glands [7, 8]. Adrenal androgens might influence bone development and behaviour, but nevertheless physiological significance of adrenarche remains unknown [9, 10].

Adrenarche is independent of gonadal development and could occur even in patients with gonadal dysgenesis [11]. However, patients with Turner syndrome and ovarian failure showed earlier onset of adrenarche contrasting with significantly delayed pubarche in comparison to healthy girls [12]. These results demonstrate that pubic hair growth depends not only on adrenal hormonal production but also on the gonadal function, and thus terms *adrenarche* and *pubarche* could not be used interchangeably [2, 12]. Adrenal gland maturation is not crucial for puberty, and patients with central precocious puberty could undergo sexual development before the onset of adrenarche [13].

Gonadarche

The pubertal key step is the reactivation of gonadotropin-releasing hormone (GnRH) pulse generator leading to the increased gonadotropin levels and subsequent activation of ovarian or testicular hormonal production. The complex neuroendocrine mechanisms that trigger the GnRH neuron function in the hypothalamus result in the development of gametogenesis and fertility during pubertal maturation [reviewed in 14–18]. The physical expression of HPG reactivation is the enlargement of testicular and ovarian volume (*gonadarche*). The elevated steroid hormones in girls induce the onset of breast development (*thelarche*).

Profound changes in hypothalamus–pituitary–gonadal system, activation of adrenal glands as well as stimulation of somatotrophic axis are the main factors responsible for physical changes in boys and girls during puberty.

Physical Changes in Girls

Breast Development

During puberty, the system and local effects of estrogens, growth hormone (GH) and insulin-like growth factor-1 (IGF1) stimulate the breast cell proliferation in maturing healthy girls [19]. Endocrine and paracrine interrelations induce mammary gland development that progresses through several stages from preadolescent state to mature breast (Fig. 4.1).

Usually, the phenotypic changes are evaluated by a visual rating method developed in the late 1960s and widely known as "Tanner stages" [20]. The long preadolescent period (Stage B1) is followed by an initial breast development at the onset of puberty (Stage B2) characterized by a specific mound-like elevation of the breast and papilla as well as slight areolar enlargement. Further growth of the breast and areola without separation of their contours is typical for stage B3. The progression through B4 stage is marked by a formation of secondary mound due to areola and papilla elevation above the breast level. Restoration of areola to the general contour as well as overall breast enlargement indicates adult breast development (Stage B5) [20–22].

Thelarche is an important sign of the puberty onset and it is usually observed in girls at the age of 10 years. However, progression toward Tanner B2 stage could occur at different time in girls from diverse racial and ethnic groups and from various geographic locations (Table 4.1) [22–33]. A Johannesburg study (1976–1977) showed that thelarche occurred at similar mean age of 11.5 years for black and white girls [34]. Twenty years later in the USA, the mean age of breast development onset was strikingly decreased especially in African-American girls (8.87 ± 1.93 years) [26]. Similar secular trend was observed in European countries, but 15 years later [35]. Danish girls examined in 1990s developed B2 stage at the age of 10.88 years, not earlier than their peers investigated in 1960s [29]. However, a study conducted in 2006–2008 within the same geographical region showed significantly earlier breast development (mean age 9.86 years) [36]. The same process of earlier female pubertal development was observed also in Asian countries in the last 50 years [37, 38], but the reasons remained unexplained. Obesity and endocrine-disrupting chemicals could affect pubertal maturation; however, other factors including ethnic differences, psychosocial environment and family conditions might be also of clinical importance [33, 39–41].

The transition from one breast stage to another takes about 12–18 months, while the whole breast maturation continues approximately 4–4.5 years [22, 25, 32, 33]. The appearance of pubertal signs in girls less than 8 years is traditionally considered as precocious sexual development, while the lack of breast development by 13 years is a sign of delayed or absent sexual maturation [42, 43].

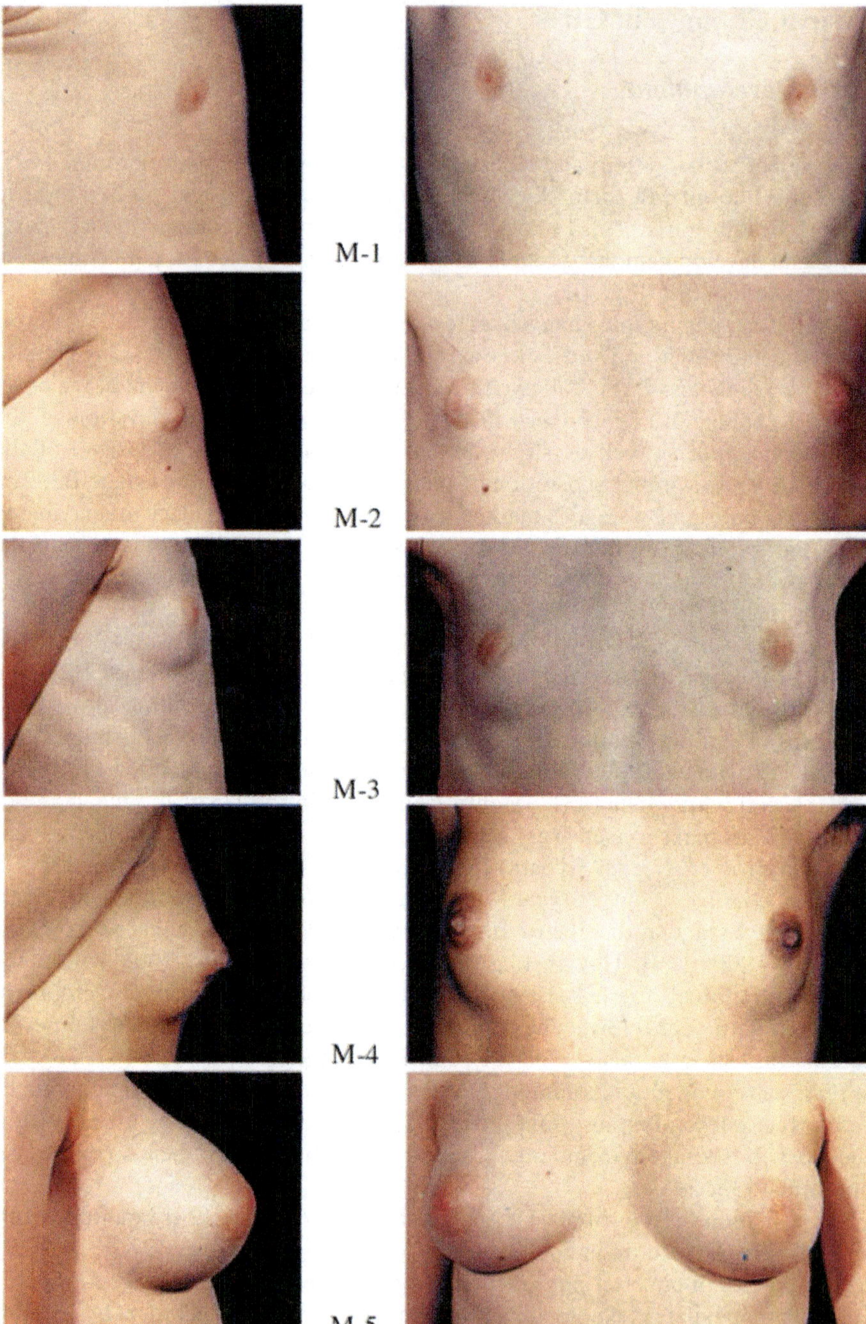

Fig. 4.1 Breast development in girls. M1–M5 correspond to breast stages B1–B5 in the text. [Reprinted from Biro F, Dorn L. Issues in Measurement of Pubertal Development. In: Preedy VR, editor. Handbook of Anthropometry: Physical Measures of Human Form in Health and Disease. New York, NY: Springer Science + Business Media; 2012:237–251. With permission from Springer Science + Business Media]

Table 4.1 Average age (mean or median) of breast (B2–B5) and pubic hair (PH2–PH5) development as well as peak height velocity (PHV) and menarche (M) in girls from different countries [22–33, 57]

Country	Authors	B2	B3	B4	B5	PH2	PH3	PH4	PH5	PHV	M
USA	Reynolds and Wines (1948) (l)	10.8	11.4	12.2	13.7	11.0	11.9	12.5	13.9		12.90
UK	Marshall and Tanner (1969) (l)	11.15	12.15	13.11	15.33	11.69	12.36	12.95	14.41	12.14	13.47
UK	Billewicz et al. (1981) (l)	10.78	12.04	13.07	13.97					12.16	13.37
Sweden	Lindgren (1996) (c)	10.8	11.7	13.0	14.8	11.2	12.3	13.4	14.9		
USA	Herman-Giddens et al. (1997) (c)[a]	9.96	11.30			10.51	11.53				12.88
USA	Herman-Giddens et al. (1997) (c)[b]	8.87	10.19			8.78	10.35				12.16
USA	Sun et al. (2002)[a] (c)	10.38	11.75	13.29	15.47	10.57	11.80	13.0	16.33		
Lithuania	Zukauskaite et al. (2005) (c)	10.2	11.3	13.9		11.2					
Denmark	Juul et al. (2006) (c)	10.88	12.40	13.54	14.66	11.29	12.39	13.51	14.49		13.42
Turkey	Bundak et al. (2008) (l)	10.3	11.7	12.3	12.8	11.2	11.8	12.3	12.8	11.3	12.2
Bulgaria	Tomova et al. (2009) (c)										12.0
Iran	Rabbani et al. (2010) (c)	10.10	11.62	13.55	14.92	9.83	11.60	13.27	14.96		12.55
UK	Christensen et al. (2010a) (l)	10.19	11.66	13.19		10.95	11.99	12.88			12.87
USA	Susman et al. (2010) (l)	9.8	11.3	12.7	14.2	10.2	11.5	12.7	14.2		

c cross-sectional, *l* longitudinal
[a]White
[b]Afro-Americans

Androgen-Dependent Hair Growth

Androgen-dependent hair growth in women results from the neuroendocrine hypothalamic–pituitary–adrenal and gonadal changes leading to increased DHEAS and testosterone levels [33].

Pubarche

Pubic hair (PH) growth is an important phenotypic sign of sexual maturation. Magnetic resonance imaging data has shown an increase of adrenal volume in accordance with the chronological age and pubic hair stages in children [44]. However, adrenal androgen levels are not associated with adrenal size, and no hormonal cut-off values specific for pubarche have been estimated, because of pronounced interindividual variability [44, 45].

The widely accepted method for evaluation of pubic hair development is Tanner staging (Fig. 4.2) [20–22]. Stage PH1 indicates preadolescent state without pubic hair, while the sparse growth of straight slightly pigmented hair mainly along the labia characterized next pubic hair stage PH2. The progression of puberty is marked by the growth of darker, coarser and curled hair that spreads over the junction of the pubes and could be detected on white–black photographs (PH3). Stage PH4 resembles the adult pattern, but the covered area is still considerably smaller than in grown-up women, and it does not spread over the inner thighs. The adult female pubic hair is distributed in the form of an inverse triangle (PH5) [21, 22].

Usually, initial breast development occurs several months earlier than pubic hair growth, but in some girls pubarche could be the first sign of true sexual maturation [2, 22]. According to the study of Biro et al., 58.6 % of the investigated female participants showed synchronous breast and pubic hair development, while in the rest separate "thelarche" or "pubarche" pathway of pubertal onset occurred [2]. The Avon Longitudinal Study of Parents and Children reported that in 46.3 % of girls, breast and pubic hair development began at the same time, while in 42.1 % of participants, B2 stage preceded pubic hair development (thelarche pathway), and in 11.6 % of girls, the opposite sequence of events was observed (pubarche pathway) [46]. According to other authors, only 17.1 % of girls underwent synchronous breast and pubic hair development, while most of the girls (66.2 %) developed breast stage 2 before pubic hair growth [33]. The pubarche pathway of sexual development was rarely found in North Europe, but not so unusual in the USA and Turkey [30, 33, 45]. Thelarche pathway in girls was associated with increased weight gain during early childhood, increased prevalence of obesity at the age of 8 years, greater proportion of body fat at the onset of puberty and increased prevalence of obese mothers [2, 46, 47]. The pubarche pathway was related to significantly increased DHEAS levels, while no differences in estradiol and testosterone levels in comparison to the thelarche

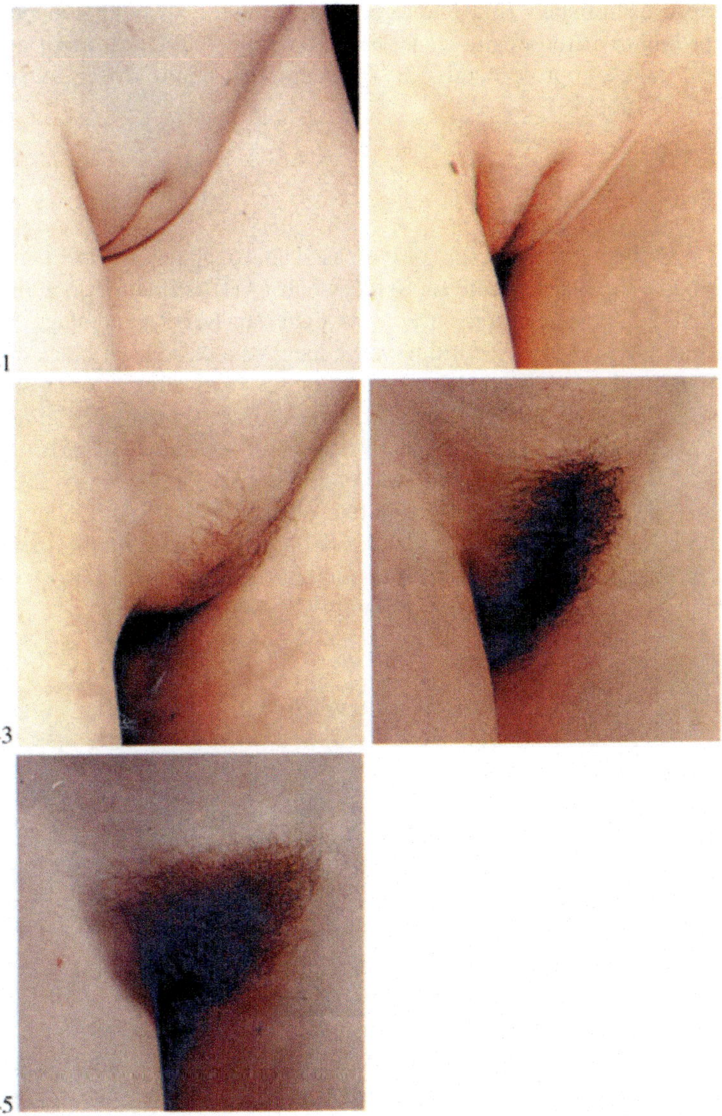

Fig. 4.2 Pubic hair development stages (P-1–P-5). [Reprinted from Biro F, Dorn L. Issues in Measurement of Pubertal Development. In: Preedy VR, editor. Handbook of Anthropometry: Physical Measures of Human Form in Health and Disease. New York, NY: Springer Science+Business Media; 2012:237–251. With permission from Springer Science+Business Media]

pathway were established [2]. The age of progression through the pubic hair stages according to different studies is shown on Table 4.1. Duration of pubic hair development takes approximately 3.5–4 years but could differ substantially among studies (Table 4.1).

Axillarche

Axillarche is another important sign of increased androgen levels. Herman-Giddens et al. described a three-level scale for axillary hair (AH) estimation including stage 1, no hair (AH1); stage 2, sparse curly or straight hair (AH2); and stage 3, mature adult-type hair (AH3) [26]. Accordingly, the mean age of AH2 in black and white girls was 10.08 and 11.80 years, respectively, or 1.3 years after entering stage PH2 for both races [26]. Axillary hair appeared later in English and Lithuanian girls at the age of 12.53 and 12.7 years, respectively [24, 28]. Lithuanian girls developed axillarche 1.5 years after pubarche, while in Turkish girls axillary hair (AH2) emerged only several months after pubic hair onset (PH2) [28, 30]. The transition between the initial stage AH2 and mature axillary hair (AH3) took about a year (0.9–1.22 years) [24, 30]. In some populations, full axillary hair growth was observed in only 75 % of girls within B5 and PH5 stages [48].

Internal and External Genitalia Development

Internal Genitalia

The average ovarian volume rises from 1.01 cm^3 in prepubertal girls to 2.60 cm^3 in Tanner stage 2, while in the Tanner stage 5, it reaches 7.24 cm^3 [49]. Significant changes in ovarian morphology with increased prevalence of polycystic ovaries during puberty have been described by some but not all authors [50, 51].

The uterine volume in newborns regresses postnatally in accordance with the cessation of placental estrogens and remains consistently small until the age of 7 years [52, 53]. Thereafter, it increases gradually in accordance to age, pubertal stages and estradiol levels [50, 52, 53]. The change in uterine volume could be considered as the earliest pubertal event in girls, since it occurs before the appearance of breast development or pubic hair [50, 52]. The female maturation is associated also with a concomitant increase of uterine fundo-cervical ratio and mean endometrial thickness [54].

Menarche

The pubertal hormonal changes ensure the adequate development of internal genitalia and lead to the appearance of the first menstrual bleeding in healthy girls (*menarche*). Usually, menarche occurs between 12.0 and 13.5 years of age, but it could vary among ethnical groups and in different study periods [55]. In the nineteenth and twentieth centuries, the mean age of menarche has decreased significantly, while nowadays the secular trend begins to slow down [56–59]. According to Marshall and Tanner, menarche is a late pubertal event occurring about 2.3 years after the onset of breast development mostly during stage B4 [22]. Interestingly, in recent studies menarche appears between stages B3 and B4, but again about two and a half years after the onset of puberty [30–32]. A lack of menarche by the age of 15 years as well as more than 3 years after thelarche could be accepted as abnormality and needs clinical evaluation [60].

The median length of the first cycle after menarche is shown to be approximately 34 days, and the first few postmenarcheal years are characterized by a pronounced irregularity with mixed short and long intervals between menstrual cycles [61, 62]. Different studies conducted in the second half of the twentieth century have found that a transition toward more regular menstrual pattern occurs about 5–7 years after menarche at the chronological age of approximately 20 years [61, 63, 64]. A study measuring 24-h urine pregnanediol output as a marker of luteal activity found that the presence of ovulatory cycles depended on the postmenarcheal age. Ovulation was observed in 22.9 % of girls in the first postmenarcheal year, but in 71.8 % of adolescents 5–8 years from the menarche [64]. However, recent studies showed that 65 % of adolescent girls had an established adult-type pattern (10 or more menstruations) even in the first postmenarcheal year [65]. Regular ovulatory cycles in some girls soon after menarche suggest faster HPG maturation in contemporary environment [66].

External Genitalia

Female external genitalia undergo significant transformation during puberty such as deposition of subcutaneous fat in the mons pubis and labia majora and enlargement of the labia minora, introitus, vagina, vaginal fornices and cervix [67, 68]. A small increase in clitoral dimensions was also observed during puberty [69]. The vaginal changes include thickening and stratification of the epithelium, hormone-dependent deposition of intracellular glycogen, increase in cervico-vaginal secretion as well as a shift in vaginal biocoenosis with raised prevalence of lactobacilli and acidification of the vaginal milieu [67, 68, 70]. The complex pubertal transformation of internal and external genitalia allows the achievement of full sexual maturity and ability to reproduce.

Growth and Skeletal Maturation

Pubertal Height Spurt

The pubertal growth spurt is an important event during the complex maturation process between infancy and adulthood. Growth velocity is low in the preadolescent years but accelerates rapidly during midpuberty due to increased interaction between growth hormone (GH), insulin-like growth factor 1 (IGF-1), gonadal steroid hormones and insulin [71, 72]. GH pulse amplitude increases significantly before pubertal onset in girls and reaches a peak at midpubertal stages [73]. Thereafter, GH secretion rate declines to prepubertal values at breast stage 5 [74]. Pubertal development is associated also with increased growth hormone receptor gene expression and decreased levels of growth hormone-binding protein [75]. In healthy girls, IGF-1 and insulin levels show a parallel stepwise increase between each Tanner stage from prepuberty to breast stage 4, and decline afterward [76].

In accordance with the hormonal changes, normal pubertal growth is characterized by acceleration, deceleration and cessation leading to a total height gain of approximately 25 cm during female puberty [71, 77]. The height velocity begins to rise at the mean age of 9 years and peaks in 11–12-year-old girls at Tanner breast stage 3 [22, 30, 77]. After reaching the maximal value of average 8.3 cm/year, the growth velocity decreases to nearly zero at the age of 16 years [77, 78]. Peak height velocity (PHV) is achieved approximately 1 year before the onset of menstruation [22, 30].

Pubertal Weight Changes

The pubertal growth spurt is accompanied by an increased bone mineralization as well as a significant weight gain. The bone mineral density shows a significant raise in girls during Tanner stage B3 and continues to increase in stages B4 and B5 [79]. The peak weight velocity reaches 7.81 kg/year and occurs several months after the PHV at the average age of 12.78 years [80]. The changes in body composition shape a specific for adult women fat distribution. Bioelectrical impedance analysis revealed a constant increase in fat mass percentage in adolescent girls that was independent of their initial body weight and corresponded with a stable increase of leptin levels during pubertal transition [81]. Magnetic resonance imaging showed that intra-abdominal and subcutaneous fat areas increased in adolescent girls, while their intra-abdominal to subcutaneous ratio decreased [82]. Beyond fat tissue distribution, different musculoskeletal changes in laxity, flexibility and strength of lower limbs during the female adolescent growth have been observed [83].

Physical Changes in Boys

Testicular Development and Spermarche

Testicular Development

Reactivation of HPG axis in boys stimulates the endocrine and exocrine testicular functions leading to increased steroid hormone production from the Leydig cells as well as spermatogenesis. An adequate development of secondary sexual characteristics indicates the presence of sufficient testosterone concentrations, while an increase of testicular volume reflects the enlargement of the seminiferous tubules following the follicle-stimulating hormone (FSH) concentration raise [84, 85]. Tanner stages are widely accepted as a visual rating method for evaluation of pubertal male genitalia: G1 reflects the preadolescent state, while the G2 stage shows the initial pubertal development with an increase of the testicular volume and scrotum as well as a discrete scrotal skin reddening; G3 stage is characterized by penile growth and further enlargement of the testis and scrotum; G4 stage is distinguished by the enlargement of the penis with a glance shaping; and further testis and penile growth leads to the adult appearance of male genitalia known as G5 stage [86].

The increase of testicular volume is the first physically detectable sign of puberty in boys and could be manually measured by Prader or other type of orchidometer (see Chap. 15: Fig. 15.2) [84, 87, 88]. Such objective measurement of the testicular increase can detect more precisely the onset and development of puberty compared to subjective estimation of the Tanner genital stages. Testicular volumes evaluated by orchidometer have shown high correlation coefficients with ultrasonographic measurements as well as with the actual size of testes from orchidectomized patients determined by the gold standard (water displacement of the surgical specimen) [88, 89]. Determining of the gonadal size is more accurate using ultrasound technique, but the latter is rarely used in epidemiological studies because of the greater cost and complexity [88, 89].

A testicular volume of 3 ml or greater is usually considered as a hallmark of pubertal transition, even though some authors use the volume of 4 ml [90–92]. According to longitudinal data of Bulgarian boys, the mean age of reaching testicular volume of 3 ml is 11.50 (9–14) years for the right testis and 11.63 (9–14) years for the left testis [93]. Thus, the development of the right testis overtakes that of the left testis with approximately 1–2 months. Similarly, the boys in neighbouring Greece started pubertal transition at the mean age of 11 years, while the corresponding age in Turkish children was 11.6 years [91, 94].

The sexual development in North-European children began at the mean age of 11.92 years in 1991–1993, but significantly earlier at the mean age of 11.66 years in children investigated 15 years later [95]. A pronounced secular trend was described recently in a US study [92]. Gonadal enlargement begins earlier in boys who are overweight and obese than in normal weight children, while the slowest pubertal development was observed in underweight boys [96]. Thus, the increased prevalence of overweight nowadays could be one of the most important reasons for the earlier pubertal development of both sexes. Different other factors might influence the maturation process, such as heredity, general health condition, nutrition, physical activity, habits, environmental pollution and socio-economic state [35, 97–100].

Usually, the increase of the testicular volume precedes the development of pubic hair as the first sign of sexual maturation in boys (testicular pathway), but in some adolescents the opposite sequence of events have been observed (pubarche pathway). According to a transversal study in Bulgarian boys, pubarche occurred at the average age of 11.40 years, several months after gonadarche (mean age of 11.23 years)

[96]. A Danish longitudinal study showed that 59 % of boys entered puberty by the usual testicular pattern, 24.6 % by the pubarche pathway, and in 16.4 % pubic hair and testicular enlargement appeared synchronously [45]. According to other studies, only 1.4–3.8 % of US boys underwent synchronous pubertal development, 91.1–95.1 % entered puberty by the testicular pathway and 1.1–7.5 % by the pubarche pathway [33, 101]. On the contrary, the Fels longitudinal study reported synchronous pattern of development in 75.3 % of investigated boys [47]. Distinct pathways of maturation in boys were not associated with differences in the pubertal body mass index or androgen levels [45, 47].

The gonadal development continues approximately 4.5–5 years, and boys reach genital stage 5 at the mean age of 15 years. Unlike pubertal onset, the age at stage G5 has not been changed in the last 50 years [85]. The appearance of genital stages according to various studies in different countries is shown at Table 4.2 [25, 29, 33, 86, 90, 92, 94–96, 101–108]. Sexual development before 9 years is considered precocious, while the lack of testicular enlargement by the age of 14 years indicates a pubertal delay [42, 43].

Spermarche

Maturation of germ cells during puberty is associated with a first appearance of spermatozoa in the urine (*spermarche*) as well as with onset of ejaculation (*ejacularche* or *oigarche*). The sperm in the urine (*spermaturia*) could be observed in the earlier stages of male pubertal development and even in prepubertal boys [103, 109]. Spermatozoa were found more frequently in urine samples collected in early than in late puberty suggesting different underlying mechanisms [110]. According to Pedersen et al., spermaturia might result from a spontaneous flow to the urethra in the beginning adolescence in contrast to postejaculatory peristaltic flow observed in late pubertal boys and adults [110].

The average age of spermarche varies between 13.4 and 14.5 years according to different studies [103, 111–113]. However, the passive spermatozoa flow in urine does not reflect the profound psychosomatic changes leading to a conscious ejaculation. According to some authors, the first conscious ejaculation (FCE) is the pubertal milestone in boys corresponding to menarche in girls [114]. The FCE occurs at the mean chronological age of 13.17–14.25 years and at the average bone age of 13.5 years [108, 114, 115].

Data from primate species show that first pubertal ejaculates might not contain spermatozoa. During the maturation process, the ejaculate volume as well as sperm count and motility increases [116]. The low quality of sperm in pubertal chimpanzee has been associated with insufficient epididymal maturation as well as impaired balance between seminal and prostatic secretions [116]. Similar data in boys was reported by Janczewski and Bablok: first ejaculations were characterized by small volumes and very high prevalence of azoospermia (over 80 %) [117]. During pubertal development sperm characteristics improved in parallel with the increase of testicular volume and androgen-dependent hair growth. An optimal spermatozoa quality was reached approximately 21 months after the first ejaculation [117, 118]. Thus,

Table 4.2 Average age (mean or median) of genital (G2–G5) and pubic hair (PH2–PH5) development as well as gonadarche (Go), peak height velocity (PHV) and spermarche/ejacularche (Sp/Ej) in boys from different countries [25, 29, 33, 86, 90, 92, 94–96, 101–108]. *c* – cross-sectional; *l* – longitudinal. Gonadarche (Go) – development of testicular volume ≥ 3 ml (* >3 ml)

Country	Authors	Go	G2	G3	G4	G5	PH2	PH3	PH4	PH5	PHV	Sp/Ej
USA	Reynolds and Wines (1951) (l)		11.5	12.7	13.4	17.3	12.2	13.3	13.9	16.1		
UK	Marshall and Tanner (1970) (l)		11.64	12.85	13.77	14.92	13.44	13.90	14.36	15.18	14.06	
Switzerland	Largo and Prader (1983) (l)	11.8	11.2	12.9	13.8	14.7	12.2	13.5	14.2	14.9		
UK	Nielsen et al. (1986) (l)										13.80	13.4
Turkey	Yenioğlu et al. (1995) (c)		11.6	13.3	14.4	15.8	12.2	13.3	14.6	15.8		
USA	Biro et al. (1995) (l)	12.18					12.79	13.74	14.63	15.19		
Sweden	Lindgren (1996) (c)		11.6	13.5	14.1	15.1	12.7	13.5	14.3	15.5		
Greece	Papadimitriou et al. (2002) (c)	11.0	11.0	12.2	13.3	14.2	11.5	12.7	13.4	14.1		
USA	Karpati et al. (2002) (c)		9.9	12.2	13.6	15.8	11.9	12.6	13.6	15.7		
Denmark	Juul et al. (2006) (c)*	11.92	11.83	13.30	14.31	15.39	11.88	13.45	14.28	15.56		
Greece	Pantsiotou (2007) (l)		10.3	11.9	12.9		10.8	12.4	13.0		13.2	
USA	Susman et al. (2010) (l)		10.3	12.3	13.4	14.8	11.3	12.6	13.6	15.0		

(continued)

Table 4.2 (continued)

Country	Authors	Go	G2	G3	G4	G5	PH2	PH3	PH4	PH5	PHV	Sp/Ej
Denmark	Sørensen et al. (2010) (c)*	11.66	11.59	13.13	13.61	14.31	12.38	13.25	13.67	14.45		
Bulgaria	Tomova et al. (2011, 2015) (c)	11.23					11.40	12.60	13.93	15.82		13.27
USA	Herman-Giddens et al. (2012) (c) /White/	9.95	10.14	12.49	13.72	15.57	11.47	12.89	13.76	15.83		
USA	Herman-Giddens et al. (2012) (c) /Afro-americans/	9.71	9.14	11.58	13.04	15.51	10.25	11.79	13.06	15.72		

spermarche and ejacularche are not completely identical events, and the presence of first conscious ejaculation is not equal to mature spermatogenesis.

Androgen-Dependent Hair Growth, Voice Changes and Penile Development

Pubarche

The gradual increase of androgen levels in pubertal boys ensures the development of secondary sexual characteristics including pubic, axillary and facial hair growth. The pubic hair pattern between stages PH2 and PH5 is similar in boys and girls, but in most men the triangular pubic hair typical for mature women spreads further along the linea alba (PH 6) [86]. The mean age at PH2 varies in different ethnic and racial groups: 10.9 years in German boys [119], 11.4 years in Saudi Arabia [120], 11.50 years in Italy [121], 12.0 years in Thailand [122] and 12.67 in China [123]. The latest US study has found that PH2 emerges nowadays approximately 6–12 months earlier than in the twentieth century, but definitive conclusions could not be drawn [92, 101].

The progression of pubic hair growth according to Tanner stages in several countries and in different periods is shown on Table 4.2. The duration of pubic hair development between PH2 and PH5 is about 4 years.

Axillarche

The axillary hair stages in boys might be described by the same three-level scale as in girls (AH1–AH3), although some authors have used a more complicated four-level scale [92, 99]. Axillarche emerges at the age of 12 years in Greek and Bulgarian boys (average age 12.2 and 12.28 years, respectively) [94, 124], but 1–2 years later in other ethnic groups: 13.55 years in Egypt, 14.32 and 14.4 in boys from the UK and Sweden [24, 25, 125]. The progress from the appearance of axillary hair to AH3 stage takes at least 1 year [25]. Thus, adult-type axillary hair growth is observed rarely in boys younger than 15 years, and in many adolescents this stage developed beyond the age of 17 years [94, 100].

Facial Hair Growth

Facial hair is an important secondary sexual feature of men. Development of facial hair passes through several stages from absent (FH1) to adult-type abundant hair growth on the cheeks and chin (FH4) [24, 100]. The intermediate steps include the appearance of slightly long and pigmented hair at the upper lip (FH2) and the spreading of hair growth on the upper part of the cheeks and below the lower lip (FH3) [24, 100]. FH2 occurs 6–16 months after the axillarche at the age of 14 years, while the subsequent progression toward FH3 takes about 2 years [24, 100]. Adult-type FH4 develops rarely in adolescents boys and is more typical for young men (over 18–20 years).

Voice Break

Increased androgen production in pubertal boys leads to an enlargement of the laryngeal cartilages, muscles and ligaments mainly in posterior–anterior length with protrusion of the Adam's apple resulting in a drop of the average voice pitch of about one octave [126, 127]. On the contrary, female larynx undergoes milder hormone-dependent changes predominantly in height leading to only one-third octave decrease of the lower terminal pitch in normoandrogenic girls [126, 127]. Thus, voice break (V) is an important event in the late puberty of boys. Voice change could be measured through voice recording and sound analysing computer system or simply by three- or four-level voice scales. Most pubertal studies use three-level scale describing the voice as unbroken (V1), not fully broken (V2) or completely broken (V3) [24, 128]. The onset of voice break (V2) occurs at the mean age of 13.7–14.0 years [129, 130]. Decrease of the mean speaking frequency corresponds to the pubic hair development, and the greatest change has been observed between PH2 and PH3 stages [131].

A longitudinal study of UK men born in 1946 showed that boys with more advanced voice-breaking status at the age of 14 years grew faster than the others in early infancy and maintained higher body mass index as adolescents and adults [128]. Some studies found a secular trend in the age of voice break as a marker of accelerated pubertal development [129]. Different nutritional and social factors could have influenced the voice change in modern children such as the prevalence of obesity, diet quality, maternal unhealthy habits as well as socio-economic level of the family [99, 132, 133].

Penile Growth

Normal penile growth is determined mostly by the increased androgen secretion and enhanced androgen receptor protein expression in the critical periods of male development including gestation, early postnatal months and pubertal transition [134, 135]. The penile length increases slightly during childhood, while rapid growth occurs during adolescence [107, 136]. Longitudinal data show that between 9 and 14 years, the penile length in boys increases with 60 % [93]. The highest rise in the mean penile length could be observed between pubic hair stages PH1 and PH2 in Japan children, but later (between PH2 and PH4) in Bulgarian (Fig. 4.3) and Brazilian boys [107, 136, 137]. Cross-sectional and longitudinal data in Bulgarian boys show that the maximal increase in penile size coincides with the rapid growth of testicular volumes between 12 and 14 years [93, 107]. Interestingly, the average penile size is bigger at the end of sexual maturation in rural compared to urban Bulgarian male population [107].

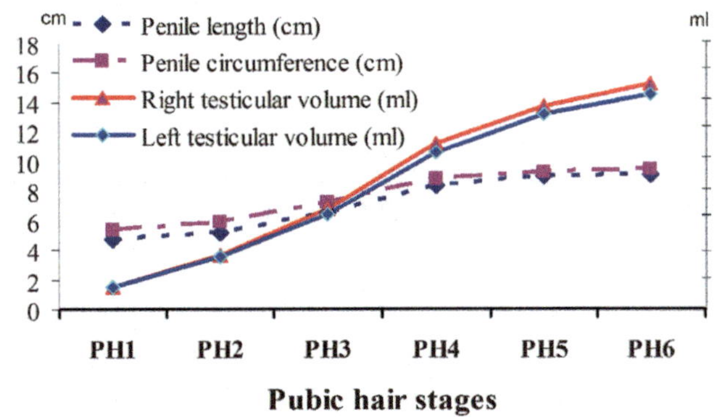

Fig. 4.3 Increase in the testicular volumes and penile size of Bulgarian boys in accordance with the progression through the Tanner pubic hair stages. [Based on data from [107]

Growth and Skeletal Maturation

Pubertal Height Spurt

The height in children is comparable in both sexes, but pubertal growth is more pronounced in boys than in girls leading to a higher adult height in men compared to women. In prepubertal children, mean growth hormone production is similar in both sexes, while during pubertal transition, GH secretion rises first in girls and then in boys [74]. Accordingly, height velocity in boys begins to increase 1–2 years later than in girls [77]. Peak height velocity in male adolescents reaches 9.79 cm/year at the mean chronological age of 14.12 years corresponding to genital stage 4 [80]. The increased growth velocity during puberty leads to an overall height gain of about 27.5–30 cm in maturing boys [77, 107]. Thereafter, the growth velocity decreases, and the epiphyseal closure limits further growth usually after the age of 17 years [71].

Pubertal Weight Gain

Pubertal weight gain in boys is associated with the accelerated linear growth and increase of bone and muscle mass, while no significant raise in percentage of fat mass has been found [81, 98]. Nevertheless, in comparison to girls, boys accumulate greater amounts of fat intra-abdominally, and their intra-abdominal to subcutaneous ratio increases during puberty leading to the sex-specific android distribution of fat tissue [82]. Peak weight velocity coincides with the peak height velocity and reaches 8.64 kg/year at the mean age of 14.27 years [80]. Thereafter, weight velocity decreases in the later stages of pubertal development [80, 81].

Other Changes

Beyond changes in growth, genital development and body composition, pubertal development in boys is associated with blood and metabolic alterations, such as increased haemoglobin and haematocrit values, as well as decreased total and high-density lipoprotein cholesterol levels [138, 139]. Sexually specific changes have been described also in brain development, cognition and behaviour of male adolescents. Especially, the brain amygdala–hippocampus complex could be significantly influenced by the steroid levels during puberty [140]. Animal studies have shown that pubertal increase of sex steroid hormones might alter the sensory associations and could induce strong motivation to seek out reproductive opportunities by modulating different brain zones including reward-related brain structures such as nucleus accumbens and dopaminergic pathways to the prefrontal cortex [reviewed in 141]. Thus, the physical changes in puberty are associated with mental alterations that both aim to create an optimal ability and willingness to reproduce.

Conclusions

The first pubertal signs appear at the mean age of 10 years in girls and approximately 1–2 years later in boys. The progression between B2 and B5 stages takes about 4 years in girls, while the genital development in boys needs a little longer (approximately 4.5 years). Most girls reach B5 stage at the age of 14, while most boys complete their genital development after the age of 15 years.

Menarche occurs at the mean age of 12.8 years, while the mean age of spermarche or ejacularche is about a year later. The peak height velocity is achieved early in girls, mostly at stage B3 or about a year before menarche. On the contrary, peak height velocity is a midpubertal event in boys occurring at the stage G4 and very close to the time of ejacularche. The appearance of menarche or ejacularche does not mean complete fertility potential, since anovulatory cycles in the first post-menarcheal year as well as low sperm quality in the first ejaculate samples are frequent. The timing and duration of pubertal events could vary among different ethnic groups, but nevertheless, the sequence of events underlying pubertal development is similar in boys and girls worldwide as shown on the classical figure by Marshall and Tanner (Fig. 4.4) [86, 107].

The transitional period is also the time of great worry. Adolescents as well as their parents and often doctors observing them are concerned if the children develop normally. Therefore on reasonable time intervals, norms for growth, weight and pubertal physical characteristics should be established as we did with our comprehensive study on boys [107] in order to have an actual basis for comparison and evaluation of the changes in every single case.

Sexual development is a complex process of specific physical and psychical changes that transform healthy children into mature men and women who are motivated and capable to create offspring.

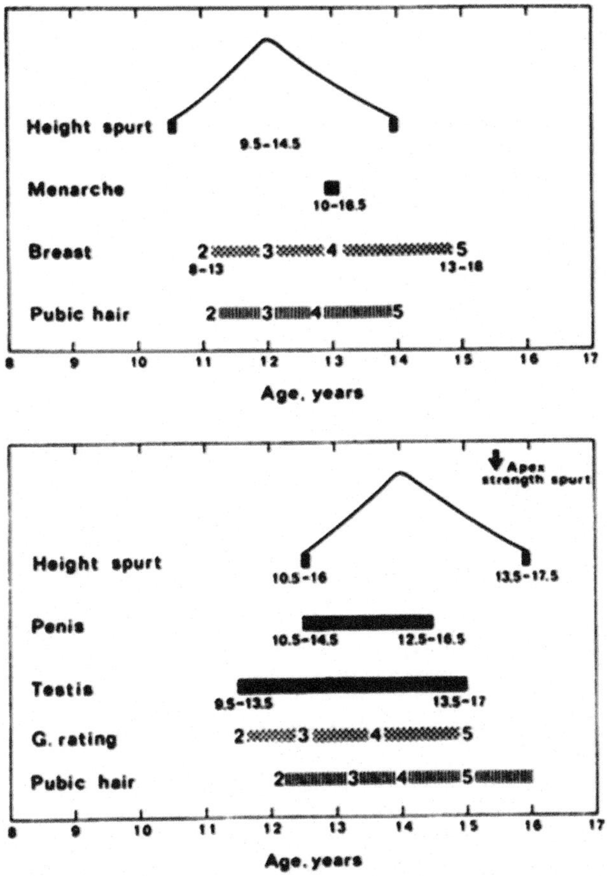

Fig. 4.4 The classical diagrams of the sequence of events at puberty created by Marshall and Tanner. [Reprinted from Marshall WA, Tanner JM. Variations in the pattern of pubertal changes in boys. Arch Dis Child. 1970; 45(239):13–23. With permission from BMJ Publishing Group Ltd]

References

1. Kuiri-Hänninen T, Sankilampi U, Dunkel L. Activation of the hypothalamic-pituitary-gonadal axis in infancy: minipuberty. Horm Res Paediatr. 2014;82(2):73–80.
2. Biro FM, Huang B, Daniels SR, Lucky AW. Pubarche as well as thelarche may be a marker for the onset of puberty. J Pediatr Adolesc Gynecol. 2008;21(6):323–8.
3. Auchus RJ, Rainey WE. Adrenarche: physiology, biochemistry and human disease. Clin Endocrinol (Oxf). 2004;60(3):288–96.
4. de Peretti E, Forest MG. Pattern of plasma dehydroepiandrosterone sulfate levels in humans from birth to adulthood: evidence for testicular production. J Clin Endocrinol Metab. 1978;47:572–77.
5. Rege J, Rainey WE. The steroid metabolome of adrenarche. J Endocrinol. 2012;214(2):133–43.
6. Utriainen P, Laakso S, Liimatta J, Jääskeläinen J, Voutilainen R. Premature adrenarche: a common condition with variable presentation. Horm Res Paediatr. 2015;83(4):221–31.

7. Cutler Jr GB, Glenn M, Bush M, Hodgen GD, Graham CE, Loriaux DL. Adrenarche: a survey of rodents, domestic animals, and primates. Endocrinology. 1978;103(6):2112–18.
8. Pignatelli D, Xiao F, Gouveia AM, Ferreira JG, Vinson GP. Adrenarche in the rat. J Endocrinol. 2006;191(1):301–8.
9. Remer T, Boye KR, Hartmann M, Neu CM, Schoenau E, Manz F, et al. Adrenarche and bone modeling and remodeling at the proximal radius: weak androgens make stronger cortical bone in healthy children. J Bone Miner Res. 2003;18(8):1539–46.
10. Havelock JC, Auchus RJ, Rainey WE. The rise in adrenal androgen biosynthesis: adrenarche. Semin Reprod Med. 2004;22(4):337–47.
11. Teller WM, Homoki J, Wudy S, Schlickenrieder JH. Adrenarche is dissociated from gonadarche: studies in patients with Turner's syndrome. Acta Endocrinol Suppl (Copenh). 1986;279:232–40.
12. Martin DD, Schweizer R, Schwarze CP, Elmlinger MW, Ranke MB, Binder G. The early dehydroepiandrosterone sulfate rise of adrenarche and the delay of pubarche indicate primary ovarian failure in Turner syndrome. J Clin Endocrinol Metab. 2004;89(3):1164–68.
13. Sklar CA, Kaplan SL, Grumbach MM. Evidence for dissociation between adrenarche and gonadarche: studies in patients with idiopathic precocious puberty, gonadal dysgenesis, isolated gonadotropin deficiency, and constitutionally delayed growth and adolescence. J Clin Endocrinol Metab. 1980;51(3):548–56.
14. Terasawa E, Fernandez DL. Neurobiological mechanisms of the onset of puberty in primates. Endocr Rev. 2001;22:111–51.
15. Grumbach MM. The neuroendocrinology of human puberty revisited. Horm Res. 2002;57 Suppl 2:2–14.
16. Plant TM, Barker-Gibb ML. Neurobiological mechanisms of puberty in higher primates. Hum Reprod Update. 2004;10(1):67–77.
17. Terasawa E, Guerrier KA, Plant TM. Kisspeptin and puberty in mammals. Adv Exp Med Biol. 2013;784:253–73.
18. Plant TM. Neuroendocrine control of the onset of puberty. Front Neuroendocrinol. 2015;38:73–88.
19. Macias H, Hinck L. Mammary gland development. Wiley Interdiscip Rev Dev Biol. 2012;1(4):533–57.
20. Biro F, Dorn L. Issues in measurement of pubertal development. In: Preedy VR, editor. Handbook of anthropometry: physical measures of human form in health and disease. New York: Springer, LLC; 2012. pp. 237–251.
21. Tanner JM. Growth at adolescence. 2nd ed. Oxford: Blackwell; 1962.
22. Marshall WA, Tanner JM. Variations in the pattern of pubertal changes in girls. Arch Dis Child. 1969;44:291–03.
23. Reynolds EL, Wines JV. Individual differences in physical changes associated with adolescence in girls. Am J Dis Child. 1948;75:329–50.
24. Billewicz WZ, Fellowes HM, Thomson AM. Pubertal changes in boys and girls in Newcastle upon Tyne. Ann Hum Biol. 1981;8(3):211–19.
25. Lindgren G. Pubertal stages 1980 of Stockholm schoolchildren. Acta Paediatr. 1996;85(11):1365–67.
26. Herman-Giddens ME, Slora EJ, Wasserman RC, Bourdony CJ, Bhapkar MV, Koch GG, et al. Secondary sexual characteristics and menses in young girls seen in office practice: a study from the Pediatric Research in Office Settings network. Pediatrics. 1997;99(4):505–12.
27. Sun SS, Schubert CM, Chumlea WC, Roche AF, Kulin HE, Lee PA, et al. National estimates of the timing of sexual maturation and racial differences among US children. Pediatrics. 2002;110:911–19.
28. Zukauskaite S, Lasiene D, Lasas L, Urbonaite B, Hindmarsh P. Onset of breast and pubic hair development in 1231 preadolescent Lithuanian schoolgirls. Arch Dis Child. 2005;90(9):932–36.

29. Juul A, Teilmann G, Scheike T, Hertel NT, Holm K, Laursen EM, et al. Pubertal development in Danish children: comparison of recent European and US data. Int J Androl. 2006;29(1):247–55.
30. Bundak R, Darendeliler F, Günöz H, Baş F, Saka N, Neyzi O. Puberty and pubertal growth in healthy Turkish girls: no evidence for secular trend. J Clin Res Pediatr Endocrinol. 2008;1(1):8–14.
31. Rabbani A, Motlagh ME, Mohammad K, Ardalan G, Maftoon F, Shahryari S, et al. Assessment of pubertal development in Iranian girls. Iran J Pediatr. 2010;20(2):160–6.
32. Christensen KY, Maisonet M, Rubin C, Holmes A, Flanders WD, Heron J, et al. Progression through puberty in girls enrolled in a contemporary British cohort. J Adolesc Health. 2010;47(3):282–89.
33. Susman EJ, Houts RM, Steinberg L, Belsky J, Cauffman E, Dehart G, et al. Eunice Kennedy Shriver NICHD Early Child Care Research Network. Longitudinal development of secondary sexual characteristics in girls and boys between ages 9 1/2 and 15 1/2 years. Arch Pediatr Adolesc Med. 2010;164(2):166–73.
34. Chaning-Pearce SM, Solomon L. Pubertal development in black and white Johannesburg girls. S Afr Med J. 1987;71(1):22–4.
35. Toppari J, Juul A. Trends in puberty timing in humans and environmental modifiers. Mol Cell Endocrinol. 2010;324(1–2):39–44.
36. Aksglaede L, Sørensen K, Petersen JH, Skakkebaek NE, Juul A. Recent decline in age at breast development: the Copenhagen Puberty Study. Pediatrics. 2009;123(5):e932–939.
37. Huen KF, Leung SS, Lau JT, Cheung AY, Leung NK, Chiu MC. Secular trend in the sexual maturation of southern Chinese girls. Acta Paediatr. 1997;86(10):1121–24.
38. Ma HM, Du ML, Luo XP, Chen SK, Liu L, Chen RM, Pubertal Study Group of the Society of Pediatric Endocrinology and Genetic Disease, Chinese Medical Association, et al. Onset of breast and pubic hair development and menses in urban Chinese girls. Pediatrics. 2009;124(2):e269–77.
39. Aksglaede L, Juul A, Olsen LW, Sørensen TI. Age at puberty and the emerging obesity epidemic. PLoS One. 2009;4(12), e8450.
40. Buck Louis GM, Gray Jr LE, Marcus M, Ojeda SR, Pescovitz OH, Witchel SF, et al. Environmental factors and puberty timing: expert panel research needs. Pediatrics. 2008;121 Suppl 3:S192–207.
41. Deardorff J, Ekwaru JP, Kushi LH, Ellis BJ, Greenspan LC, Mirabedi A, et al. Father absence, body mass index, and pubertal timing in girls: differential effects by family income and ethnicity. J Adolesc Health. 2011;48(5):441–47.
42. Dixon JR, Ahmed SF. Precocious puberty. Paediatr Child Health. 2007;17(9):343–48.
43. Dunkel L, Quinton R. Transition in endocrinology: induction of puberty. Eur J Endocrinol. 2014;170(6):R229–39.
44. Mouritsen A, Johansen ML, Wohlfahrt-Veje C, Hagen CP, Tinggaard J, Mieritz MG, et al. Determination of adrenal volume by MRI in healthy children: associations with age, body size, pubertal stage and serum levels of adrenal androgens. Clin Endocrinol (Oxf). 2014;81(2):183–89.
45. Mouritsen A, Aksglaede L, Soerensen K, Hagen CP, Petersen JH, Main KM, et al. The pubertal transition in 179 healthy Danish children: associations between pubarche, adrenarche, gonadarche, and body composition. Eur J Endocrinol. 2013;168(2):129–36.
46. Christensen KY, Maisonet M, Rubin C, Holmes A, Flanders WD, Heron J, et al. Pubertal pathways in girls enrolled in a contemporary British cohort. Int J Pediatr. 2010;2010:329261.
47. Wan W, Deng X, Archer KJ, Sun SS. Pubertal pathways and the relationship to anthropometric changes in childhood: the Fels longitudinal study. Open J Pediatr. 2012;2:118–26.
48. Fakeye O, Fagbule D. Age and anthropometric status of Nigerian girls at puberty: implication for the introduction of sex education into secondary schools. West Afr J Med. 1990;9(3):226–31.

49. Ersen A, Onal H, Yildirim D, Adal E. Ovarian and uterine ultrasonography and relation to puberty in healthy girls between 6 and 16 years in the Turkish population: a cross-sectional study. J Pediatr Endocrinol Metab. 2012;25(5–6):447–51.
50. Holm K, Laursen EM, Brocks V, Müller J. Pubertal maturation of the internal genitalia: an ultrasound evaluation of 166 healthy girls. Ultrasound Obstet Gynecol. 1995;6(3):175–81.
51. Bridges NA, Cooke A, Healy MJ, Hindmarsh PC, Brook CG. Standards for ovarian volume in childhood and puberty. Fertil Steril. 1993;60(3):456–60.
52. Haber HP, Mayer EI. Ultrasound evaluation of uterine and ovarian size from birth to puberty. Pediatr Radiol. 1994;24(1):11–3.
53. Salardi S, Orsini LF, Cacciari E, Bovicelli L, Tassoni P, Reggiani A. Pelvic ultrasonography in premenarcheal girls: relation to puberty and sex hormone concentrations. Arch Dis Child. 1985;60(2):120–25.
54. Khadilkar VV, Khadilkar AV, Kinare AS, Tapasvi HS, Deshpande SS, Maskati GB. Ovarian and uterine ultrasonography in healthy girls between birth to 18 years. Indian Pediatr. 2006;43(7):625–30.
55. Parent AS, Teilmann G, Juul A, Skakkebaek NE, Toppari J, Bourguignon JP. The timing of normal puberty and the age limits of sexual precocity: variations around the world, secular trends, and changes after migration. Endocr Rev. 2003;24(5):668–93.
56. Wyshak G, Frisch R. Evidence for a secular trend in age of menarche. N Engl J Med. 1982;306:1033–103.
57. Tomova A, Genov N, Kumanov F, Robeva R. Menarche in Bulgarian-secular trend in twenty century. Akush Ginekol (Sofiia). 2009;48(3):10–4. Bulgarian.
58. Karapanou O, Papadimitriou A. Determinants of menarche. Reprod Biol Endocrinol. 2010;8:115.
59. Papadimitriou A, Fytanidis G, Douros K, Bakoula C, Nicolaidou P, Fretzayas A. Age at menarche in contemporary Greek girls: evidence for levelling-off of the secular trend. Acta Paediatr. 2008;97(6):812–15.
60. ACOG Committee on Adolescent Health Care. ACOG Committee Opinion No. 349, November 2006: menstruation in girls and adolescents: using the menstrual cycle as a vital sign. Obstet Gynecol. 2006;108(5):1323–28.
61. Treloar AE, Boynton RE, Behn BG, Brown BW. Variation of the human menstrual cycle through reproductive life. Int J Fertil. 1967;12:77–126.
62. World Health Organization multicenter study on menstrual and ovulatory patterns in adolescent girls. II. Longitudinal study of menstrual patterns in the early postmenarcheal period, duration of bleeding episodes and menstrual cycles. World Health Organization Task Force on Adolescent Reproductive Health. J Adolesc Health Care. 1986;7(4):236–44.
63. Flug D, Largo RH, Prader A. Menstrual patterns in adolescent Swiss girls: a longitudinal study. Ann Hum Biol. 1984;11(6):495–508.
64. Metcalf MG, Skidmore DS, Lowry GF, Mackenzie JA. Incidence of ovulation in the years after the menarche. J Endocrinol. 1983;97(2):213–19.
65. Legro RS, Lin HM, Demers LM, Lloyd T. Rapid maturation of the reproductive axis during perimenarche independent of body composition. J Clin Endocrinol Metab. 2000;85(3):1021–25.
66. Zhang K, Pollack S, Ghods A, Dicken C, Isaac B, Adel G, et al. Onset of ovulation after menarche in girls: a longitudinal study. J Clin Endocrinol Metab. 2008;93(4):1186–194.
67. Farage M, Maibach H. Lifetime changes in the vulva and vagina. Arch Gynecol Obstet. 2006;273(4):195–202.
68. Farage MA, Maibach HI. Morphology and physiological changes of genital skin and mucosa. Curr Probl Dermatol. 2011;40:9–19.
69. Sane K, Pescovitz OH. The clitoral index: a determination of clitoral size in normal girls and in girls with abnormal sexual development. J Pediatr. 1992;120:264–66.
70. Matytsina LA, Greydanus DE, Gurkin YA. Vaginal microbiocoenosis and cytology of prepubertal and adolescent girls: their role in health and disease. World J Pediatr. 2010;6(1):32–7.

71. Rogol AD, Clark PA, Roemmich JN. Growth and pubertal development in children and adolescents: effects of diet and physical activity. Am J Clin Nutr. 2000;72:521–28.
72. Rogol AD. Sex steroids, growth hormone, leptin and the pubertal growth spurt. Endocr Dev. 2010;17:77–85.
73. Rose SR, Municchi G, Barnes KM, Kamp GA, Uriarte MM, Ross JL, et al. Spontaneous growth hormone secretion increases during puberty in normal girls and boys. J Clin Endocrinol Metab. 1991;73(2):428–35.
74. Albertsson-Wikland K, Rosberg S, Karlberg J, Groth T. Analysis of 24-hour growth hormone profiles in healthy boys and girls of normal stature: relation to puberty. J Clin Endocrinol Metab. 1994;78(5):1195–201.
75. Pagani S, Meazza C, Gertosio C, Bozzola E, Bozzola M. Growth hormone receptor gene expression in puberty. Horm Metab Res. 2015;47(8):581–4.
76. Sørensen K, Aksglaede L, Petersen JH, Andersson AM, Juul A. Serum IGF1 and insulin levels in girls with normal and precocious puberty. Eur J Endocrinol. 2012;166(5):903–10.
77. Abbassi V. Growth and normal puberty. Pediatrics. 1998;102:507–11.
78. Tanner JM, Davies PSW. Clinical longitudinal standards for height and height velocity for North American children. J Pediatr. 1985;107:317–29.
79. Moretto MR, Silva CC, Kurokawa CS, Fortes CM, Capela RC, Teixeira AS, et al. Bone mineral density in healthy female adolescents according to age, bone age and pubertal breast stage. Open Orthop J. 2011;5:324–30.
80. Buckler JM, Wild J. Longitudinal study of height and weight at adolescence. Arch Dis Child. 1987;62(12):1224–32.
81. Xu L, Li M, Yin J, Cheng H, Yu M, Zhao X, et al. Change of body composition and adipokines and their relationship with insulin resistance across pubertal development in obese and nonobese chinese children: the BCAMS Study. Int J Endocrinol. 2012;2012:389108.
82. Fox KR, Peters DM, Sharpe P, Bell M. Assessment of abdominal fat development in young adolescents using magnetic resonance imaging. Int J Obes Relat Metab Disord. 2000;24(12):1653–59.
83. Wild CY, Steele JR, Munro BJ. Musculoskeletal and estrogen changes during the adolescent growth spurt in girls. Med Sci Sports Exerc. 2013;45(1):138–45.
84. Zachmann M, Prader A, Kind HP, Hafliger H, Budliger H. Testicular volume during adolescence: cross-sectional and longitudinal studies. Helv Paediatr Acta. 1974;29(1):61–72.
85. Euling SY, Herman-Giddens ME, Lee PA, Selevan SG, Juul A, Sørensen TI, et al. Examination of US puberty-timing data from 1940 to 1994 for secular trends: panel findings. Pediatrics. 2008;121:172–91.
86. Marshall WA, Tanner JM. Variations in the pattern of pubertal changes in boys. Arch Dis Child. 1970;45(239):13–23.
87. Prader A. Testicular size: assessment and clinical importance. Triangle. 1966;7(6):240–43.
88. Lin CC, Huang WJ, Chen KK. Measurement of testicular volume in smaller testes: how accurate is the conventional orchidometer? J Androl. 2009;30(6):685–89.
89. Sakamoto H, Saito K, Oohta M, Inoue K, Ogawa Y, Yoshida H. Testicular volume measurement: comparison of ultrasonography, orchidometry, and water displacement. Urology. 2007;69(1):152–7.
90. Largo RH, Prader A. Pubertal development in Swiss boys. Helv Paediatr Acta. 1983;38(3):211–28.
91. Bundak R, Darendeliler F, Gunoz H, Bas F, Saka N, Neyzi O. Analysis of puberty and pubertal growth in healthy boys. Eur J Pediatr. 2007;166(6):595–600.
92. Herman-Giddens ME, Steffes J, Harris D, Slora E, Hussey M, Dowshen SA, et al. Secondary sexual characteristics in boys: data from the Pediatric Research in Office Settings Network. Pediatrics. 2012;130(5):1058–68.
93. Kumanov P, Yordanov Y, Robeva R, Tomova A. Anthropometrical indices and pubertal maturation of boys in Bulgaria. Acta Morphol Anthropol. 2010;16:96–101.

94. Papadimitriou A, Stephanou N, Papantzimas K, Glynos G, Philippidis P. Sexual maturation of Greek boys. Ann Hum Biol. 2002;29(1):105–8.
95. Sørensen K, Aksglaede L, Petersen JH, Juul A. Recent changes in pubertal timing in healthy Danish boys: associations with body mass index. J Clin Endocrinol Metab. 2010;95(1): 263–70.
96. Tomova A, Robeva R, Kumanov P. Influence of the body weight on the onset and progression of puberty in boys. J Pediatr Endocrinol Metab. 2015;28(7–8):859–65.
97. Lall KB, Singhi S, Gurnani M, Singhi P, Garg OP. Somatotype, physical growth, and sexual maturation in young male smokers. J Epidemiol Community Health. 1980;34(4):295–98.
98. Rogol AD, Roemmich JN, Clark PA. Growth at puberty. J Adolesc Health. 2002;31:192–200.
99. Davis EM, Peck JD, Peck BM, Kaplan HB. Associations between early alcohol and tobacco use and prolonged time to puberty in boys. Child Care Health Dev. 2015;41(3):459–66.
100. Neyzi O, Alp H, Yalcindag A, Yakacikli S, Orphon A. Sexual maturation in Turkish boys. Ann Hum Biol. 1975;2(3):251–59.
101. Biro FM, Lucky AW, Huster GA, Morrison JA. Pubertal staging in boys. J Pediatr. 1995;127(1):100–2.
102. Reynolds EL, Wines JV. Physical changes associated with adolescence in boys. AMA Am J Dis Child. 1951;82(5):529–47.
103. Nielsen CT, Skakkebaek NE, Richardson DW, Darling JA, Hunter WM, Jørgensen M, et al. Onset of the release of spermatozoa (spermarche) in boys in relation to age, testicular growth, pubic hair, and height. J Clin Endocrinol Metab. 1986;62(3):532–5.
104. Yenioğlu H, Güvenç H, Aygün AD, Kocabay K. Pubertal development of Turkish boys in Elaziğ, eastern Turkey. Ann Hum Biol. 1995;22(4):337–40.
105. Karpati AM, Rubin CH, Kieszak SM, Marcus M, Troiano RP. Stature and pubertal stage assessment in American boys: the 1988–1994 Third National Health and Nutrition Examination Survey. J Adolesc Health. 2002;30(3):205–12.
106. Pantsiotou K. Data on pubertal development in Greek boys. A longitudinal study. Hormones (Athens). 2007;6(2):148–51.
107. Tomova A, Deepinder F, Robeva R, Lalabonova H, Kumanov P, Agarwal A. Growth and development of male external genitalia. A cross-sectional study of 6200 males aged 0 to 19 years. Arch Pediatr Adolesc Med. 2010;164(12):1152–7.
108. Tomova A, Lalabonova C, Robeva RN, Kumanov PT. Timing of pubertal maturation according to the age at first conscious ejaculation. Andrologia. 2011;43(3):163–6.
109. Nysom K, Pedersen JL, Jørgensen M, Nielsen CT, Müller J, Keiding N, et al. Spermaturia in two normal boys without other signs of puberty. Acta Paediatr. 1994;83(5):520–1.
110. Pedersen JL, Nysom K, Jørgensen M, Nielsen CT, Müller J, Keiding N, et al. Spermaturia and puberty. Arch Dis Child. 1993;69(3):384–7.
111. Schaefer F, Marr J, Seidel C, Tilgen W, Schärer K. Assessment of gonadal maturation by evaluation of spermaturia. Arch Dis Child. 1990;65(11):1205–7.
112. Guízar-Vázquez JJ, Rosales-López A, Ortiz-Jalomo R, Nava-Delgado SE, Salamanca-Gómez F. Age of onset of spermaturia (spermache) in 669 Mexican children and its relation to secondary sexual characteristics and height. Bol Med Hosp Infant Mex. 1992;49(1):12–7.
113. Hirsch M, Shemesh J, Modan M, Lunenfeld B. Emission of spermatozoa, age of onset. Int J Androl. 1979;2:289–98.
114. Carlier JG, Steeno OP. Oigarche: the age at first ejaculation. Andrologia. 1985;17:104–6.
115. Laron Z, Arad J, Gurewitz R, Grunebaum M, Dickerman Z. Age at first conscious ejaculation: a milestone in male puberty. Helv Paediatr Acta. 1980;35(1):13–20.
116. Marson J, Meuris S, Cooper RW, Jouannet P. Puberty in the male chimpanzee: progressive maturation of semen characteristics. Biol Reprod. 1991;44(3):448–55.
117. Janczewski Z, Bablok L. Semen characteristics in pubertal boys. I. Semen quality after first ejaculation. Arch Androl. 1985;15(2–3):199–205.
118. Janczewski Z, Bablok L. Semen characteristics in pubertal boys. III. Semen quality and somatosexual development. Arch Androl. 1985;15(2–3):213–8.

119. Kahl H, Schaffrath Rosario A, Schlaud M. Sexual maturation of children and adolescents in Germany. Results of the German Health Interview and Examination Survey for Children and Adolescents (KiGGS). Bundesgesundheitsblatt Gesundheitsforschung Gesundheitsschutz. 2007;50(5–6):677–85. German.
120. Al Alwan I, Felimban N, Altwaijri Y, Tamim H, Al Mutair A, Shoukri M, et al. Puberty onset among boys in Riyadh. Saudi Arabia Clin Med Insights Pediatr. 2010;4:19–24.
121. De Simone M, Danubio ME, Amicone E, Verrotti A, Gruppioni G, Vecchi F. Age of onset of pubertal characteristics in boys aged 6–14 years of the Province of L'Aquila (Abruzzo, Italy). Ann Hum Biol. 2004;31(4):488–93.
122. Jaruratanasirikul S, Yuenyongwiwat S, Kreetapirom P, Sriplung H. Age of onset of pubertal maturation of Thai boys. J Pediatr Endocrinol Metab. 2014;27(3–4):215–20.
123. Sun Y, Tao F, Su PY, China Puberty Research Collaboration. National estimates of pubertal milestones among urban and rural Chinese boys. Ann Hum Biol. 2012;39(6):461–7.
124. Kumanov P, Yordanov Y, Robeva R, Tomova A. A longitudinal study of the pubertal maturation in Bulgarian boys. Endocrinologia. 2010;2:68–86. Bulgarian.
125. Ghaly I, Hussein FH, Abdelghaffar S, Anwar G, Seirvogel RM. Optimal age of sexual maturation in Egyptian children. East Mediterr Health J. 2008;14(6):1391–9.
126. Kadakia S, Carlson D, Sataloff R. The effect of hormones on the voice. J Sing. 2013;69(5):571–4.
127. Gackle L. The adolescent female voice. Characteristics of change and stages of development. Choral J. 1991;31(8):17–25.
128. Ong KK, Bann D, Wills AK, Ward K, Adams JE, Hardy R, et al. National Survey of Health and Development Scientific and Data Collection Team. Timing of voice breaking in males associated with growth and weight gain across the life course. J Clin Endocrinol Metab. 2012;97(8):2844–52.
129. Juul A, Magnusdottir S, Scheike T, Prytz S, Skakkebaek NE. Age at voice break in Danish boys: effects of pre-pubertal body mass index and secular trend. Int J Androl. 2007;30(6):537–42.
130. Remer T, Shi L, Buyken AE, Maser-Gluth C, Hartmann MF, Wudy SA. Prepubertal adrenarchal androgens and animal protein intake independently and differentially influence pubertal timing. J Clin Endocrinol Metab. 2010;95(6):3002–9.
131. Vuorenkoski V, Lenko HL, Tjernlund P, Vuorenkoski L, Perheentupa J. Fundamental voice frequence during normal and abnormal growth, and after androgen treatment. Arch Dis Child. 1978;53(3):201–9.
132. Günther AL, Karaolis-Danckert N, Kroke A, Remer T, Buyken AE. Dietary protein intake throughout childhood is associated with the timing of puberty. J Nutr. 2010;140(3):565–71.
133. Håkonsen LB, Brath-Lund ML, Hounsgaard ML, Olsen J, Ernst A, Thulstrup AM, et al. In utero exposure to alcohol and puberty in boys: a pregnancy cohort study. BMJ Open. 2014;4(6), e004467.
134. Husmann DA. Micropenis: an animal model and its human correlates. Adv Exp Med Biol. 2002;511:41–54.
135. Ma YM, Wu KJ, Dang Q, Shi Q, Gao Y, Guo P, et al. Testosterone regulates keratin 33B expression in rat penis growth through androgen receptor signaling. Asian J Androl. 2014;16(6):817–23.
136. Fujieda K, Matsuura N. Growth and maturation in the male genitalia from birth to adolescence. II. Change of penile length. Acta Paediatr Jpn. 1987;29(2):220–3.
137. Gabrich PN, Vasconcelos JS, Damião R, Silva EA. Penile anthropometry in Brazilian children and adolescents. J Pediatr (Rio J). 2007;83(5):441–6.
138. Willows N, Grimston S, Roberts D, Smith D, Hanley D. Iron and hematologic status in young athletes relative to puberty: a cross-sectional study. Pediatr Exerc Sci. 1993;5(4):367–76.
139. Mascarenhas LP, Leite N, Titski AC, Brito LM, Boguszewski MC. Variability of lipid and lipoprotein concentrations during puberty in Brazilian boys. J Pediatr Endocrinol Metab. 2015;28(1–2):125–31.

140. Neufang S, Specht K, Hausmann M, Güntürkün O, Herpertz-Dahlmann B, Fink GR, et al. Sex differences and the impact of steroid hormones on the developing human brain. Cereb Cortex. 2009;19(2):464–73.
141. Blakemore SJ, Burnett S, Dahl RE. The role of puberty in the developing adolescent brain. Hum Brain Mapp. 2010;31(6):926–33.

Chapter 5
Growth in Childhood and Puberty

Michael Hermanussen

Introduction

After birth, the human development progresses through several states of maturation [1]. The transition from *infancy* to *childhood* by about age 3 years is characterised by the termination of maternal lactation, eating of soft and nutrient dense foods and the completion of deciduous tooth eruption. The *juvenile stage* spans from age 7 years to onset of the adolescent growth spurt at approximately age 10 for healthy girls and age 12 for boys. Juveniles are sexually immature, but physically and mentally capable of providing for much of their own food and care. The juvenile stage starts with a change in cognitive function, a shift from the preoperational to concrete operational stage. Near the end of the juvenile stage, sexual maturation begins, and one measurable effect is the adolescent growth spurt. The *adolescent stage* is the period from around the age of 13–14 years in boys, and 11–12 years in girls, to the end of the spurt and the almost complete termination of growth of the skeleton. The end of adolescence usually coincides with the eruption of the third molar (if present). *Adulthood* and reproductive maturity follow. Body height, weight, BMI and other anthropometric parameter can be plotted on *distance curves*. Distance curves indicate the amount of height, weight, BMI, etc. achieved at a given age; *velocity curves*, or *rate of growth*, indicate the annual increment at a given age. Velocity curves best coincide with the stages of maturation. *Age at take-off (ATO)* is the age just prior to the onset of the adolescent growth spurt; *adolescent growth* is the height increment between the ATO and final height.

Some children are short, others are tall. But what is short and tall? *Short and tall are statistical terms*; their definition is arbitrary. Conventionally a child is considered short, when height is below the third centile, and tall when height is above the 97th centile. The term *centile* indicates how many percent of the observations have

M. Hermanussen (✉)
Aschauhof 3, 24340 Altenhof, Germany
e-mail: michael.hermanussen@gmail.com

P. Kumanov, A. Agarwal (eds.), *Puberty*, DOI 10.1007/978-3-319-32122-6_5

lower values. The third centile indicates that 3 % are smaller/shorter/lighter than children of a reference population. Shortness and tallness per se do not imply a pathological condition, but children with growth disorders are more often found among children who are short or tall. Centiles can be converted into standard deviation scores (SDS). SDS or Z-values are the differences between the individual measurements and the age- and sex-specific mean values of the reference population, divided by the standard deviation (SD) of the reference population. SDS or Z-values should be given preference over centiles.

At this point it appears necessary to briefly mention a very common, but ill-recognised dilemma. A *short child* is a child who is short. The statement is trivial and can be made after a single measurement. But a dilemma occurs when a child is repeatedly measured. Children never grow exactly parallel to their centiles. They can be short at one occasion and normal when measured later. When screening for short stature, up to 10 % of longitudinally measured children are temporarily caught at the third centile.

Growth is a *target-seeking process* [2]. Parental height strongly determines this target and, thus, can be used to predict this target. Tanner et al. [3] defined target height (TH) in centimetres as the *sex-corrected mean parental height*:

$$\text{TH} = \text{mean parental height } \pm 6.5\text{cm}$$

As the mean sex difference is typically 13 cm, +6.5 cm should be added for boys and –6.5 cm subtracted for girls. Tanner suggested a 95 % confidence interval of TH ± 10 cm for boys and TH ± 9 cm for girls, independent of the population height. Yet, this approach ignores the parent–parent correlation with $r = 0.27$: assortative mating describes that tall women tend to choose tall men and vice versa and short women rather tend to choose short men. The approach also ignores that the parent–offspring correlation is not 1.0, but $r = 0.57$ [4]. It is therefore recommended to replace the traditional Tanner approach by a formula that allows for assortative mating and the parent–offspring correlation.

We propose calculating the *conditional target height SDS* (cTHSDS) as follows [5]:

$$\text{cTHSDS} = 0.72 \times (\text{fatherSDS} + \text{motherSDS}) / 2.$$

This estimate of target height has a 95 % confidence interval of ±1.64 SDS. The formula is independent of sex, and if parental height SDS is obtained from growth charts dating back one generation, the formula is also independent of secular height trends.

Growth is a dynamic process and shows a characteristic pattern with three major growth spurts: the *postnatal spurt* followed by rapid growth deceleration during infancy and early childhood; the mild *mid-growth spurt* around the age of 6–7 years that however remains invisible in most velocity charts, this spurt possibly relating to adrenarche and the rise in adrenal steroids; and the *adolescent growth spurt* that parallels full sexual maturation. The maximum peak in height velocity (*peak height velocity*) of the adolescent spurt tends to be higher in early than in late-maturing individuals. Body weight follows a very similar pattern. The majority of children grow non-linearly, but documenting non-linearity is not trivial. Children should preferably be measured at annual or semi-annual intervals, but reality usually differs. In addition semi-annual intervals are still too long to describe *short-term growth*. Short-term growth is growth at much shorter, *at weekly or even daily intervals*. Short-term growth patterns are characterised by irregular sequences of mini growth spurts. Measurements at intervals of less than 24 h are affected by circadian variation. *Circadian variation* by far surpasses the average 24-h increments in height and weight. Height measurements are most reliable when performed in the evening hours; weight measurements are most reliable in the morning shortly after getting up.

Mini growth spurts are chaotic series of rapid height changes [6, 7]. In the American literature, this characteristic pattern of steep rises in height velocity followed by stagnation has been named *saltation and stasis* [8]. Time series analysis confirmed that mini growth spurts do not occur at strictly periodic intervals but at random intervals of a few days.

The analysis of short-term growth is difficult. It either requires highly accurate measuring techniques such as knemometry (lower leg length measurements [9, 10] for measuring child and infant growth [11]), or in case of conventional height measurements, it requires series of measurements and appropriate statistical analyses. It is good to know that increasing the number of measurements is trivial and that measurements can be obtained at home. Parents are usually very cooperative, and serial *home-made measurements* [12] are amazingly accurate. Figure 5.1 illustrates daily measures in a growth hormone (GH) deficient girl successfully treated with GH. Recent advances in statistics suggest using jump-preserving smoothing techniques for the analysis of serial height data [13].

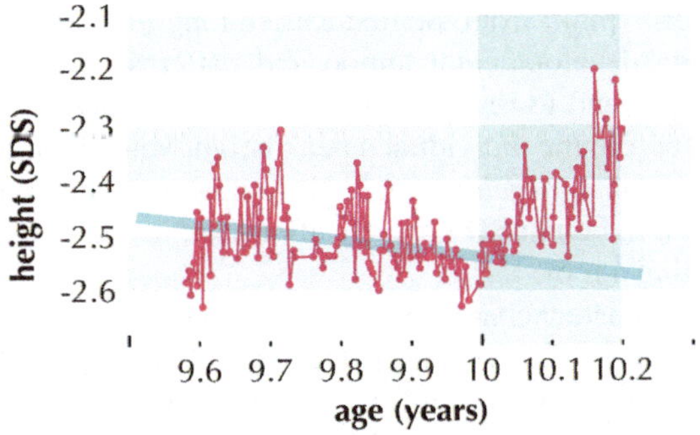

Fig. 5.1 Growth in a growth hormone (GH) deficient girl successfully treated with GH, measured daily by her parents. (Reprinted from Hermanussen M (ed). Auxology—studying human growth and development. Schweizerbart, Stuttgart, 2013 with kind permission of Schweizerbart, www.schweizerbart.de)

Tempo and Amplitude

Growth is the increase of size (*amplitude*) over time. But physical time is not directly relevant to the internal dynamics of growth. Individuals differ in *developmental tempo*: their *calendar age* may not parallel their *biological age*. A slow-maturing child needs more; a fast-maturing child needs less calendar years for reaching the same stage of maturity. The slow-maturing child appears younger and temporarily short; the fast-maturing child appears older and temporarily tall. Good clinical practice attempts to separately assess tempo and amplitude, but developmental tempo is *an auxiliary construct*. Whereas physical size is immediately measurable in absolute terms by metric scales (centimetres, kilogram, kg/m^2, etc.), and physical time by calendars and clocks, there is no apparent metric scale for maturity. Three techniques are currently available to assess the physical aspect of tempo: (1) assessing skeletal maturity, (2) assessing the state of pubertal maturity, and (3) analysing multiple records of height standard deviation scores (SDS).

Skeletal maturity of the bones of the hand and wrist is assessed by several methods; the Greulich–Pyle method [14] in combination with the growth prediction tables of Bayley and Pinneau [15] and the Tanner–Whitehouse method [16, 17] are the most commonly used. Thodberg [18] suggested replacing the manual assessment of skeletal maturity by automatic techniques.

Pubertal maturity can be rated by pubertal signs but only in healthy individuals. In disorders of sexual development, these signs often fail to reflect the tempo of maturation.

Height measurements can be described in absolute terms, or they can be related to a reference population. This can be done by plotting measurements on *centile charts* or by transforming measurements into *standard deviation or Z-scores (SDS)* [12]. A suitable reference population may be the same ethnic group, or people from the same regional area, or a population that lives under similar conditions.

Multiple records of height standard deviation score (SDS) allow rough, but quick estimates of tempo. Figure 5.2 illustrates the height SDS of nine healthy boys (blue) and nine healthy girls (pink) from the first Zürich longitudinal study and shows the association between developmental tempo and patterns of SDS [19]. *Delays in developmental tempo* tend to result in steadily declining height SDS and a downward peak shortly before the individual's peak height velocity and a rise thereafter, resembling a flat V. *Tempo acceleration* leads to upward rising in height SDS, with a characteristic peak in height SDS shortly after peak height velocity and a decline thereafter, resembling a roof.

Tempo is a very persistent characteristic throughout an individual's development: fast-maturing children tend to be fast from early childhood onwards and remain accelerated until maturity. Slow-maturing children tend to be slow from the very beginning and usually remain delayed. Differences in developmental tempo become particularly apparent during adolescence—40 % (girls) and 50 % (boys) of adolescent height variation is variation in tempo [20, 21]. The tempo of physical maturation may grossly differ from the tempo of mental, emotional or social maturation.

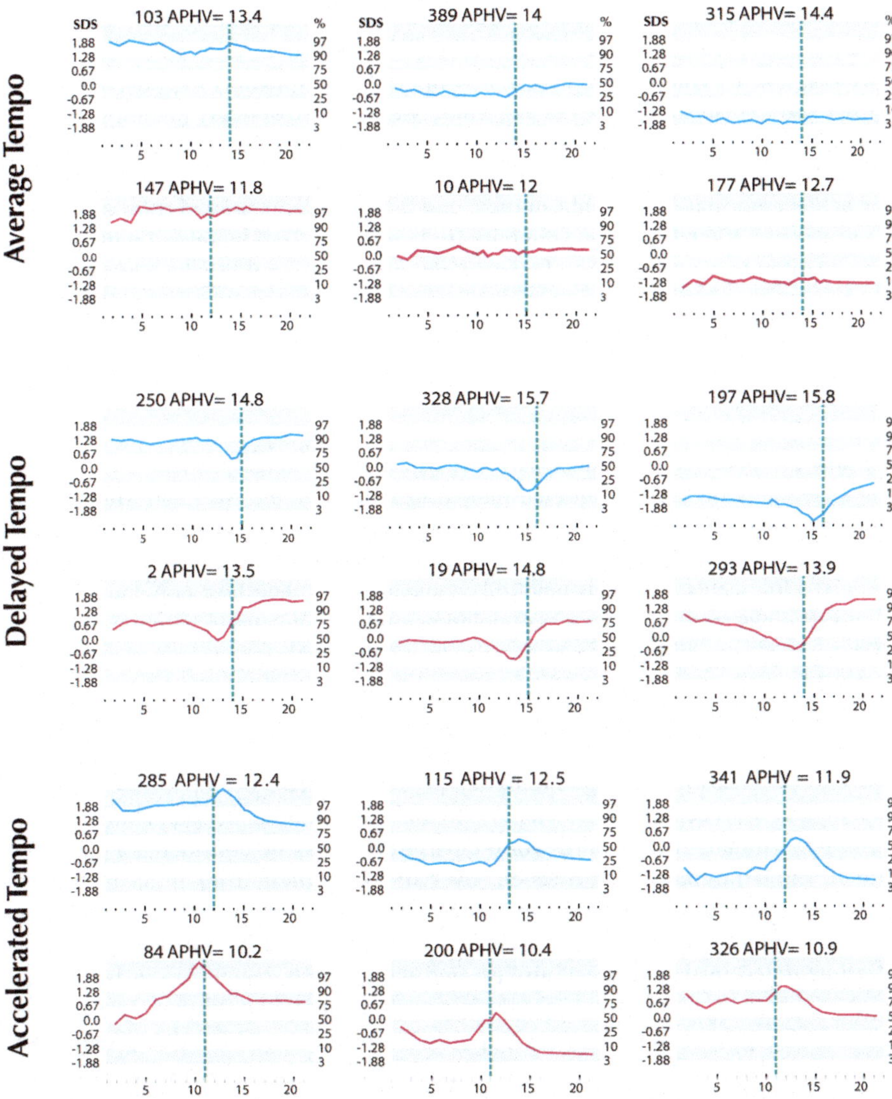

Fig. 5.2 Height SDS of nine healthy boys (*blue colour*) and nine healthy girls (*pink colour*) from the Zürich study (numbers correspond to the original numbering of the study population). The upper two rows of the graphs indicate children with average developmental tempo, the central rows show children with delayed developmental tempo, and the lower rows show children with accelerated developmental tempo. Vertical bars denote the age at peak height velocity (APHV) in years. (Reprinted from Hermanussen M (ed). Auxology—studying human growth and development. Schweizerbart, Stuttgart, 2013 with kind permission of Schweizerbart, www.schweizerbart.de)

Developmental tempo is influenced by a variety of factors of which malnutrition, illness and stress are only a few. Catch-up growth after short intermittent illnesses in otherwise healthy children is *catch up in tempo*. Even chronically *ill patients* are usually not short because of losses in amplitude, but because of delay in tempo. Aswani et al. [22] provide an excellent example in patients suffering from cystic fibrosis (CF). CF patients grow poorly at all ages, they are short up to early adulthood, but they achieve normal final height in their mid-20s. Wiedemann et al. [23] stated that in a group of 4306 CF patients, the initially low height SDS increased with age and normal height was achieved by almost all patients when reaching the adult age.

Migrants and Adoptees

Migrants are persons who transitorily or permanently *change residency*. In Europe, migrants mainly originate from the Mediterranean region, the Near and Middle East, and Africa. Migration occurs in the direction of improvement in socioeconomic circumstances and usually exhibits significant effects on growth and development in children and adolescents. Migrants tend to become as tall as their host population. When two populations merge, the shorter population tends to catch up in height towards the taller target. Maya children born to families from Guatemala who migrated to the USA are 11.5 cm taller than Maya children living in Guatemala [24]. Non-adult migrants tend to mature early and reach taller adult height than their nonmigrant relatives. Migrants are prone to obesity [25, 26]. Growth references need to consider migration. Separate references for native and migrant populations have been published, e.g. for Turkish- and Moroccan-born Dutch [27, 28] and Turkish-born German children [29].

Adopting infants from a third-world environment may be considered a particular form of child migration. In Sweden, over 6800 children from India have been adopted during the last four decades [30]. Many were severely undernourished and suffered from infectious illnesses upon arrival, but their health improved when they were integrated in their foster families, and they usually caught up in height and weight. Only the severely stunted children caught up less. Low birth weight appears to be a limiting factor for later catch-up growth. Adopted girls tend to *prematurely start pubertal development* at 11.6 years (range of 7.3–14.6) which was earlier than Swedish (13.0 years) and wealthy Indian girls (12.4–12.9 years). The adolescent growth component was on average 1.5 years earlier, but the final height was reduced to 154 cm. Eight percent of the adopted Indian girls even remained 145 cm or shorter. It is not known why this phenomenon is not so frequently observed in adopted boys.

Proportions

Humans follow a *cephalocaudal (head-to-tail) gradient of growth*. A special feature of the human pattern is that between birth and puberty, legs grow relatively faster than other body segments. This gives the human species a distinctive body shape.

Adolescent growth proceeds in a *distal-to-proximal pattern*. Body proportions change with age. First, the feet, the hands and the distal parts of the lower and upper extremities start to grow, thereafter the proximal, then the central parts of the skeleton. The peak height velocity of total body height may precede the peak height velocity of sitting height by several months. Rump growth can proceed into the third decade of life. The adolescent spurt is larger in early than in late-maturing children [31].

Proportional age defines the biological age by the change of head–trunk–extremity proportions. *Sitting height* is a useful parameter to estimate the trunk–leg proportion. Particularly in younger children, the increase in body length largely reflects the increase in leg length.

Also *skeletal robustness* (e.g. pelvic or relative elbow breadth) is subject to distinct changes both during individual life and in populations over periods of several decades. Skeletal robustness is associated with daily physical activity. A recent analysis of elbow breadth, pelvic breadth (bicristal) and thoracic depth and breadth of up to 28,975 healthy females and 28,288 healthy males aged 3–18 years from cross-sectional anthropological surveys performed between 1980 and 2012 by the Universities of Potsdam and Berlin, Germany, showed that relative elbow breadth and, to an even greater extent, absolute and relative pelvic breadth significantly decreased in both sexes since 1980 [32]. The trend towards slighter built coincides with the modern decline in physical activity and underscores the phenotypic plasticity of humans while adapting to new environmental conditions.

The Historic Aspect

The aspect of tempo and amplitude is not limited to individual growth, but it is obvious also in the population data as exemplified in Fig. 5.3. During World War II, Oslo schoolgirls suffered from marked growth impairment during the German occupation [33], but caught up later and achieved normal adult height. The *Oslo growth impairment* was impairment in tempo, limited to the time of hardship; it was not impairment in amplitude.

Measuring tempo in a population is not easy. Menarcheal age has been used for this purpose. There is a marked *secular trend in menarche*. In most European countries, the average age at menarche decreases [34] from some 18 years in the mid-nineteenth century to about 16 years around 1900 and to modern values in the urban centres already in the 1930s, e.g. in Germany: 12.6 years in Leipzig 1934 and 13.3 years in Halle 1939 [35]. At present, the mean menarcheal age in Germany is 12.7 years (low social class), 13.0 years (high class), 12.5 years (migration background) and 12.9 years (no migration background) [36]. Menarcheal age in Mediterranean countries is about 1 year earlier than in Northern Europe. Menarcheal age in the USA has mildly declined over the past 40 years, with black girls maturing 0.5–1 year earlier [37].

The average age at onset of the adolescent growth spurt may also be taken as a substitute for adolescent maturation in a population. The faster a given population matures, the earlier the adolescents start their adolescent growth spurt. Quantifying

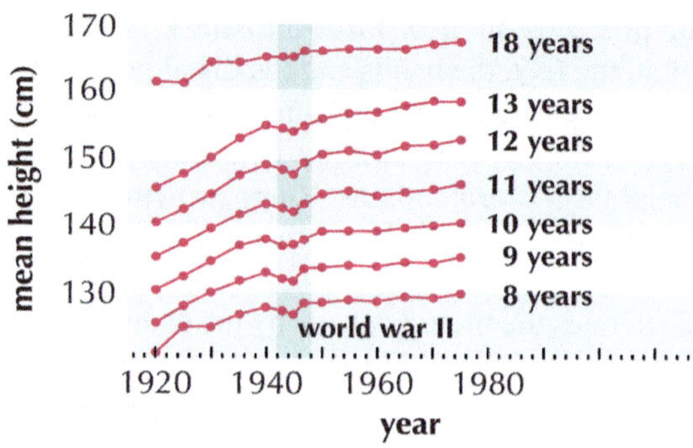

Fig. 5.3 Oslo schoolgirls suffered from marked growth impairment during the German occupation [33], but caught up later and finally achieved normal adult height. (Reprinted from Hermanussen M (ed). Auxology—studying human growth and development. Schweizerbart, Stuttgart, 2013 with kind permission of Schweizerbart, www.schweizerbart.de)

Table 5.1 Age at take-off (ATO), the rise of height at take-off (HTO), the adolescent growth (AG) and the adult height (AH) in six male Japanese growth surveys published in 1955, 1960, 1970, 1980, 1990 and 2000

	ATO (years)	HTO (cm)	AH (cm)	AG (cm)
Japan2000	8.1	125.4	171.1	45.7
Japan1990	8.3	126.3	170.5	44.2
Japan1980	8.3	125.1	169.8	44.6
Japan1970	8.7	126.0	167.5	41.5
Japan1960	9.1	124.4	165.4	41.0
Japan1955	9.3	122.9	162.6	39.7
Difference 2000–1955	1.2	2.5	8.5	6.0

Based on the data from [39, 40], Satake (2012, personal communication)

the pattern of adolescent growth in a population needs some mathematical modelling. Among several models we preferentially use the Preece–Baines model [38] for this purpose. The model explicitly calculates the *height and age at take-off (HTO* and *ATO)* and *age at peak height velocity (APHV)* and thus provides two useful parameters for estimating the state of maturation. The Preece–Baines model can be applied to population data, and it is mathematically not very sophisticated.

Table 5.1 illustrates the forward displacement of ATO, the rise of HTO, the adolescent growth and the adult height in six male Japanese growth surveys published in 1955, 1960, 1970, 1980, 1990 and 2000. Japanese boys in 2000 spurt about 1 year earlier than in 1955, and their adolescent growth is 6 cm larger than in 1955. The table illustrates that the secular trend in height is both a trend in tempo and a trend in amplitude.

The intermingling of tempo and amplitude often leads to misinterpretation when analysing secular trends in populations. When depicting differences between average height and a reference for height, for the same populations at different historic moments, populations behave similar to individuals. Figure 5.4 exemplifies the differences between average height and the WHO standards/references for height [41] in modern and historic Japanese children [39, 40] (Satake, 2012, personal communication). At all ages, Japanese are shorter than WHO standards/references—Japanese differ in amplitude at all ages. But the patterns also show that the historic cohorts steadily decline in height compared with WHO height, with a downward peak at mid-adolescence and a rise thereafter, and that the modern cohorts (though still shorter than the reference at all ages) partially resemble the accelerated pattern in Fig. 5.2, with a characteristic peak in height SDS at mid-adolescence. Modern children are taller and they mature faster. At 12 years, modern boys are taller and biologically older than their fathers at age 12. The

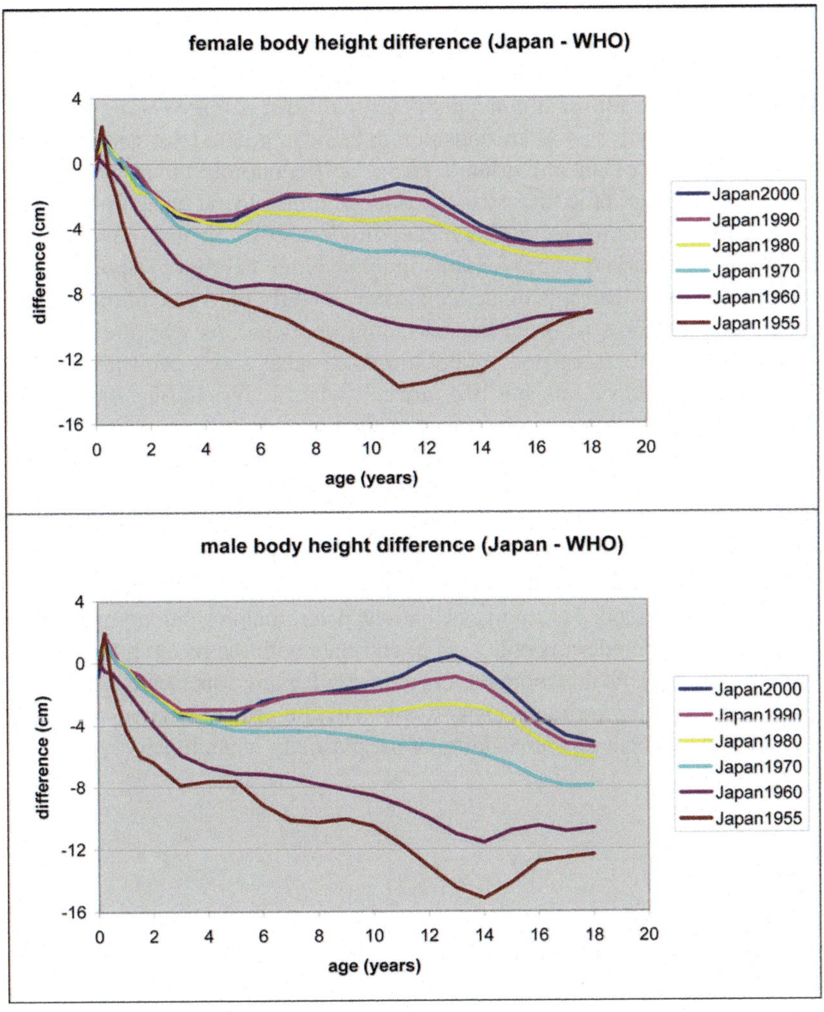

Fig. 5.4 Height difference between modern and historic Japanese children (Based on data from: [39, 40], Satake (2012, personal communication); WHO standards/references [41])

trend in tempo superimposes the trend in amplitude. The superimposition of the two trends needs to be disentangled. This is important for the understanding of secular changes in growth.

The rise in adult height observed in recent history is spectacular. Old World Europeans increased in height by some 11–19 cm since the mid-nineteenth century [42]. Interestingly this was different in Europeans who lived abroad. Late-nineteenth century white US conscripts were already almost as tall as today [43]. White South African males reached an average body height of near 172 cm at the turn of the nineteenth to twentieth century, with no remarkable trend since [44]. European Australians reached 175 cm at the beginning of the twentieth century [45]. The discrepancy in growth of white Europeans born within and outside the European continent strongly contrasts the notion that adult height is *one of the most heritable human phenotypes* [46]. The data rather support the vision that adult height depends on environmental cues.

This contradicts traditional concepts of *growth as a target-seeking process* [2]. Since decades, growth has been considered being regulated by genes, nutrition, health and the state of an individual's social and economic environment. Social, economic and demographic history has produced multiple evidence for interactions between living conditions, technology, economy and body height [43, 47]: optimal conditions lead to marked improvements in the average height of populations; poor populations are short. But this evidence appears to only hold true at the population level. This concept fails to provide convincing explanations why the healthy and well-nourished members of poor populations are also short. Well-nourished and healthy people should be tall, but they are not when living among short and poor people. *Growth appears to seek its target at the community level. Tall stature communities appear to generate tall people*; *short stature communities appear to generate short people*. We named this the *community effect in height* [48–50].

At first view this idea appears bizarre, and it has already generated vivid debates. But evidence has accumulated that social and psychological phenomena are directly involved in the regulation of adult height. The pathomechanism of this regulation is still far from being understood. But it appears that self-determination, autonomy, democracy and happiness of the modern people tend to correlate with the recent trends in adolescent growth (Fig. 5.4). At this moment it is too early for any conclusive statements, but new evidence may provide more insights into the complex regulation of adolescent growth and lead to a better understanding of the plasticity of adult height [49].

References

1. Bogin BA. Patterns of human growth. 2nd ed. Cambridge: Cambridge University Press; 1999.
2. Tanner JM. Growth as a mirror of the condition of society: secular trends and class distinctions. In: Demirjian A, editor. Human growth: a multidisciplinary review. London: Taylor & Francis; 1986. pp. 3–34.
3. Tanner JM, Goldstein H, Whitehouse RH. Standards for children's height at age 2–9 years allowing for height of parents. Arch Dis Child. 1970;45:755–62.

4. Luo ZC, Albertsson-Wikland K, Karlberg J. Target height as predicted by parental heights in a population- based study. Pediatr Res. 1998;44:563–71.
5. Hermanussen M, Cole TJ. The calculation of target height reconsidered. Horm Res. 2003;59:180–3.
6. Hermanussen M, Rol de Lama MA, F-Tresguerres JA, Grasedyck L, Burmeister J. Short-term growth: evidence for chaotic series of mini growth spurts in rat growth. Physiol Behav. 1998;64:7–13.
7. Hermanussen M. The analysis of short-term growth. Horm Res. 1998;49:53–64.
8. Lampl M, Johnson ML, Frongillo Jr EA. Mixed distribution analysis identifies saltation and stasis growth. Ann Hum Biol. 2001;28:403–11.
9. Hermanussen M, Geiger-Benoit K, Burmeister J, Sippell WG. Knemometry in childhood: accuracy and standardization of a new technique of lower leg length measurement. Ann Hum Biol. 1988;15:1–16.
10. Hermanussen M, Geiger-Benoit K, Burmeister J, Sippell WG. Periodical changes of short term growth velocity ("mini growth spurts") in human growth. Ann Hum Biol. 1988;15:103–9.
11. Kaempf DE, Pflüger MS, Thiele AM, Hermanussen M, Linderkamp O. Influence of nutrition on growth in premature infants: assessment by knemometry. Ann Hum Biol. 1998;25:127–36.
12. Hermanussen M (ed). Auxology: studying human growth and development. Stuttgart: Schweizerbart; 2013.
13. Caino S, Kelmansky D, Adamo P, Lejarraga H. Short-term growth in healthy infants, schoolchildren and adolescent girls. Ann Hum Biol. 2006;33:213–26.
14. Greulich WW, Pyle SI. Radiographic atlas of skeletal development of the hand and wrist. 2nd ed. Stanford: Stanford. Stanford University Press; 1959.
15. Bayley N, Pinneau SR. Tables for predicting adult height from skeletal age: revised for use with the Greulich-Pyle hand standards. J Pediatr. 1952;40:423–41, Erratum J Pediatr. 41:371.
16. Tanner JM, Goldstein H, Cameron N, Saunders WB, Healy MJR. Assessment of skeletal maturity and prediction of adult height. 3rd ed. Philadelphia: WB Saunders; 2001.
17. Tanner JM, Whitehouse RH, Marshall WA, Healy MJR, Goldstein H. Assessment of skeletal maturity and prediction of adult height (TW2 method). 2nd ed. London, New York, Paris, San Diego, San Francisco, Sidney, Tokyo, Toronto: Academic; 1983.
18. Thodberg HH. Clinical review: an automated method for determination of bone age. J Clin Endocrinol Metab. 2009;94:2239–44.
19. Hermanussen M. Auxology: an update. Horm Res Paediatr. 2010;74:153–64.
20. Hermanussen M, Meigen C. Phase variation in child and adolescent growth. Int J Biostat. 2007;3:1–16.
21. Molinari L, Hermanussen M. The effect of variability in maturational tempo and midparent height on variability in linear body measurements. Ann Hum Biol. 2005;32:679–82.
22. Aswani N, Taylor CJ, McGaw J, Pickering M, Rigby AS. Pubertal growth and development in cystic fibrosis: a retrospective review. Acta Paediatr. 2003;92:1029–32.
23. Wiedemann B, Steinkamp G, Sens B, Stern M. German cystic fibrosis quality assurance group: the German cystic fibrosis quality assurance project: clinical features in children and adults. Eur Respir J. 2001;17:1187–94.
24. Bogin B, Smith P, Orden AB, Varela Silva MI, Loucky J. Rapid change in height and body proportions of Maya American children. Am J Hum Biol. 2002;14:753–61.
25. Fredriks AM, van Buuren S, Hira Sing RA, Wit JM, Verloove-Vanhorick SP. Alarming prevalence of overweight and obesity for children of Turkish, Moroccan and Dutch origin in The Netherlands according to international standards. Acta Paediatr. 2005;94:496–8.
26. Kirchengast S, Schober E. Obesity among female adolescents in Vienna, Austria: the impact of childhood weight status and ethnicity. Br J Obstet Gynaecol. 2006;113:1188–94.
27. Fredriks AM, Buuren SV, Burgmeijer RJF, Meulmeester JF, Beuker RJ, Brugman E, Roede MJ, Verloove-Vanhorick SP, Wit JM. Continuing positive secular growth change in the Netherlands 1955–1997. Pediatr Res. 2000;47:316–23.
28. Fredriks AM. Growth diagrams. Fourth Dutch nation-wide survey. Doctorial dissertation. Leiden; 2004. pp. 91–104.

29. Redlefsen T, Commentz J, Meigen C, Hermanussen M. Reference values for height, weight and body mass index of German born Turkish children. Anthropol Anz. 2007;65:263–74.
30. Proos LA. Growth and development of Indian children adopted in Sweden. Indian J Med Res. 2009;130:646–50.
31. Shuttleworth FK. Sexual maturation and the physical growth of girls age six to nineteen. Monogr Soc Res in Child Develop. vol 2, no 5. Washington, DC: National Research Council; 1937.
32. Scheffler C, Hermanussen M. Is there an influence of modern life style on skeletal build? Am J Hum Biol. 2014;26:590–7.
33. Brundtland GH. Height, weight and menarcheal age of Oslo schoolchildren during the last 60 years. Ann Hum Biol. 1980;7:307–22.
34. van Wieringen JC. Secular growth changes. In: Falkner F, Tanner JM, editors. Human growth. vol 3, 2nd ed. New York, London: Plenum Press; 1986. pp. 307–31.
35. Lehmann A, Scheffler C, Hermanussen M. Evidence of seasonal variation in longitudinal growth of height in a sample of boys from Stuttgart Carlsschule, 1771–1793, using combined principal component analysis and maximum likelihood principle. Homo. 2010;61:59–63.
36. Kahl H, Schaffrath Rosario A, Schlaud M. Sexual maturation of children and adolescents in Germany. Results of the German. Health Interview and Examination Survey for Children and Adolescents (KiGGS). Bundesgesundheitsblatt Gesundheitsforschung Gesundheitsschutz. 2007;50:677–85.
37. Kaplowitz P. Pubertal development in girls: secular trends. Curr Opin Obstet Gynecol. 2006;18:487–91.
38. Preece MA, Baines MJ. A new family of mathematical models describing the human growth curve. Ann Hum Biol. 1978;5:1–24.
39. Takahashi E, Atsumi H. Age differences in thoracic form as indicated by thoracic index. Hum Biol. 1955;27:65–74.
40. Technology. Report on school health survey 2003. Tokyo: National Printing Bureau; 2004. pp. 130–3.
41. WHO multicentre growth reference study group. WHO child growth standards. Acta Paediatr Suppl. 2006;95 Suppl 450:1–104.
42. Bodzsar BE, Susanne C. Secular growth changes in Europe. Budapest: Eotvos University Press; 1998.
43. Komlos J. Height and social status in eighteenth-century Germany. J Interdisciplinary Hist. 1990;20:607–21.
44. Henneberg M, van den Berg ER. Test of socioeconomic causation of secular trend: stature changes among favored and oppressed South Africans are parallel. Am J Phys Anthropol. 1990;83:459–65.
45. Henneberg M. Possible causes of secular trends in body size: lessons from the Southern Hemisphere. In: Schulze M, et al. editors. Homo: unsere Herkunft und Zukunft. Goettingen: Cuvillier Verlag; 2001. pp. 234–7.
46. Lettre G. Recent progress in the study of the genetics of height. Hum Genet. 2011;129:465–72.
47. Fogel RW. The escape from hunger and premature death, 1700–2100. Cambridge, New York, Melbourne: Cambridge University Press; 2004.
48. Aßmann C, Hermanussen M. Modeling determinants of growth: evidence for a community-based target in height? Pediatr Res. 2013;74:88–95.
49. Bogin B, Hermanussen M, Blum WF, Aßmann C. Sex, sport, IGF-1 and the community effect in height hypothesis. Int J Environ Res Public Health. 2015;12:4816–32.
50. Hermanussen M, Alt C, Staub K, Aßmann C, Groth D. The impact of physical connectedness on body height in Swiss conscripts. Anthropol Anz. 2014;71:313–27.

Chapter 6
Bone Development in Children and Adolescents

Mihail A. Boyanov

Introduction

Bone is a living tissue and integrated into the compact skeleton it has to fulfill a number of vital functions: (1) to provide a mechanical barrier for the protection of soft tissues and internal organs; (2) to allow movement, together with muscles (the so-called muscle–bone unit); (3) to store calcium and other molecules involved in the equilibrium of the extracellular space; and (4) to protect the bone marrow and to interact with its cell lines, as well as many other functions. Bone development during childhood and adolescence is a process of great complexity and can be viewed from many aspects [1–3]. Among the most debated ones are the development and maintenance of the growth plate, the bone mineral accrual at the different skeletal parts, and the factors contributing to the regulation of all these events. The implementation of bone age is another interesting point combining classical clinical use with up-to-date computerized applications. These aspects will be commented below.

Mechanisms of Bone Development: The Role and Structure of the Growth Plate

The bone tissue is derived from different parts of the mesoderm. Craniofacial elements develop through the process of intramembranous ossification, while long bones are the product of endochondral ossification. In the latter type of ossification, the mesodermal stem cells form condensed groups and differentiate into chondrocytes

M.A. Boyanov (✉)
Department of Internal Medicine, Clinic of Endocrinology and Metabolism, University Hospital Alexandrovska, Medical University Sofia,
1, Georgi Sofiyski Street, 1431 Sofia, Bulgaria
e-mail: mihailboyanov@yahoo.com

P. Kumanov, A. Agarwal (eds.), *Puberty*, DOI 10.1007/978-3-319-32122-6_6

producing an extracellular matrix, rich in collagen type 2. The chondrocytes in the midportion become hypertrophic and start to secrete collagen type 10, which can be then mineralized. Cells from the perichondrium can differentiate into osteoblasts providing the basis for the so-called bone collar—the initiation site for the cortical envelope. A critical step in this process is the invasion by blood vessels, followed by apoptosis of terminally differentiated chondrocytes and resorption of the calcified cartilage matrix. The cartilage is replaced by bone and vascular elements, building the primary ossification center.

The remaining chondrocytes at both ends of the long bones provide the basis for further bone growth—the growth plate. The growth plate is entrapped between the epiphyseal and metaphyseal bone and consists of distinct layers with different functions. The most superficial layer (adjacent to the epiphysis) is built by round chondrocytes (resting zone), followed by more mature and strongly proliferating columnar ones (proliferation zone). They further mature to the so-called hypertrophic chondrocytes (which build the differentiation zone). The chondrocytes adjacent to the metaphysis are subjected to apoptosis and cell death. The junction between the growth plate and the metaphysis is the site for invasion of new vessels, osteoclasts, and osteoblasts. The osteoclasts resorb the calcified cartilage matrix, while the osteoblasts deposit mineralized bone matrix on the remnants. So, the chondrocytes in the growth plate are both spatially and temporarily differentiated. The linear bone growth, in its turn, leads to an age gradient in the metaphysis [4]. The newest part of the metaphysis is adjacent to the growth plate, while the oldest one—to the epiphysis. During childhood, the growth plate matures and it fuses (closes) at the end of puberty under the influence of gonadal steroids and other specific factors. A very comprehensive depiction of these processes might be found elsewhere [1–3].

Modern molecular biology allows a closer look into the mechanisms of bone development and the key regulating factors. A number of questions concerning the growth plate maturation and fusion, as well as growth factors and local regulators, are still being debated. Most data come from mice. A very comprehensive picture of all these factors is provided in the review by Emons et al. [5]. Chondrocytes receive a variety of signals from the perichondrial cells, including bone morphogenetic proteins (BMPs), fibroblast growth factors (FGFs), and other highly conserved secreted signaling molecules that regulate cell-to-cell interactions during development and adult tissue homeostasis such as Wnt signaling. BMP signaling is essential for converting the mesenchymal cells into chondrocytes, as well as in the later stages of cartilage development. BMPs have distinct and sometimes opposing effects in the different chondrocytic zones (agonistic in the hypertrophic and antagonistic in the resting and proliferative zones) [6]. The Wnt signaling pathway is a conserved pathway in animals: the name Wnt being resultant from a fusion of the name of the *Drosophila* segment polarity gene *wingless* and the name of the vertebrate homolog *integrated or int-1*.

FGF-18 and FGF-9 are considered important in regulating chondrogenesis [7, 8]. FGFs may act as antagonists to BMPs. Activating mutations in FGF-3 receptor may lead to achondroplasia or hypochondroplasia, while loss-of-function mutations in the responsible gene are accompanied by tall stature in humans [9, 10]. The activation of the canonical Wnt pathway results in activation of β-catenin and induction of osteoblast, instead of chondrocyte formation [11]. A number of transcription factors (such as Runx2, Sox9, and others) and growth factors (such as transforming growth factor-beta, TGF-β) are also implicated in the complex regulatory processes. Vascular endothelial growth factor (VEGF) is a potent stimulator of blood vessel invasion and expansion. It is also considered crucial for the estrogen-driven growth plate fusion. A study in rats found that the expression of VEGF in the growth plate was stimulated by estradiol, although the precise role of VEGF in estrogen-mediated growth plate fusion could not be demonstrated [12]. Key factors in the regulation of the growth plate are also the hormonal and paracrine factors, such as parathyroid hormone (PTH), parathyroid hormone-related peptide (PTHrp), vitamin D, and Indian hedgehog (Ihh). Ihh and PTHrp form a negative feedback loop regulating the hypertrophic differentiation of chondrocytes. Ihh, produced by the early hypertrophic chondrocytes, stimulates the expression of PTHrp, which in turn slows down the differentiation and keeps the chondrocytes in the proliferative stage [13]. A homozygous mutation in the Ihh gene may lead to disproportional short stature, brachydactyly, and premature fusion of the growth plates [14]. An inactivating mutation in the PTH receptor may lead to chondrodysplasia with advanced bone maturation (Blomstrand chondrodysplasia), while an activating mutation leads to short stature and delay in bone maturation in Jansen chondrodysplasia [15, 16]. Vitamin D deficiency is known to result in increased width of the hypertrophic chondrocytic zone due to decreased cell death and in delayed invasion by angiogenic and bone cells [17]. All these hormonal, transcriptional, and other regulating factors have their origins in distinct patterns of gene expression. A recent study, looking for evolutionary conserved networks, identified a number of growth pathways (Notch, VEGF, TGF-β, Wnt, and glucocorticoid receptor) [18].

The classical model of growth plate maturation and epiphyseal fusion involves the sex steroids—estrogens and androgens. It is derived from the observation that precocious puberty is accompanied by early skeletal maturation and early growth stop, while delayed puberty or hypogonadism leads to slow skeletal maturation and excessive growth of the long bones. There was active debate on the relative contributions of estrogens and androgens in both sexes. A role has been clearly attributed to the estrogen receptor-α (ER-α), while the role of the estrogen receptor-β (ER-β) remains to be elucidated [19, 20]. Estrogen is thought to accelerate growth plate senescence (maturation and aging), in addition to a genetically programmed mechanism intrinsic to the growth plate itself [21]. Estrogens can also be produced locally in the growth plate. Androgens were thought to act mainly via conversion into estrogens, but recent work has shown an independent pathway for androgenic substances, since androgen receptors are found in the human growth plate, as well as on human osteoblasts [22, 23].

While sexual maturation and puberty progress, the growth plate is a subject of structural and functional changes—the so-called senescence. It is partly due to genetic programming and finite proliferative capacity. The classical hypothesis is that of apoptosis resulting in cell shrinkage, DNA fragmentation, and degradation of the cytoplasm and nucleus in the absence of signs of inflammation. Other suggested mechanisms include autophagy, *trans*-differentiation of hypertrophic chondrocytes into osteoblasts (the oldest hypothesis), hypoxia, and others. However, human studies focused on the growth plate have not provided conclusive evidence for all these hypotheses [24].

Osteoclastogenesis and Osteoblastogenesis

Two cell types are indispensable for the development of mature bone tissue—osteoblasts and osteoclasts. Once the hypertrophic cartilage is invaded by blood vessels and VEGF is secreted, it is the osteoclasts that resorb cellular and matrix debris to free space for the newly built bone. Osteoblasts, in their turn, react to signals such as BMPs, TGF-β, and others and start building collagen and non-collagen proteins, which further become mineralized. A number of regulating factors are key players for osteoclast recruitment, differentiation, and survival. Both macrophages and osteoclast precursor cells originate from a common myeloid precursor under the action of transcription factor PU [25]. This factor also enhances the transcription of the receptor for another crucial regulator, the so-called receptor activator of nuclear factor-k-β (RANK) [26]. The ligand of this receptor (RANKL), together with the macrophage colony-stimulating factor (M-CSF), is critical for osteoclastogenesis. The M-CSF acts in the earlier stages of osteoclastogenesis, while the RANKL is responsible for osteoclast recruitment, differentiation, maturation, and survival [27]. The activation of the nuclear factor-k-β by the binding of RANKL to the membrane-bound receptor leads to c-*fos* expression and induction of osteoclast-specific genes [28]. RANKL is secreted by the osteoblasts in response to different cellular signals. RANKL is regulated negatively by a soluble decoy receptor called osteoprotegerin (OPG), which is also secreted by the osteoblasts [29, 30]. Thus, one of the key regulating cells for the osteoclastogenesis and survival is the osteoblast itself. The osteoblast is the primary target for different signals to the bone in physiological and pathological conditions, such as vitamin D, parathyroid hormone, PTHrp, different cytokines—interleukins (in inflammatory and immune diseases)—and many others [31–33]. It is interesting to note that the osteoclast gives signals back to the osteoblast, thus modulating the equilibrium between RANKL and OPG. Among these are different BMPs, TGF-β, and others [34]. The discovery of RANKL led to the development of a targeted, fully human antibody, used in the treatment of postmenopausal osteoporosis [35]. The scientific work in the field of postmenopausal osteoporosis led to the discovery of the third important cell type in the development of bone. Osteocytes, previously thought to be aging and exhausted osteoblasts, play an important role in the suppression of bone formation and the induction of resorption. Through their dendritic processes, they sense mechanical forces, communicate with each other, and send signals to the bone-forming cells, such as the inhibitor of the canonical Wnt pathway—osteosclerostin (SOST) [36, 37]. SOST binds two synergistically acting receptor families and stabilizes the so-called β-catenin protein, which regulates the expression of downstream target genes

[38]. The homozygous loss-of-function mutation in SOST may lead to sclerosteosis, while mutations, affecting its transcription, cause van Buchem disease—both associated with high bone mass phenotypes [39]. The discovery of SOST gave way to the development of antagonistic antibodies, which promise to become one of the most potent bone-forming agents under study [40].

At the structural level, bone development during childhood and adolescence is the net result of two processes—bone modeling and bone remodeling [41]. The evolutionary role of bone modeling is to build new bone, while during bone remodeling, damaged bone is first removed and the resorption cavities are subsequently mineralized [1]. Bone modeling is typical for the growing bone and results in bone mineral apposition and bone size increases. During bone modeling, osteoclasts and osteoblasts are uncoupled; they act separately at different sites of the bone. Bone modeling is most active until skeletal maturity and was believed to stop at skeletal maturity, although recent work has shown some modeling to occur at later ages at a very modest rate [42]. Bone remodeling is characterized by the coupling of osteoblasts and osteoclasts, which build the so-called bone remodeling unit (BMU) [43]. The osteoclasts first excavate a resorption lacuna, which is then filled by the osteoblasts and subjected to a slow process of mineralization. The frequency of activation of the BMU and the depth of the resorption cavities are among the key factors determining the bone loss in adulthood and senescence [44].

During childhood and adolescence, bones grow in both length and width. Periosteal apposition is responsible for the growth in width, while endochondral ossification for the growth in length. Resorption occurs inside the bone, while new bone is deposited on the outer surface (subperiosteal apposition driven mainly by osteoblasts and bone modeling). Bones are subject to constant changes in shape and size. This process terminates around the time of skeletal maturity with the bone resorption continuing throughout life at different rates according to age [1, 45].

Bone Mineral Accretion in Children and Adolescents

The question of bone mineral accrual during adolescence and of the timing of peak bone mass is very difficult to address. Firstly, bone mass can be measured at different sites—the vertebrae, femur, radius, tibia, and whole body—which grow and develop at different rates and time scales. The different skeletal parts are affected by different factors (e.g., weight-bearing activities). Secondly, there is a great variety of measuring techniques—dual-energy X-ray absorptiometry (DXA), quantitative computed tomography (QCT), high-resolution computed tomography, and magnetic resonance imaging (hr-pQCT, hr-MRI). The most widely used technique, DXA, provides data on bone mineral content (BMC) and bone mineral density (BMD). DXA-derived BMD is bidimensional; it is called areal BMD and does not properly reflect the contribution of the third dimension (bone depth or the anteroposterior diameter). BMC and aBMD change rapidly during growth because of bone size increases. An attempt to overcome this intrinsic methodological problem is to measure the true volumetric BMD by QCT or its peripheral modification, pQCT. Volumetric BMD can also be calculated if bone density scans in two planes are available, such as vBMD of the vertebrae derived from anteroposterior and lateral spine scans. In a previous study, an algorithm for calculation of forearm vBMD has been proposed, although the accuracy of all calculated parameters is debatable [46]. The third problem is due to the different proportions of cortical and trabecular bone in the skeletal parts. Cortical and trabecular bone might be regarded as two distinct components and their interaction determines the net effect on bone development. In an experimental model, calculated cortical and trabecular forearm BMD showed a distinct pattern of changes over time in adult women [47]. Only the QCT, pQCT, and high-resolution techniques are capable of distinguishing both components of the bone. And fourth, a large number of factors are affecting bone growth and development, such as heredity, age, sex, race, physical activity, nutrition, pubertal stage, etc. It is almost impossible to dissect a single factor and define its contribution to the whole. To summarize, the problem of different skeletal sites, measurement techniques, and biological factors should be kept in mind, when interpreting data about bone mineral changes during childhood and adolescence.

A DXA-based study in healthy Italian children showed that before puberty, boys and girls had equal BMD at the lumbar spine, while the femoral neck BMD was higher in boys [48]. In the areas rich of cortical bone, the boys showed higher values before puberty, while trabecular bone was equivalent until the age of 9 and increasing more steeply in girls thereafter. The authors concluded that male sex and lean mass were predictors for the higher cortical bone mass in boys, while female sex and pubertal stage predicted the higher trabecular bone accrual in girls [48]. Another DXA-based study explained the differences in BMC as mainly due to the differences in body size [49]. Body size was held responsible for most of the racial/ethnic differences in BMC. In a cohort of Spanish adolescents, females had higher values of the DXA-derived BMC and BMD at most of the sites, probably due to the smaller diameters of bones [50]. Bone growth from 11 to 17 years was studied by pQCT at the distal forearm [51]. This study showed that bone width and mineral content increased with age albeit independently, which resulted in a modest decrease of vBMD during early puberty followed by a rapid increase. Physical growth occurred at a higher tempo than bone growth. By the age of 17, boys had attained 86 % of the reference adult BMC and vBMD, while girls had attained 93 and 94 %, respectively [51]. A very interesting study assessed the structural and biomechanical basis for sexual dimorphism at the hip by using the DXA-derived FN areal BMD and measured the periosteal diameter to estimate the endocortical diameter, cortical thickness, section modulus (a measure of bending strength), and buckling ratio (indices for structural stability) [45]. In this study, FN cortical thickness or volumetric density did not differ in young adult women and men after adjustment for height and weight. The sex differences in geometry were best described by the further displacement of the cortex from the FN neutral axis in young men, which produced a 13.4 % greater bending strength than in young women. The changes in FN diameters, cortical thickness, and geometry during puberty are presented in Fig. 6.1 according to [45].

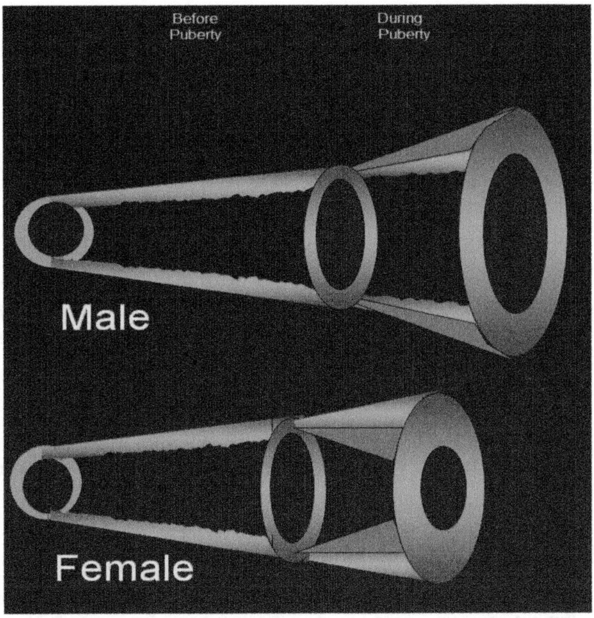

Fig. 6.1 Changes in FN diameters, cortical thickness, and geometry during puberty. Cortical thickness or volumetric density does not differ in young adult women and men; the sex differences in geometry are best described by the further displacement of the cortex from the FN neutral axis in young men [45]. This is now thought to be partly due to the longer prepubertal growth and intrapubertal growth in males than females (Courtesy of Prof. E. Seeman)

The effects of sex, race, and puberty on cortical bone were examined by pQCT of the distal tibia [52]. This study found higher cortical measures in blacks than whites in Tanner stages 1–4; however, differences were negligible in Tanner stage 5. Cortical BMC, periosteal and endosteal circumferences, and section modulus were higher in pubertal males than females; however, cortical BMD was higher in Tanner 3–5 females. The authors were unable to explain maturation-specific differences in cortical BMD and dimensions solely by differences in bone length or muscle [52]. Cortical porosity at the distal radius and tibia was studied during pubertal growth by hr-pQCT [53]. At the radius, girls had higher cortical density and lower cortical porosity than boys, while boys had higher trabecular bone volume ratios and larger cortical cross-sectional areas. These results could provide a solid basis for the sex- and maturity-related differences in bone microarchitecture and strength [53].

The task of describing bone changes is further complicated by the contribution of muscle development to the so-called muscle–bone unit. Bone and muscle properties were studied prospectively by tibial DXA and pQCT—the growth velocity of the muscle cross-sectional area peaked earlier than tibial BMC and later than tibial outer dimensions [54]. Tibial length was the first to stop increasing 2 years after menarche, while all other muscle and bone parameters continued to increase even at the age of 18 years. This study corroborated the hypothesis that the development of lean mass precedes that of bone mass but did not support the role of the muscles as the central driving force for bone growth during puberty [54]. In summary, all the data coming from bone measurement techniques show an absence of gender-specific differences in bone mass until the onset of puberty. The bone maturation period seems longer in males than females, and the increase in bone size is greater in males. Changes in vBMD between sexes are negligible at the end of puberty; the differences in BMD are due mainly to the differences in bone size and architecture, as stated by other authors [1, 55].

Peak bone mass (PBM) is essential for the future risk of osteoporosis and fragility fractures. The exact age, at which PBM is attained, remains a matter of debate. A DXA-based study found that in males, bone mass at different skeletal sites continued to increase between 15 and 18 years, while in girls, it slowed down at the levels of both lumbar spine and femoral neck (FN) at 15–16 years of age [56]. Girls attained values near PBM at an earlier age than boys. In the 14–15-year-old female group, BMD in L2–L4, FN, and femoral shaft corresponded to 99.2, 105.1, and 94.1 %, respectively, and BMC in L2–L4 to 97.6 % of the mean values for 20–35-year-old women [56]. In a similar study, the contribution of the third decade of life to BMD in women was found to be only 6.8 % at the LS and 4.8 %—at the forearm [57]. The authors located the end of bone mass acquisition around the age of 28.3 and 29.5 years. The sex differences in bone mass acquisition during growth were estimated in the Fels Longitudinal Study [58]. This study showed that PBM and density are attained generally between the ages of 20 and 25 years and occur earlier in females than males. vBMD was shown to rise much slower than BMC and aBMD, due to the different contributions of bone size and density [59]. Peak vBMD of the lumbar vertebrae was reached between 22 and 29 years of age, while peak values were reached substantially earlier for the femoral neck (around 12 years of age) and ultradistal radius (around 19 years of age) [59].

Factors Contributing to Bone Development in Children and Adolescents

Bone development occurs under the influence of many contributing factors—age, sex, race, pubertal development, body weight and height (size), physical activity, nutrition, and many others. Age, sex, and pubertal stage also affect the skeleton by supporting a specific hormonal milieu. Some of these factors have been extensively studied in the last decades.

The influence of being overweight was studied in 11–13-year-old boys by DXA at the LS, FN, and whole body (WB) [60]. Overweight boys displayed similar values for LS and WB and lower for the FN, compared to normal-weight controls. In normal-weight boys, fat-free mass was the major determinant of bone mineral indices, while in overweight boys, it correlated only with the FN; the LS and WB BMD correlating better with the fat mass [60]. This study showed that the influence of body weight on BMD is not uniform and cannot be explained as putting more mechanical stress on the skeleton and thus stimulating the growth of the muscle–bone unit. Another study tested the association of lean and fat body mass with bone mass during pre- and midpuberty and found appendicular lean mass to be the strongest determinant [61]. These associations were also studied by tibial pQCT in the Avon Longitudinal Study of Parents and Children [62]. Lean mass showed a positive

Table 6.1 The correlation coefficients (R-square) from curve estimation analyses with lumbar spine BMD (as the dependent variable) and body weight, % body fat, and fat and lean mass (as the independent variables) are in the same magnitude

Model	R-square			
Equation	Fat mass	Lean mass	Total body weight	% Body fat
Linear	0.181	0.160	0.231	0.106
Logarithmic	0.207	0.177	0.258	0.095
Inverse	0.209	0.190	0.275	0.077
Quadratic	0.226	0.202	0.280	0.117
Cubic	0.229	0.202	0.280	0.112
Compound	0.181	0.154	0.232	0.109
Power	0.212	0.174	0.265	0.097
S	0.220	0.191	0.288	0.079
Exponential	0.181	0.154	0.232	0.109

The significance was $p<0.001$ for all equations including body weight, fat, and lean mass and $0.01>p>0.001$ for the % of body fat (Reprinted from Boyanov M. Body fat, lean mass and bone density of the spine and forearm in women. Central European Journal of Medicine 2014;9(1): 121–125. With permission from Springer Science+Business Media)

correlation with cortical BMC in both boys and girls and its correlation with periosteal circumference was stronger in girls. Fat mass showed a stronger correlation with cortical BMC and periosteal circumference and a negative one with endosteal circumference in girls. The authors concluded that lean mass stimulated the development of cortical bone mass in a similar way in boys and girls, while fat mass was a stronger stimulus only in girls [62]. The difficulty in differentiating the relative contributions of lean and fat mass to the BMD values was confirmed in adult women also (see Table 6.1) [63].

Physical activity is a crucial activator of skeletal modeling and remodeling. The effect of physical activity early in life was tested at ages 5, 13, and 15 years in the Iowa Bone Development Study [64]. In boys, physical activity predicted later spine BMC, while this was not the case in girls. In another longitudinal study in boys, vigorous physical activity and sedentary time had a significant effect only on FN BMD [65]. The negative influence of sedentary time on bone mineral parameters was tested prospectively in peripubertal boys and was confirmed for all areas of interest (WB, LS, FN) with the strongest negative effect on FN BMD [66]. The type of sport or vigorous physical activity should also be kept in mind. The influence of different sports on bone mass was studied in girls [67]. In the pubertal group, arms BMD, pelvis BMD, and FN BMD were higher in soccer and handball players than in the control group, while swimmers had significantly higher values in the arms BMD. The authors recommended sport activities that support body weight as an important factor for achieving an optimal peak bone mass [67]. A meta-analysis of the effect of exercise on pediatric bone and fat revealed a small positive effect of bone-targeted exercise on WB, FN, LS BMC, and fat mass [68]. Another meta-analysis examined the effects of weight-bearing exercise in girls and found that these were site specific and affected primarily LS BMD, while BMC was increased at both LS and FN [69]. The authors also noted that physical activity for more than 3 days per week resulted in significantly greater values [69]. All these studies support the beneficial effect of exercise on bone development and health. The importance of mechanical influences for bone development in children has led to the formulation of a "mechanostat paradigm" [70].

Nutrition is another important aspect for optimal bone health. International and national agencies have adopted recommendations for optimal daily calcium and vitamin D intake at different ages. An epidemiological study in women aged 20–49 years revealed that milk consumption during childhood and adolescence was correlated with bone density and fracture risk later in life [71]. The positive association of calcium intake with bone mass was displayed in another study in adolescents [72]. The effect of calcium supplementation was more pronounced in cortical-rich (radius and femur) than in trabecular-rich bone (LS) [72]. An interventional study in 8-year-old prepubertal girls showed an increase in bone mass by 0.25 standard deviations only in those with very low-calcium intake at baseline [73]. A more recent study examined the interaction of low-calcium diet and low 25(OH)D levels in late-pubertal girls and found that LS BMC and BMD were not associated with 25(OH)D, except when calcium intake was below 600 mg/day [74]. The response to calcium intake interacts also with physical activity: the higher the calcium intake, the more pronounced is the effect of physical activity on bone growth [75, 76]. In two other studies (a cross-sectional and longitudinal one) the effect of physical activity on WB BMC accrual varied only among Tanner stages after adjustment for calcium intake [77, 78]. The positive interaction of high-protein intake and physical activity on bone strength and microstructure from prepuberty to mid-to-late adolescence was shown in a study using hr-pQCT of the tibia [79]. Bone mass accrual might be influenced also by harmful habits, such as early initiation of smoking and alcohol drinking, as shown in a cohort study in late adolescent girls [80].

Puberty is one of the main driving forces of bone development. The timing of puberty was shown to be inversely associated with peak bone mass, e.g., individuals with late puberty had lower bone mass in young adulthood [81, 82]. In Tanner stage 5, height growth was found to exert a more pronounced effect on bone accrual than at puberty start [81, 82]. It is intuitive to make the assumption that puberty acts on bone through a variety of mechanisms, among which the hormonal ones play a leading role [83, 84]. However, it is very difficult to dissect (discern) the relative contribution of every single hormone or factor. BMD, bone markers, and gonadal steroids were studied in girls and boys in different pubertal stages [85]. BMD significantly increased until Tanner stage 4 in girls, while in boys at Tanner stage 4, it was higher than in all other pubertal stages. There was a modest correlation of BMD with testosterone (T) and estrogen (E) in boys and only with estrogen in girls. Bone alkaline phosphatase was a better predictor of bone mass in girls than in boys [85]. In another study, estradiol was the most significant determinant of bone mass only during mid-puberty and not before that [61]. A similar result was obtained in boys with constitutional delay of growth and puberty [86]. In this study, the strongest correlation coefficients were found between BMD and serum estradiol levels among hormones, with estradiol being the most potent determinant in pubertal boys. Puberty also interacts with the influence of physical activity on bone. A meta-analysis found gains in BMC due to exercise only in prepubertal subjects [87]. The efficacy of training in terms of bone mineral accrual was substantially affected only by the maturational status of the participants [87].

At the cellular level, it is well known that testosterone and estradiol are very potent stimulators of bone formation, and this knowledge will not be further discussed into detail. Testosterone exerts its effect on bone cells in boys mainly through conversion to estradiol, with its direct actions being more important for the muscle growth and development. A steep rise in testosterone levels in boys and girls was shown to precede the pubertal increase in bone mass [85]. A relationship between polymorphisms of the aromatase gene and BMD was described in young men [88]. The role of androgens for the stimulation of muscle growth, independent of other hormones such as IGF-1, was summarized in reviews by Vanderschueren et al. (2004) and de Oliveira et al. (2012), while the actions of estrogens were described in the review by Clarke et al. (2010) [22, 23, 89]. The role of androgen aromatization was further emphasized in a randomized trial of the nonaromatizable androgen dihydrotestosterone (DHT) in healthy adult men [90]. In this study, DHT treatment suppressed serum testosterone resulting in bone loss at the lumbar spine as no estradiol was formed [90].

Another hormonal group, well known for its leading role in the development of the muscle–bone unit, comprises growth hormone (GH) and IGF-1. GH can stimulate longitudinal bone growth and increase the effect of physical stress on bone formation [91]. At the cellular level, it stimulates bone formation on endosteal and subperiosteal surfaces. For many years it has been thought that GH exerts its effect on bone mainly through IGF-1 [1]. IGF-1 is involved in direct actions on growth plate chondrocytes and osteogenic cells, building the cortical and trabecular bone. IGF-1 can modulate the production of 1,25$(OH)_2$-vitamin D and the transport system of inorganic phosphate [1]. A recent study has shown, however, that growth hormone can mediate pubertal skeletal development separately from hepatic IGF-1 production [92]. In this study, liver-specific IGF-1-deficient mice were treated with pegvisomant (a GH antagonist), separating the role of GH from IGF-1, whose production by the liver was basically reduced. The amount of cortical tissue formed in the treated mice was substantially lower, showing an independent contribution of GH to the effects of the GH–IGF-1 axis [92]. The strength of the association of IGF-1 versus 25(OH)D with BMC accrual was tested in prepubertal females followed up for a period of up to 9 years [93]. IGF-1 was more strongly associated with BMC accrual than vitamin D at the total body, proximal femur, radius, and lumbar spine. In multistep regression analysis, 25(OH)D did not have a predictive effect on BMC accrual beyond that of IGF-1 [93]. The expression of IGF-1 and its contribution to bone acquisition in mice have been related to the presence of thyroid hormones [94]. Other insulin-like growth factors may also contribute to the acquisition and maintenance of bone mass. In an experimental study, mutations in the insulin-like factor 3 receptor were associated with decreased bone mass in both mice and men (by dual X-ray bone densitometry), as well as with reduced mineralizing surface, bone formation, and osteoclast surface in mice (dynamic histomorphometric and micro-CT analyses) [95].

Adiponectin and leptin are among the other hormones that were studied for their associations with bone growth. The association of adiponectin with bone mass was studied by using DXA and pQCT in the Avon Longitudinal Study of Parents and Children [96]. Adiponectin was found to be inversely related with DXA-derived bone parameters (BMC, bone area) as well as with endosteal relative to periosteal expansion (from pQCT) resulting in increased cortical thickness [96]. The associations of leptin with tibial speed of sound (tSoS) were tested in early and late-pubertal girls [97]. In this study, adiposity and leptin were both negative predictors of tSoS, with leptin being specifically predictive in the postmenarcheal group [97]. Osteosclerostin levels were also studied in relation to bone development during childhood. They were measured in 6–21-year-old girls and boys and related to trabecular and cortical bone microarchitectural parameters using hr-pQCT [98]. Serum sclerostin levels were higher in boys as compared to girls and declined in both sexes following the onset of puberty. The authors found no consistent relationship between sclerostin levels and trabecular bone parameters in either sex, in contrast with an inverse association with cortical vBMD and cortical thickness in girls and a positive one with the cortical porosity index in both girls and boys [98].

In conclusion, bone development during childhood and adolescence is under the influence of so many hormonal factors, whose actions cannot always be differentiated from one another. On the other hand, bone itself may act as an independent endocrine organ, modulating the insulin resistance and secretion, gonadal function, and others [99, 100]. It should also be noted that the pubertal growth spurt is an event typical for the human species, which cannot be fully reproduced in animal models. Different hypotheses explaining that observation have been proposed, but the evolutionary meaning of these particular time events is not fully understood.

The Use of Bone Age (BA) in Clinical Practice

Skeletal development and maturity have been traditionally studied by the use of bone age (BA) based on hand and wrist radiographs. Two methods are most widely used: the Greulich and Pyle atlas and the Tanner–Whitehouse method [101]. The former is based on comparisons with reference images while the latter—on scores applied to the maturity indicators. At the end of the 1980s, another method was developed—the FELS method [102]. There are many good editions depicting those and other methods for BA assessment [103]. The inter- and intra-observer variability of BA assessment has been a major concern for many years. A recent study in four ethnicities from Los Angeles found a mean standard error of 0.45 years, which is slightly better than the figures reported by older studies [104]. This error might seem significant from a scientific point of view, but is negligible in everyday clinical practice. In recent years, the use of automatic BA assessment has gained more and more followers. For instance, a fully automated computer-based system, which was the first to be introduced in Europe, was the BoneXpert (Visiana, Denmark) [105]. The advantage of this system is the practical lack of variance between readings.

BA is used as the main indicator of skeletal maturity and is routinely compared to chronological age. However, bone mineral accrual and muscle development, height velocity, and others might better correlate with BA than just chronological age. BA is used in a variety of clinical situations [106, 107]. In precocious puberty BA is a part of the routine work-up and is performed at regular intervals thereafter. It is very useful in decisions regarding treatment. BA is assessed also in cases of premature adrenarche. A recent study found that bone age advancement by 2 or more years is common in children with premature adrenarche and is generally benign [108]. BA is also used in children with unknown chronological age, as well as in delayed puberty. In delayed puberty, BA can help to differentiate between reversible and permanent hypogonadism. Children with skeletal dysplasia remain a difficult population in BA assessment. The hand and wrist radiographs might also be used for other diagnostic purposes, such as in rickets, hypothyroidism, hypochondroplasia, and many others as well as in sports medicine.

Comparisons of different cohorts by the use of BA provided information on secular trends in skeletal maturity. A 35-year difference between the years of birth (1930–1964 versus 1965–2001) resulted in more advanced skeletal maturity (maximum difference of 5 months at age 13 years for girls and 4 months at age 15 years for boys) [109].

Conclusions

Bone development during childhood and adolescence is a very complex process. This complexity mirrors the important evolutionary and biological role of the skeleton. There is a long way to go to the full understanding of all processes implicated in bone growth and development.

References

1. Bonjour J-P, Chevalley T, Ferrari S, Rizzoli R. Bone and its characteristics during childhood and adolescence up to peak bone mass. In: Roux C, editor. The living skeleton. Wolters Kluwer Health/Les Laboratories Servier; Rueuil Malmaison, 2007. pp. 1–26.
2. Maes C, Kronenberg HM. Bone development and remodeling. In: Potts JT Jr, volume editor, Endocrinology: adult and pediatric. 6th ed. The parathyroid gland and bone metabolism. Philadelphia: Elsevier Saunders; 2013. pp. e72–e96.
3. Provot S, Schipani E, Wu JY, Kronenberg H. Development of the skeleton. In: Marcus R, Feldman D, Dempster DW, Lucky M, Cauley JA, editors. Osteoporosis. 4th ed. Elsevier/Academic Press; Oxford, 2013. pp. 97–126.
4. Rauch F. The dynamics of bone structure development during pubertal growth. J Musculoskeletal Neuronal Interact. 2012;12(1):1–6.
5. Emons J, Chagin AS, Sävendahl L, Karperien M, Wit JM. Mechanisms of growth plate maturation and epiphyseal fusion. Horm Res Paediatr. 2011;75(6):383–91.
6. Yoon BS, Pogue R, Ovchinnikov DA, Yoshii I, Mishina Y, Behringer RR, et al. BMPs regulate multiple aspects of growth-plate chondrogenesis through opposing actions on FGF pathways. Development. 2006;133(23):4667–78.

7. Liu Z, Xu J, Colvin JS, Ornitz DM. Coordination of chondrogenesis and osteogenesis by fibroblast growth factor 18. Genes Dev. 2002;16(7):859–69.
8. Hung IH, Yu K, Lavine KJ, Ornitz DM. FGF-9 regulates early hypertrophic chondrocyte differentiation and skeletal vascularization in the developing stylopod. Dev Biol. 2007;307(2):300–13.
9. Pannier S, Mugniery E, Jonqoy A, Benoist-Lasselin C, Odent T, Jais JP, et al. Delayed bone age due to a dual effect of FGFR3 mutation in achondroplasia. Bone. 2010;47(5):905–15.
10. Toydemir RM, Brassington AE, Barak-Toydemir P, Krakowiak PA, Jorde LB, Whitby FG, et al. A novel mutation in FGFR3 causes camptodactyly, tall stature and hearing loss (CATSHL) syndrome. Am J Hum Genet. 2006;79(5):935–41.
11. Day TF, Day BS, Yang Y. Wnt and hedgehog signaling pathways in bone development. J Bone Joint Surg Am. 2008;90 Suppl 1:19–24.
12. Emons J, Chagin AS, Malmlöf T, Lekman M, Tivesten A, Ohlsson C, et al. Expression of vascular endothelial growth factor in the growth plate is stimulated by estradiol and increases during pubertal development. J Endocrinol. 2010;205(1):61–8. doi:10.1677/JOE-09-0337.
13. Kobayashi T, Chung UI, Schipani E, Starbuck M, Karsenty G, Katagiri T, et al. PTHrp and Indian hedgehog control differentiation of growth plate chondrocytes at multiple steps. Development. 2002;129(12):2977–86.
14. Hellemans J, Coucke PJ, Giedion A, De Paepe A, Kramer P, Beemer F, et al. Homozygous mutations in IHH cause acrocapitofemoral dysplasia, an autosomal recessive disorder with cone-shaped epiphyses in hands and hips. Am J Hum Genet. 2003;72(4):1040–6.
15. Risom L, Christoffersen L, Daugaard-Jensen J, Hove HD, Andersen HS, Andresen BS, et al. Identification of six novel PTH1R mutations in families with a history of primary failure of tooth eruption. PLoS One. 2013;8(9), e74601.
16. Bastepe M, Raas-Rothschild A, Silver J, Weissman I, Wientroub S, Jüppner H, et al. A form of Jansen's metaphyseal chondrodysplasia with limited metabolic and skeletal abnormalities is caused by a novel activating parathyroid hormone (PTH)/PTH-related peptide receptor mutation. J Clin Endocrinol Metab. 2004;89(7):3595–600.
17. Idelevich A, Kerschnitzki M, Shahar R, Monsonego-Ornan E. 1,25$(OH)_2D_3$ alters growth plate maturation and bone architecture in young rats with normal renal function. PLoS One. 2011;6(6), e20772. doi:10.1371/journal.pone.0020772.
18. Stevens A, Hanson D, Whatmore A, Destenaves B, Chatelain P, Clayton P. Human growth is associated with distinct patterns of gene expression in evolutionarily conserved networks. BMC Genomics. 2013;14:547. doi:10.1186/1471-2164-14-547.
19. Börjesson AE, Windahl SH, Karimian E, Eriksson EE, Lagerquist MK, Engdahl C, et al. The role of estrogen receptor-α and its activation function-1 for growth plate closure in female mice. Am J Physiol Endocrinol Metab. 2012;302(11):E1381–9. doi:10.1152/ajpendo.00646.2011.
20. Börjesson AE, Lagerquist MK, Windahl SH, Ohlsson C. The role of estrogen receptor α in the regulation of bone and growth plate cartilage. Cell Mol Life Sci. 2013;70(21):4023–37. doi:10.1007/s00018-013-1317-1.
21. Börjesson AE, Lagerquist MK, Liu C, Shao R, Windahl SH, Karlsson C, et al. The role of estrogen receptor α in growth plate cartilage for longitudinal bone growth. J Bone Miner Res. 2010;25(12):2690–700. doi:10.1002/jbmr.156.
22. Vanderschueren D, Vandenput L, Boonen S, Lindberg MK, Bouillon R, Ohlsson C. Androgens and bone. Endocr Rev. 2004;25(3):389–425.
23. De Oliveira DH, Fighera TM, Bianchet LC, Kulak CA, Kulak J. Androgens and bone. Minerva Endocrinol. 2012;37(4):305–14.
24. Emons J, Chagin AS, Hultenby K, Zhivotovsky B, Wit JM, Karperien M, et al. Epiphyseal fusion in the human growth plate does not involve classical apoptosis. Pediatr Res. 2009;66(6):654–9. doi:10.1203/PDR.0b013e3181beaa8c.
25. De la Rica L, Rodríguez-Ubreva J, García M, Islam AB, Urquiza JM, Hernando H, et al. PU.1 target genes undergo Tet2-coupled demethylation and DNMT3b-mediated methylation in monocyte-to-osteoclast differentiation. Genome Biol. 2013;14(9):R99.

26. Kwon OH, Lee CK, Lee YI, Paik SG, Lee HJ. The hematopoietic transcription factor PU.1 regulates RANK gene expression in myeloid progenitors. Biochem Biophys Res Commun. 2005;335(2):437–46.
27. Stanley ER, Chitu V. CSF-1 receptor signaling in myeloid cells. Cold Spring Harb Perspect Biol. 2014;6(6):pii: a021857. doi:10.1101/cshperspect.a021857.
28. Leibbrandt A, Penninger JM. RANK(L) as a key target for controlling bone loss. Adv Exp Med Biol. 2009;647:130–45.
29. Schneeweis LA, Willard D, Milla ME. Functional dissection of osteoprotegerin and its interaction with receptor activator of NF-κB ligand. J Adv Exp Med Biol. 2009;647:130–45. doi:10.1007/978-0-387-89520-8_9.
30. Zhao H, Liu X, Zou H, Dai N, Yao L, Gao Q, et al. Osteoprotegerin induces podosome disassembly in osteoclasts through calcium, ERK, and p38 MAPK signaling pathways. Cytokine. 2015;71(2):199–206. doi:10.1016/j.cyto.2014.10.007.
31. Souza PP, Lerner UH. The role of cytokines in inflammatory bone loss. Immunol Invest. 2013;42(7):555–622. doi:10.3109/08820139.2013.822766.
32. Wang Y, Qin QH, Kalyanasundaram S. A theoretical model for simulating effect of parathyroid hormone on bone metabolism at cellular level. Mol Cell Biomech. 2009;6(2):101–12.
33. Takahashi N, Udagawa N, Suda T. Vitamin D endocrine system and osteoclasts. Bonekey Rep. 2014;3:495. doi:10.1038/bonekey.2013.229.
34. Sims NA, Vrahnas C. Regulation of cortical and trabecular bone mass by communication between osteoblasts, osteocytes and osteoclasts. Arch Biochem Biophys. 2014;561:22–8. doi:10.1016/j.abb.2014.05.015.
35. Luis Neyro J, Jesús Cancelo M, Palacios S. Inhibition of RANK-L in the pathophysiology of osteoporosis. Clinical evidences of its use. Ginecol Obstet Mex. 2013;81(3):146–57.
36. Bonewald LF, Johnson ML. Osteocytes, mechanosensing and Wnt signaling. Bone. 2008;42(4):606–15. doi:10.1016/j.bone.2007.12.224.
37. Galli C, Passeri G, Macaluso GM. Osteocytes and WNT: the mechanical control of bone formation. J Dent Res. 2010;89(4):331–43. doi:10.1177/0022034510363963.
38. Kubota T, Michigami T, Ozono K. Wnt signaling in bone. Clin Pediatr Endocrinol. 2010;19(3):49–56. doi:10.1297/cpe.19.49.
39. Baron R, Kneissel M. WNT signaling in bone homeostasis and disease: from human mutations to treatments. Nat Med. 2013;19(2):179–92. doi:10.1038/nm.3074.
40. Yavropoulou MP, Xygonakis C, Lolou M, Karadimou F, Yovos JG. The sclerostin story: from human genetics to the development of novel anabolic treatment for osteoporosis. Hormones (Athens). 2014;13(4):323–37. doi:10.14310/horm.2002.1552.
41. Seeman E. Bone modeling and remodeling. Crit Rev Eukaryot Gene Expr. 2009;19(3):219–33.
42. Briot K, Kolta S, Fechtenbaum J, Said-Nahal R, Benhamou CL, Roux C. Increase in vertebral body size in postmenopausal women with osteoporosis. Bone. 2010;47(2):229–34. doi:10.1016/j.bone.2010.03.020.
43. Sims NA, Martin TJ. Coupling the activities of bone formation and resorption: a multitude of signals within the basic multicellular unit. Bonekey Rep. 2014;3:481. doi:10.1038/bonekey.2013.215.
44. Feng X, McDonald JM. Disorders of bone remodeling. Annu Rev Pathol. 2011;6:121–45. doi:10.1146/annurev-pathol-011110-130203.
45. Duan Y, Beck TJ, Wang X-F, Seeman E. Structural and biomechanical basis of sexual dimorphism in femoral neck fragility has its origins in growth and aging. J Bone Miner Res. 2003;18(10):1766–74.
46. Boyanov M, Popivanov P, Gentchev G. Assessment of forearm volumetric bone mineral density from standard areal densitometry data. J Clin Densitom. 2002;5(4):391–402.
47. Boyanov M, Popivanov P, Roux C. Separate assessment of forearm cortical and trabecular bone density from standard densitometry data. Ann Med. 2001;33(7):497–506.
48. Ausili E, Rigante D, Salvaggio E, Focarelli B, Rendeli C, Ansuini V, et al. Determinants of bone mineral density, bone mineral content, and body composition in a cohort of healthy

children: influence of sex, age, puberty, and physical activity. Rheumatol Int. 2012;32(9):2737–43. doi:10.1007/s00296-011-2059-8.
49. Weaver CM, McCabe LD, McCabe GP, Novotny R, Van Loan M, Going S, et al. Bone mineral and predictors of bone mass in white, Hispanic, and Asian early pubertal girls. Calcif Tissue Int. 2007;81(5):352–63.
50. Gracia-Marco L, Vicente-Rodríguez G, Valtueña J, Rey-López JP, Díaz Martínez AE, Mesana MI, et al. Bone mass and bone metabolism markers during adolescence: the HELENA Study. Horm Res Paediatr. 2010;74(5):339–50. doi:10.1159/000314965.
51. Magarey AM, Boulton TJ, Chatterton BE, Schultz C, Nordin BE, Cockington RA. Bone growth from 11 to 17 years: relationship to growth, gender and changes with pubertal status including timing of menarche. Acta Paediatr. 1999;88(2):139–46.
52. Leonard MB, Elmi A, Mostoufi-Moab S, Shults J, Burnham JM, Thayu M, et al. Effects of sex, race, and puberty on cortical bone and the functional muscle bone unit in children, adolescents, and young adults. J Clin Endocrinol Metab. 2010;95(4):1681–9. doi:10.1210/jc.2009-1913.
53. Nishiyama KK, Macdonald HM, Moore SA, Fung T, Boyd SK, McKay HA. Cortical porosity is higher in boys compared with girls at the distal radius and distal tibia during pubertal growth: an HR-pQCT study. J Bone Miner Res. 2012;27(2):273–82. doi:10.1002/jbmr.552.
54. Xu L, Nicholson P, Wang Q, Alén M, Cheng S. Bone and muscle development during puberty in girls: a seven-year longitudinal study. J Bone Miner Res. 2009;24(10):1693–8. doi:10.1359/jbmr.090405.
55. Naganathan V, Sambrook P. Gender differences in volumetric bone mineral density: a study of opposite-sex twins. Osteoporos Int. 2003;14(7):564–9.
56. Bonjour JP, Theintz G, Buchs B, Slosman D, Rizzoli R. Critical years and stages of puberty for spinal and femoral bone mass accumulation during adolescence. J Clin Endocrinol Metab. 1991;73(3):555–63.
57. Recker RR, Davies KM, Hinders SM, Heaney RP, Stegman MR, Kimmel DB. Bone gain in young adult women. JAMA. 1992;268(17):2403–8.
58. Nguyen TV, Maynard LM, Towne B, Roche AF, Wisemandle W, Li J. Sex differences in bone mass acquisition during growth. The Fels longitudinal study. J Clin Densitom. 2001;4(2):147–57.
59. Henry YM, Fatayerji D, Eastell R. Attainment of peak bone mass at the lumbar spine, femoral neck and radius in men and women relative contributions of bone size and volumetric bone mineral density. Osteoporos Int. 2004;15(4):263–73.
60. Ivuskans A, Lätt E, Mäestu J, Saar M, Purge P, Maasalu K, et al. Bone mineral density in 11–13-year-old boys: relative importance of the weight status and body composition factors. Rheumatol Int. 2013;33(7):1681–7. doi:10.1007/s00296-012-2612-0.
61. Csakvary V, Erhardt E, Vargha P, Oroszlan G, Bodecs T, Torok D, et al. Association of lean and fat body mass, bone biomarkers and gonadal steroids with bone mass during pre- and midpuberty. Horm Res Paediatr. 2012;78(4):203–11. doi:10.1159/000342335.
62. Sayers A, Tobias JH. Fat mass exerts a greater effect on cortical bone mass in girls than boys. J Clin Endocrinol Metab. 2010;95(2):699–706. doi:10.1210/jc.2009-1907.
63. Boyanov M. Body fat, lean mass and bone density of the spine and forearm in women. Cent Eur J Med. 2014;9(1):121–5. doi:10.2478/s11536-013-0259-1.
64. Francis SL, Letuchy EM, Levy SM, Janz KF. Sustained effects of physical activity on bone health: Iowa Bone Development Study. Bone. 2014;63:95–100. doi:10.1016/j.bone.2014.03.004.
65. Vaitkeviciute D, Lätt E, Mäestu J, Jürimäe T, Saar M, Purge P, Maasalu K, Jürimäe J. Physical activity and bone mineral accrual in boys with different body mass parameters during puberty: a longitudinal study. PLoS One. 2014;9(10), e107759. doi:10.1371/journal.pone.0107759.
66. Ivuškāns A, Mäestu J, Jürimäe T, Lätt E, Purge P, Saar M. Sedentary time has a negative influence on bone mineral parameters in peripubertal boys: a 1-year prospective study. J Bone Miner Metab. 2015;33(1):85–92. doi:10.1007/s00774-013-0556-4.
67. Ubago-Guisado E, Gómez-Cabello A, Sánchez-Sánchez J, García-Unanue J, Gallardo L. Influence of different sports on bone mass in growing girls. J Sports Sci. 2015;21:1–9.
68. Nogueira RC, Weeks BK, Beck BR. Exercise to improve pediatric bone and fat: a systematic review and meta-analysis. Med Sci Sports Exerc. 2014;46(3):610–21. doi:10.1249/MSS.0b013e3182a6ab0d.

69. Ishikawa S, Kim Y, Kang M, Morgan DW. Effects of weight-bearing exercise on bone health in girls: a meta-analysis. Sports Med. 2013;43(9):875–92. doi:10.1007/s40279-013-0060-y.
70. Schoenau E, Fricke O. Mechanical influences on bone development in children. Eur J Endocrinol. 2008;159 Suppl 1:S27–31. doi:10.1530/EJE-08-0312.
71. Kalkwarf KJ, Khoury JC, Lanphear BP. Milk intake during childhood and adolescence, adult bone density and osteoporotic fractures in US women. Am J Clin Nutr. 2003;77(1):257–65.
72. Wosje KS, Specker BL. Role of calcium in bone health during childhood. Nutr Rev. 2000;58(9):253–68.
73. Bonjour JP, Carrie AL, Ferrari S, Clavien H, Slosman D, Theintz G, et al. Calcium-enriched foods and bone mass growth in prepubertal girls: a randomized, double-blind, placebo-controlled trial. J Clin Invest. 1997;99(6):1287–94.
74. Esterle L, Nguyen M, Walrant-Debray O, Sabatier JP, Garabedian M. Adverse interaction of low-calcium diet and low 25(OH)D levels on lumbar spine mineralization in late-pubertal girls. J Bone Miner Res. 2010;25(11):2392–8. doi:10.1002/jbmr.134.
75. Specker B, Binkley T. Randomized trial of physical activity and calcium supplementation on bone mineral content in 3- to 5-year old children. J Bone Miner Res. 2003;18(5):885–92.
76. Iuliano-Burns S, Saxon L, Naughton G, Gibbons K, Bass SL. Regional specificity of calcium and exercise during skeletal growth in girls: a randomized controlled trial. J Bone Miner Res. 2003;18(1):156–62.
77. Dogan M, Derman O, Oksüz-Kanbur N, Akgül S, Kutluk T. The effects of nutrition and physical activity on bone development in male adolescents. Turk J Pediatr. 2009;51(6):545–50.
78. Lappe JM, Watson P, Gilsanz V, Hangartner T, Kalkwarf HJ, Oberfield S, et al. The longitudinal effects of physical activity and dietary calcium on bone mass accrual across stages of pubertal development. J Bone Miner Res. 2015;30(1):156–64. doi:10.1002/jbmr.2319.
79. Chevalley T, Bonjour JP, van Rietbergen B, Ferrari S, Rizzoli R. Tracking of environmental determinants of bone structure and strength development in healthy boys: an eight-year follow up study on the positive interaction between physical activity and protein intake from prepuberty to mid-late adolescence. J Bone Miner Res. 2014;29(10):2182–92. doi:10.1002/jbmr.2247.
80. Lucas R, Fraga S, Ramos E, Barros H. Early initiation of smoking and alcohol drinking as a predictor of lower forearm bone mineral density in late adolescence: a cohort study in girls. PLoS One. 2012;7(10), e46940. doi:10.1371/journal.pone.0046940.
81. Zemel B. Bone mineral accretion and its relationship to growth, sexual maturation and body composition during childhood and adolescence. World Rev Nutr Diet. 2013;106:39–45. doi:10.1159/000342601.
82. Gilsanz V, Chalfant J, Kalkwarf H, Zemel B, Lappe J, Oberfield S, et al. Age at onset of puberty predicts bone mass in young adulthood. J Pediatr. 2011;158(1):100–105.e2. doi:10.1016/j.jpeds.2010.06.054.
83. Schoenau E. Bone mass increase in puberty: what makes it happen? Horm Res. 2006;65 Suppl 2:2–10.
84. Pérez-López FR, Chedraui P, Cuadros-López JL. Bone mass gain during puberty and adolescence: deconstructing gender characteristics. Curr Med Chem. 2010;17(5):453–66.
85. Yilmaz D, Ersoy B, Bilgin E, Gümüşer G, Onur E, Pinar ED. Bone mineral density in girls and boys at different pubertal stages: relation with gonadal steroids, bone formation markers, and growth parameters. J Bone Miner Metab. 2005;23(6):476–82.
86. Doneray H, Orbak Z. Association between anthropometric hormonal measurements and bone mineral density in puberty and constitutional delay of growth and puberty. West Indian Med J. 2010;59(2):125–30.
87. Behringer M, Gruetzner S, McCourt M, Mester J. Effects of weight-bearing activities on bone mineral content and density in children and adolescents: a meta-analysis. J Bone Miner Res. 2014;29(2):467–78. doi:10.1002/jbmr.2036.
88. Riancho JA. Polymorphisms in the CYP19 gene that influence bone mineral density. Pharmacogenomics. 2007;8(4):339–52.
89. Clarke BL, Khosla S. Female reproductive system and bone. Arch Biochem Biophys. 2010;503(1):118–28.

90. Sartorius GA, Ly LP, Handelsman DJ. Male sexual function can be maintained without aromatization: randomized placebo-controlled trial of dihydrotestosterone (DHT) in healthy, older men for 24 months. J Sex Med. 2014;11(10):2562–70.
91. Forwood MR, Li L, Kelly WL, Bennet MB. Growth hormone is permissive for skeletal adaptation to mechanical loading. J Bone Miner Res. 2001;16(12):2284–90.
92. Courtland H-W, Sun H, Beth-On M, Wu Y, Elis S, Rosen CJ, et al. Growth hormone mediates pubertal skeletal development independent of hepatic IGF-1 production. J Bone Miner Res. 2011;26(4):761–8. doi:10.1002/jbmr.265.
93. Breen ME, Laing EM, Hall DB, Hausman DB, Taylor RG, Isales CM, Ding KH, Pollock NK, Hamrick MW, Baile CA, Lewis RD. 25-hydroxyvitamin D, insulin-like growth factor-I, and bone mineral accrual during growth. J Clin Endocrinol Metab. 2011;96(1):E89–98. doi:10.1210/jc.2010-0595.
94. Xing W, Govoni KE, Donahue LR, Kesavan C, Wergedal J, Long C, Bassett JH, Gogakos A, Wojcicka A, Williams GR, Mohan S. Genetic evidence that thyroid hormone is indispensable for prepubertal insulin-like growth factor-I expression and bone acquisition in mice. J Bone Miner Res. 2012;27(5):1067–79. doi:10.1002/jbmr.1551.
95. Ferlin A, Pepe A, Gianesello L, Garolla A, Feng S, Giannini S, et al. Mutations in the insulin-like factor 3 receptor are associated with osteoporosis. J Bone Miner Res. 2008;23(5):683–93.
96. Sayers A, Timpson NJ, Sattar N, Deanfield J, Hingorani AD, Davey-Smith G, et al. Adiponectin and its association with bone mass accrual in childhood. J Bone Miner Res. 2010;25(10):2212–20. doi:10.1002/jbmr.116.
97. Klentrou P, Ludwa IA, Falk B. Factors associated with bone turnover and speed of sound in early and late-pubertal females. Appl Physiol Nutr Metab. 2011;36(5):707–14. doi:10.1139/h11-085.
98. Kirmani S, Amin S, McCready LK, Atkinson EJ, Melton III LJ, Müller R, et al. Sclerostin levels during growth in children. Osteoporos Int. 2012;23(3):1123–30. doi:10.1007/s00198-011-1669-z.
99. Guntur AR, Rosen CJ. Bone as an endocrine organ. Endocr Pract. 2012;18(5):758–62.
100. Zofkova I. Bone tissue as a systemic endocrine regulator. Physiol Res. 2014;3 [Epub ahead of print].
101. Martin DD, Wit JM, Hochberg Z, Sävendahl L, van Rijn RR, Fricke O, Cameron N, Caliebe J, Hertel T, Kiepe D, Albertsson-Wikland K, Thodberg HH, Binder G, Ranke MB. The use of bone age in clinical practice: part 1. Horm Res Paediatr. 2011;76(1):1–9.
102. De Sanctis V, Di Maio S, Soliman AT, Raiola G, Elalaily R, Millimaggi G. Hand X-ray in pediatric endocrinology: Skeletal age assessment and beyond. Indian J Endocrinol Metab. 2014;18 Suppl 1:S63–71.
103. Gilsanz V, Ratib O. Hand bone age. A digital atlas of skeletal maturity. 2nd ed. Berlin: Springer; 2012.
104. Thodberg HH, Sävendahl L. Validation and reference values of automated bone age determination for four ethnicities. Acad Radiol. 2010;17(11):1425–32. doi:10.1016/j.acra.2010.06.007.
105. Thodberg HH, Kreiborg S, Juul A, Pedersen KD. The BoneXpert method for automated determination of skeletal maturity. IEEE Trans Med Imaging. 2009;28(1):52–66.
106. Martin DD, Wit JM, Hochberg Z, van Rijn RR, Fricke O, Werther G, Cameron N, Hertel T, Wudy SA, Butler G, Thodberg HH, Binder G, Ranke MB. The use of bone age in clinical practice: part 2. Horm Res Paediatr. 2011;76(1):10–6.
107. Lazar L, Phillip M. Pubertal disorders and bone maturation. Endocrinol Metab Clin North Am. 2012;41(4):805–25.
108. DeSalvo DJ, Mehra R, Vaidyanathan P, Kaplowitz PB. In children with premature adrenarche, bone age advancement by 2 or more years is common and generally benign. J Pediatr Endocrinol Metab. 2013;26(3-4):215–21. doi:10.1515/jpem-2012-0283.
109. Duren DL, Nahhas RW, Sherwood RJ. Do secular trends in skeletal maturity occur equally in both sexes? Clin Orthop Relat Res. 2015;473:2559–67.

Chapter 7
Body Weight and Puberty

Analia Tomova

Introduction

In mammals, reproduction is acutely regulated by metabolic status [1]. The body weight is an important factor that influences on the initiation and progression of puberty. In the childhood the overweight as well as the underweight could influence the development of puberty. In recent years excessive food consumption and sedentary behavior in developed societies are the cause of overweight and obesity. The lower intake of food and increased physical activity induce unfavorable energy balance and underweight, which also may disturb the sexual function.

Globally, about 10 % of school-age children are obese or overweight, and this percentage is highest in the USA (32 %), followed by Europe (20 %) and the Middle East (16 %) [2]. The worldwide prevalence of childhood obesity increased from 4.2 to 6.7 % between 1990 and 2010 [3].

In the USA, the 85th and 95th percentiles of body mass index (BMI) for age and sex based on nationally representative survey data have been recommended as cut-off points to identify overweight and obesity, respectively, which are the same as those, proposed by the Expert Committee [4].

In most publications, the underweight is defined within different limits: 5th or 15th percentile of BMI for given age. According to World Health Organization's cutoff points, BMI of 18.5 kg/m^2 in young adults is equivalent to the 12th percentile in children [5].

Unfortunately, the data on children with underweight and its effect on sexual development are scarce. But underweight can negatively affect both the onset and progression of puberty, and also the reproductive capacity later in adulthood, especially in girls. The publications on this subject are mainly related to patients with anorexia nervosa.

A. Tomova (✉)
Clinical Center of Endocrinology, Medical Faculty, Medical University of Sofia,
2, Zdrave Street, 1431 Sofia, Bulgaria
e-mail: a.kirilova@lycos.com

P. Kumanov, A. Agarwal (eds.), *Puberty*, DOI 10.1007/978-3-319-32122-6_7

Pubertal maturation consists of two associated processes: adrenarche, the increase of adrenal androgen production, and gonadarche, the pubertal reactivation of hypothalamic-pituitary-gonadal (HPG) axis. The development of breast tissue in girls (thelarche) and testicular growth in boys are signs of the onset of puberty. Typically, adrenarche occurs before gonadarche. Some authors believe that adrenal androgens may be one of the factors necessary for the reactivation of the hypothalamic-pituitary-gonadal axis [6].

The severity of the disturbances in sexual sphere depends on the degree of the variations in body weight as more severe deviations in body weight cause more prominent abnormalities in sexual function.

Body Weight and Puberty in Girls

The adiposity in early childhood is probably linked to advanced puberty in girls [7, 8]. It is generally accepted that overweight and obesity are related with early appearance of menarche [7, 9]. Multiple studies from several continents have demonstrated that levels of childhood obesity in girls are associated with earlier onset of puberty or menarche: in the USA [10–14], in South America [3], in Europe [15, 16], and in Asia [17]. Nevertheless there are some authors who suggested that the population-level shifts in BMI and the timing of menarche are largely independent processes, although sometimes they coincide [18].

Data from several epidemiological studies in the past 30 years present a link between the earlier onset of puberty in girls and increased BMI, which is the most available method for indirectly determining body fat stores [19]. Girls with greater BMI reach breast stage 2 at younger ages. Higher BMI is the strongest predictor of earlier age at breast stage 2 in the study of Biro et al. [14]. Pubertal signs occur before 8.0 years of age in <5 % of the normal BMI female population in the USA [20]. Breast and sexual pubic hair developments are premature before 8 years of age in girls with normal BMI in general population. Girls with excessive BMI have significantly higher prevalence of breast appearance from ages 8.0–9.6 years and pubarche from ages 8.0–10.2 years than those with normal BMI [20]. Menarche is also significantly more likely to occur in preteen girls with an elevated BMI [20]. A study in Denmark found that early-matured girls had higher BMI, but similar body fat percentage, compared with late-matured similarly aged girls [21]. Results of a study in Brazil indicate that early sexual maturation is associated with a higher prevalence of excessive body weight in girls. Compared to the reference group (normal sexual maturation), early-maturing females have higher prevalence of excess body weight and increased height for age [3]. Lee et al. found a strong association between elevated body weight at all ages and the early onset of puberty as determined by breast development and the onset of menstruation [13]. Fat mass at age 8 years is strongly associated with stage and onset of puberty in both sexes. However, by age 11 year, lean mass accretion is more closely associated with more advanced puberty [22]. Four-year longitudinal study in China demonstrated that childhood obesity contributes to an earlier onset of puberty, and the mean estradiol concentration is higher in obese girls in comparison to normal or underweight girls during this period [17].

The increased incidence of childhood obesity in recent decades may be responsible for dramatic increase in early puberty in girls. From the late nineteenth century, evidence from several European countries shows a decrease in the age of menarche—as a result of the earlier achievement of the required weight for the initiation of menarche [23]. The age of the onset of menses (menarche) declined in North America and Europe from age 17 years in the mid-nineteenth century to less than 14 years in the mid-twentieth century. In a study in Bulgaria, done by the beginning of twentieth century (1904–1906), the mean age of menarche was 15 years, while at the end of the century, it was 12 years [24]. Similar trends also occurred in the age of onset of breast development (thelarche) and pubic hair development (pubarche) [25]. Moreover, in recent years an inverse correlation of BMI was found with the age of onset of menarche [26, 27]. The nutrition in the postnatal period and rapid weight gain can predict the onset of earlier puberty [28, 29].

For the changes in reproductive axis in girls with underweight can be judged mainly on the studies done in adolescents with anorexia nervosa, where the considerable weight reduction causes delay in puberty or its discontinuation. This disease is associated with unfavorable changes in the reproductive axis—hypogonadotropic hypogonadism. The degree of weight loss is associated with the degree of hormonal disturbances in the gonadal axis. The basal levels of gonadotropins are lower, and the responses of luteinizing hormone (LH) to gonadotropin-releasing hormone (GnRH) are diminished, but those of follicle-stimulating hormone (FSH) are exaggerated. The basal levels of LH are significantly correlated with body weight, BMI, and percentage of weight loss [30]. The changes in the gonadal axis are due to disturbances in the hypothalamus, and all hormonal alterations are in relationship with the degree of weight loss. The severe weight loss is mainly associated with the reduced amount of adipose tissue and with considerably decreased leptin levels [31]. Several other hormones and mediators are implicated in this process and can send signals to the hypothalamus that influence on its activity.

Body Weight and Puberty in Boys

Data from studies on the influence of body weight (especially overweight and obesity) on the onset and development of the puberty in boys are controversial. In some studies male obesity was associated with delayed pubertal development [11, 32, 33], while in others earlier start of puberty in overweight boys was found [34, 35]. In a small study Laron has not observed any difference in pubertal development between boys with obesity and those with normal weight [8]. Some authors found that earlier sexual maturation in boys was associated with greater height for age [3, 36], but not with the weight. Others considered that in contrast to the girls, there was no evidence of an association between adiposity and pubarche in boys [20]. The analyses of National Health and Nutrition Examination Survey (NHANES) III data by Karpati et al. [37] and by Wang [11] suggested that overweight and obesity might result in delayed instead of advanced puberty in boys. However, these studies have some limitations as the authors evaluated the genital stages only visually, without measuring the testicular volumes and penis sizes. With these methods the data could be more difficult for interpretation, because of the subjective evaluation of early stages and subsequent physical progression through puberty. It is not possible to define exactly the pubertal events in boys without assessment of testicular volumes. Perhaps for this reason, the influence of body weight and BMI on sexual maturation in males has not been clarified for a long period of time.

A volume of 3 ml is considered the most reliable and valid marker of male pubertal onset generally accepted to date [38–40]. According to Tanner and Whitehouse [41], a mean testicular volume of 12 ml indicates that adolescent is proceeding toward the late stage of pubertal development.

Results from study of Tomova et al. [42], based on objective data obtained by determining testicular volume, found earlier enlargement of the testicular volume in overweight and obese boys as well as earlier pubertal maturation in comparison to normal-weight children. The increase in testicular volume begins initially in boys with obesity, but subsequently overweight children have the fastest pubertal development in comparison to these with obesity and those with normal weight. Delayed pubertal development was observed in underweight boys, who were clearly behind at every stage of puberty relative to the normal-weight children (Fig. 7.1). At the beginning of the puberty at the age of 11 years, the testicular volume of 3 ml has been found in 69.6 % of the boys with overweight and obesity, in 51.5 % of the boys with normal weight and only in 29.7 % in those who were underweight. The results concerning the late stage of puberty (testicular volume $\geq$12 ml) were similar. At the age 13 the percentage of the boys with overweight and obesity, who had testicular volume of 12 ml or more, was 43.5 %, whereas in the group of underweight children, it was only 2.70 %. An early increase of penis length as well as of penis circumference was found in overweight children, while a significant delay was observed in boys with underweight and obesity [42]. From this data it is clear that the boys with overweight and obesity start puberty development earlier and finished it faster in comparison to those who are underweight [42]. In all investigated groups, it has been established a positive significant correlation of the body weight and BMI with the indices of pubertal development: pubic hair, penis length, and circumference as well as with the volume of the testes. Moreover, according to this study, the onset of puberty is expected at a certain threshold of the body weight (40.17 ± 9.10 kg) (median 39.0 kg) [42].

Similar are the observations of Vizmanos and Martí-Henneberg [35] that reveal a positive relationship between BMI and the initiation of sexual development in boys as well as the findings of Juul et al. [43] of the association of prepubertal BMI

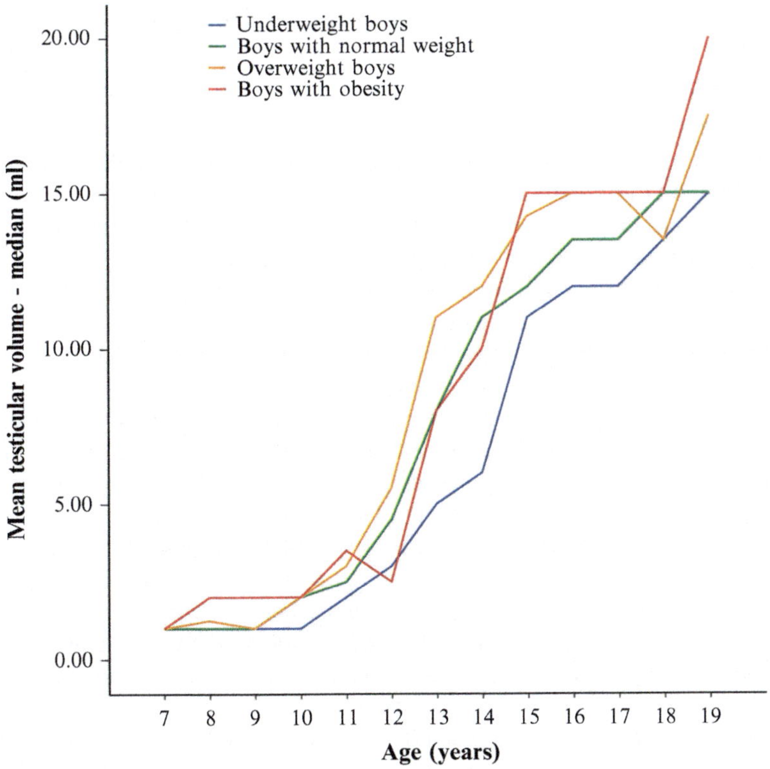

Fig. 7.1 Mean testicular volume (ml) in boys with underweight, normal weight, overweight, and obesity ($p > 0.05$ for age groups 7, 10, 18 years; $p < 0.05$ for age groups 8, 9, 15, 16, 17, 19; $p < 0.001$ for age groups 11, 12, 13, 14)

with earlier age at voice break. The other study in Denmark found that early-matured boys had higher BMI, but similar body fat percentage, compared with late-matured similarly aged boys [21]. Boyne et al. reported that fat mass at age of 8 was strongly associated with the stage and onset of puberty in both sexes. Birth size and growth through infancy and childhood were significantly associated with testicular size. Pooling both sexes together, growth in infancy, late infancy, and childhood is associated with more advanced puberty [22]. Supportive evidence was found also by Fu et al. [44], who observed an earlier activation of the inhibin B/follicle-stimulating hormone axis in boys with obesity during puberty. These authors found significantly greater testicular volume as well as advanced bone age and increased values of dehydroepiandrosterone and dehydroepiandrosterone sulfate (DHEAS) in obese prepubertal boys compared to age-matched controls [44]. Sørensen at al. reported that the mean age at onset of male puberty has declined significantly during period of 15 years, and this decline was associated with the coincident increase in BMI [45]. All these data support the hypothesis for a close relationship between body weight and maturation of the boys.

Links Between Body Weight and Puberty Development

Overweight and Obesity

According to many studies, there are clear associations between childhood obesity and earlier onset of puberty and pubertal development in both sexes.

Puberty is initiated in the late childhood through a cascade of endocrine changes that lead to sexual maturation and reproductive capability [7, 46]. It begins with increasing of GnRH secretion from the hypothalamus, which gains rhythmic, pulsatile character and in turn leads to release of gonadotropins, activation of gonadal axis, and beginning of the puberty. The gonadotropins regulate both steroidogenesis and gametogenesis. The large variability between individuals in the onset and progression of puberty indicates that the timing of puberty is not simply a function of chronological age. The neurotransmitter and neuromodulatory systems that impact upon the GnRH secretory network convey information about metabolic fuels, energy stores, and somatic development [47].

Growth and development are extremely complex processes that are regulated from many humoral and neural factors acting on the genetic basis. The secretion of GnRH is under the control of the so-called hypothalamic pulse generator which is located in the nucleus arcuatus [48, 49]. The physiological mechanisms that trigger activation of the hypothalamic-pituitary gonadal axis are still unknown, but attainment of a set point in growth, body composition, and energy balance seems important [40]. A lot of neurotransmitters, adipocytokines, and hormones, such as leptin, kisspeptin, neuropeptide Y, insulin, and opioids, which control food intake, also have a link to the release of GnRH.

Despite many human and animal studies, it is still unclear how the GnRH pulse generator manages to provoke the onset of puberty in both sexes. However, there are clear evidences that a critical amount of fat during the childhood is necessary to provoke revival of hypothalamic secretory function. Alwis et al. [50] reported that bone mass, lean body, and fat mass, measured by dual-energy X-ray absorptiometry, increased at a constant rate from age 6 until the puberty, when all these indexes showed a rapid increase in both sexes. Total lean body mass increased with 21.2 % in the boys and with 18.4 % in the girls at age 6 to 8 years, while the total amount of fat mass enhanced with 34.5 % in the boys and with 28.6 % in the girls [50]. During the growth spurt at the age of 7 years in both sexes, the rate of fat tissue accumulation was found to be at least 10 % greater than that of the lean mass [50].

After the initiation of this process neurotransmitter systems, which stimulate (neuropeptide Y and noradrenaline) and inhibit (opioids) the gonadal axis, are involve in the control of the GnRH release. During this period gonadal steroids also influence these mechanisms. For the initiation of the puberty, it is necessary to gain a certain "critical" body weight, which is a limiting factor for further processes. The probable messenger between adipose tissue and the nervous system seems to be leptin. There are numerous examples of the relationship between eating behavior, leptin, and sexual maturation. In light of these data, the proposed hypothesis from Frisch and Revelle for "critical body weight" in girls, according to which a certain minimum body weight or body fat percentage is required for appearance of menarche [51], acquires a completely modern vision.

The hypothalamic nucleus arcuatus is a crucial site for the regulation of both reproduction and metabolism. The arcuate nucleus contains proopiomelanocortin/cocaine- and amphetamine-regulated transcript (POMC/CART)-expressing neurons, whose activation suppresses feeding. In contrast, the activation of another population of arcuate neurons, neuropeptide Y/agouti-related protein (NPY/AgRP)-expressing neurons, stimulates feeding [52, 53]. Although much of the cellular and molecular mechanisms associated with the energy balance and reproduction, as well as sites in the brain that mediate these functions are not completely understood, it is well known that the reproductive axis has the ability to respond to changes in the metabolic state of the body.

There are several potential mechanisms by which body fat stores might influence onset of pubertal development as well as the progression of puberty. One is through the direct action of adipocytokines, such as leptin, signaling energy reserves as well as having other direct metabolic effects. In addition, aromatase activity is pronounced in adipose tissue, which increases androgen conversion to estrogens. Adipose tissue is also related to insulin resistance, which increases during puberty, thus lowering sex hormone-binding globulin (SHBG) levels and hence increasing bioavailability of sex steroids [54].

Adipose tissue should be considered as an endocrine organ. A wide range of different active products are released from it into blood stream. Some of them are synthesized de novo, while others are converted from already existing substances. All factors might act locally in auto-/paracrine manner or may exert metabolic, immunologic, and endocrine effects [55]. Through them the link between adipose tissue and hypothalamic-pituitary system is realized, which modulates the function of other endocrine glands. Some of these adipocytokines are actively involved in the function of the reproductive axis.

Leptin, an adipocyte-secreted hormone, is a metabolic factor that bridges the regulation of the fat mass with reproduction [56]. Its levels are elevated in individuals with overweight and obesity and decreased in persons with underweight. Moreover, leptin concentrations correlate with amount of fat mass, and for the timing of puberty, certain levels of this hormone are required [19]. Matkovic et al. found an inverse relation between menarche and serum leptin. An increase of 1 ng/mL in serum leptin level lowers the timing of menarche by 1 month, and a gain in body fat of 1 kg is associated with an earlier onset of menarche by approximately 13 days [57]. Sex differences are also observed in the concentrations of leptin, LH, and FSH before and during the puberty. In girls, a peak in leptin concentrations was observed at Tanner stage 2, followed by a peak in LH and FSH concentrations at Tanner stage 3. In boys, no peak in leptin levels was observed at Tanner stage 2, as leptin decreased from Tanner stage 2 onward and LH and FSH concentrations increased from Tanner stage 1–4 [58]. In girls leptin levels rise during the age, according to the changes in body weight, and this trend is maintained with age. In boys leptin concentrations are as a rule lower than in girls, but the pattern of gradual increase at an early age is similar. After 10 years of age, leptin levels decrease, and this could be coupled with a concomitant increase of testosterone [48, 59]. Testosterone inhibits differentiation of preadipocytes into mature adipocytes [60]. The net result of these androgen actions at multiple sites in the adipogenic processes is a reduction in fat mass [60]. Testosterone stimulates the weight gain through increased muscle mass but reduces the percentage of body fat, resulting in decrease levels of leptin. It is possible that in boys after the initial onset of puberty, this hormone is not more needed for the pubertal development. In girls, however, it is necessary that a certain threshold level of leptin to be maintained. Perhaps leptin signals the presence of a sufficient amount of adipose tissue, i.e., energy resources, that is necessary for the normal reproductive function [59]. In that regard, leptin may be a factor which allows the start of puberty. This thesis is supported by the fact that leptin is increased years before any other hormone associated with pubertal development [58].

The administration of leptin stimulates the growth of cells from cartilaginous tissue, which can result in epiphyseal cartilage growth in long bones [3]. Fat mass is an important determinant of bone density, and leptin acts directly on bone, influencing both osteoblasts and osteoclasts. The direct bone effects of leptin tend to reduce bone fragility and contribute to the high bone mass and low fracture rates of obesity [61]. Peripheral leptin is essential for normal bone resorption and enhances bone formation. The results indicate that leptin acting primarily through peripheral pathways increases osteoblast number and activity in mice [62].

The absence of signaling-competent leptin receptor expression on GnRH neurons strongly suggests that intermediary factor or pathway mediates the essential effects of leptin on activation of GnRH neurons [56]. The kisspeptin appears to play a role in reproductive effects of leptin. Kisspeptin stimulates the secretion of LH, after binding with the receptor GPR 54, which is located on the surface of the GnRH neurons. Inactivating gene mutations are associated with hypogonadotropic hypogonadism. In such patients, puberty does not occur. It is assumed that the system kisspeptin-GPR 54 is absolutely necessary to the activation of gonadotropin secretion in early sexual maturation and maintenance of reproductive function in adults [63–65]. It is believed that leptin stimulates expression of kisspeptin 1 (KISS-1) and thereby initiates the production of kisspeptin and subsequently stimulation of GnRH release [53]. Thus, the increased levels of leptin in obese and overweight children can be the cause of an earlier puberty start. Some authors consider that leptin serves as a metabolic signal for puberty to progress and appears to be a permissive factor rather than the trigger of the onset of puberty [66].

Discovered in 1999 galanin-like peptide (GALP) shows close structural similarity with galanin and specifically stimulates GnRH-mediated LH secretion. GALP-expressing cells are mainly found in the arcuate nucleus of the hypothalamus and the posterior pituitary, where they appear to be in contact with multiple neuromodulators, which are involved in the regulation of energy homeostasis and reproduction. GALP gene expression is regulated by several factors that reflect metabolic state including the metabolic hormones leptin and insulin, thyroid hormones, and blood glucose. Since the onset of puberty is so tightly regulated by metabolic status, it is possible that GALP plays a role in the onset of puberty [67].

Insulin is an important nutritional signal from periphery that may regulate the reproductive axis by direct effects on the GnRH neurons and specifically by stimulating GnRH gene expression [1]. Furthermore, there is clear evidence that insulin can act directly on the ovaries, since they have receptors for insulin and insulin-like growth factor (IGF) [68].

Children normally experience transient insulin resistance at puberty. Insulin resistance is increased immediately at the onset of puberty (Tanner 2) but returns to near prepubertal levels by the end of puberty (Tanner 5). The peak of insulin resistance occurs at Tanner 3 in both sexes, and girls are more insulin resistant than boys at all Tanner stages [69]. Insulin resistance is associated with compensatory hyperinsulinemia and decreased SHBG concentrations, which in turn causes increase in the bioavailability of sex steroids. In addition, hyperinsulinemia decreases hepatic production of SHBG. Insulin resistance is strongly related to BMI and waist circumference [69]. Obesity appears to be linked with marked insulin resistance, and the higher levels of insulin during this period may have more pronounced stimulatory effect on the reproductive axis. It may also increase the bioavailability of IGF-1, which is positively correlated to the level of obesity [70].

The increased amount of adipose tissue may play a crucial role also for the release of suprarenal androgens and consequently of adrenarche, which precedes the activation of gonadal axis. The role of adipocytes and their hormone leptin in the pubertal processes is shown in Fig. 7.2.

Other factor that has been implicated in the accelerated growth of obese children includes increased adipose tissue aromatization of androgens into estrogens [70]. Recently it was reported that maternal obesity before pregnancy may be related to earlier timing of pubertal milestones among sons [71]. The formula milk feeding may also have an impact on pubertal development, because it is more energy dense than breast milk, and this could explain the differences in rate of early weight gain between formula-fed and breastfed infants [29, 72]. Earlier beginning of artificial feeding of infants may be relevant to the earlier onset of puberty and to be a risk factor for childhood obesity. Exposure to other environmental agents such as phytoestrogens and endocrine disruptive chemicals can cause early pubertal development and early onset of menarche [54, 73].

Underweight

Underweight status may be related to genetic factors, acute or chronic undernutrition, or chronic diseases. It is a result of negative energy balance, which is most often due to reduced food intake, increased energy expenditure, or both together. Typically this occurs in patients with anorexia nervosa or in certain diseases which are associated with malnutrition. In recent years excessive exercise alone may be another cause of weight loss. Underweight status has been associated with higher rates of morbidity and mortality, although to a lesser extent that obesity.

Changes in reproductive axis in underweight children are poorly understood. The observations are mainly in patients with anorexia nervosa. Nutritional deprivation has a suppressive effect on gonadotropin secretion and gonads, regardless of its etiology. The main mechanism of gonadotropin suppression is inhibition of the

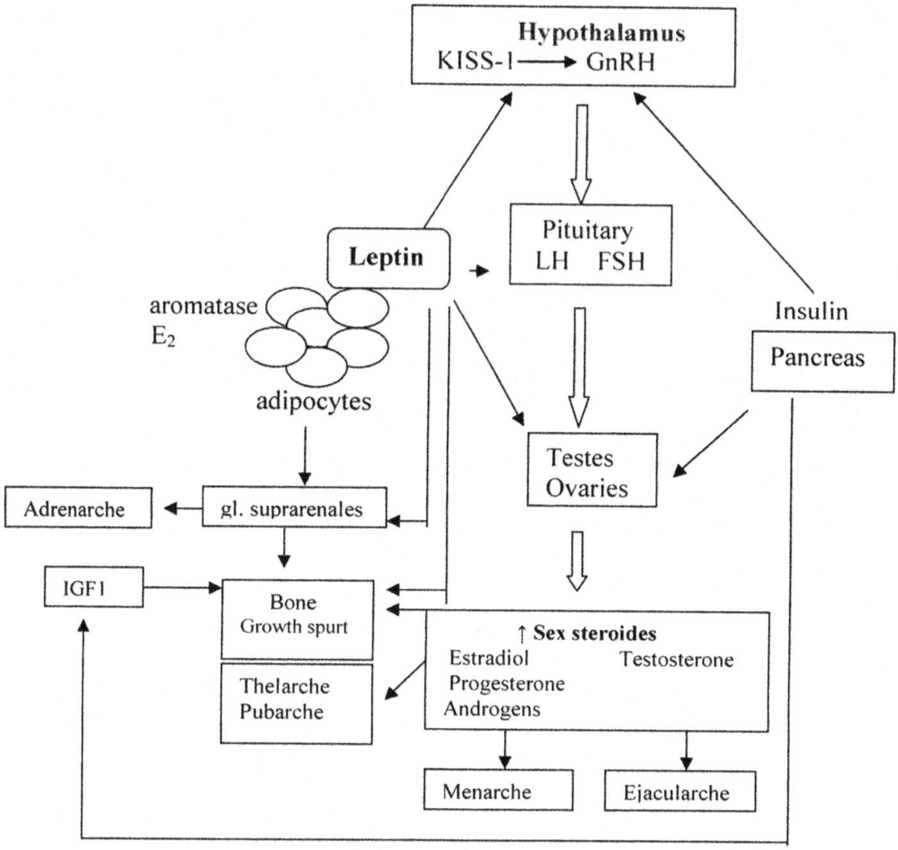

Fig. 7.2 The role of adipocytes and their hormone leptin in the pubertal processes

secretion of GnRH. Severe malnutrition leads to decreased levels of gonadotropins [30, 74], which can be increased with normalization of food imports, and this can cause a temporary increase in estrogen production [74] with the development of gynecomastia in boys (see Chap. 13). It is assumed that the decreased response of the pituitary is due to the dysfunction of the hypothalamus and the changes in the levels of certain neurotransmitters and neuropeptides. Also, some studies have found a decrease in insulin [75] and leptin [31, 74] levels and increase of SHBG concentrations [75], which may lead to disturbances in the function of gonadal axis in adolescents. Leptin stimulates the secretion of GnRH, and its lowering in conditions of negative energy balance leads to the diminish effect on the cells expressing GnRH. However, after a rise of leptin to physiological levels, its impact on GnRH is not recovered [76]. Other hormonal changes as increased levels of GH and cortisol are well described. The disturbances in patients with anorexia nervosa and malnutrition can be seen as adaptive mechanism in conditions of energy insufficiency. Increased cortisol levels intensify proteolysis in muscles to amino acids that are necessary for gluconeogenesis and for the synthesis of essential functional proteins in the liver. The increased GH on the background of reduced levels of IGF-1 does not have an anabolic effect and leads to cessation of the growth. However, lipolytic effect of GH is preserved. Gonadal axis in this extreme situation returns to prepubertal levels to keep the individual, and the reproductive function is discontinued.

Consequences of the Disturbances in Body Weight for the Pubertal Development

In girls as well as in boys, there is a positive relationship between body weight and the pubertal development. In the overweight children puberty begins and progresses earlier in comparison with the normal-weight individuals, whereas the underweight in adolescents is related to later onset and development of puberty. Early onset of puberty could have serious health and social consequences, such as increased rates of cancer in reproductive organs later in life and engagement in early sexual activity and alcohol use [34]. Overnutrition between 2 and 8 years of age will not be beneficial from a final height point of view, as the temporary increase in height gain in childhood will be compensated by an earlier maturity and subnormal height gain in adolescence. Each increased unit of BMI gained in childhood reduces the height gain in adolescence with 0.88 cm for boys and 0.51 cm for girls [77]. In recent years, the efforts have mainly focused on obesity prevention, since there is a greater risk for developing cardiovascular disease and diabetes in later life, but little attention is paid to underweight in children, which, especially in girls, can cause severe disturbances in function of gonadal axis and may affect the processes of reproduction. These data support the need of wide promotion activities regarding the optimal and healthy nutrition in children and regular physical activity.

References

1. Kim HH, DiVall SA, Deneau RM, Wolfe A. Insulin regulation of GnRH gene expression through MAP kinase signaling pathways. Mol Cell Endocrinol. 2005;242(1–2):42–9.
2. Reilly J. Obesity in childhood and adolescence: evidence based clinical and public health perspectives. Postgrad Med J. 2006;82:429–37.
3. Benedet J, da Silva Lopes A, Adami F, de Fragas Hinnig P, de Vasconcelos FA. Association of sexual maturation with excess body weight and height in children and adolescents. BMC Pediatr. 2014;14:72–8.
4. Barlow SE. Expert committee recommendations regarding the prevention, assessment, and treatment of child and adolescent overweight and obesity: summary report. Pediatrics. 2007;120 Suppl 4:S164–92.
5. Cole TJ, Bellizzi MC, Flegal KM, Dietz WH. Establishing a standard definition for child overweight and obesity worldwide: international survey. BMJ. 2000;320:1240–5.
6. Biro FM, Huang B, Daniels SR, Lucky AW. Pubarche as well as thelarche may be a marker for the onset of puberty. J Pediatr Adolesc Gynecol. 2008;21(6):323–8.

7. Burt Solorzano CM, McCartney CR. Obesity and the pubertal transition in girls and boys. Reproduction. 2010;140:399–410.
8. Laron Z. Is obesity associated with early sexual maturation? Pediatrics. 2004;113:171–2.
9. Styne DM. Puberty, obesity and ethnicity. Trends Endocrinol Metab. 2004;15(10):472–78.
10. Kaplowitz PB, Slora EJ, Wasserman RC, Pedlow SE, Herman-Giddens ME. Earlier onset of puberty in girls: relation to increased body mass index and race. Pediatrics. 2001;108(2):347–53.
11. Wang Y. Is obesity associated with early sexual maturation? A comparison of the association in American boys versus girls. Pediatrics. 2002;110:903–10.
12. Anderson SE, Dallal GE, Must A. Relative weight and race influence average age at menarche: results from two nationally representative surveys of US girls studied 25 years apart. Pediatrics. 2003;111(4 Pt 1):844–50.
13. Lee JM, Appugliese D, Kaciroti N, Corwyn RF, Bradley RH, Lumering JC. Weight status in young girls and the onset of puberty. Pediatrics. 2007;119(3):e624–30. Erratum in: Pediatrics 2007;120(1):251.
14. Biro FM, Greenspan LC, Galvez MP, Pinney SM, Teitelbaum S, Windham GC, et al. Onset of breast development in a longitudinal cohort. Pediatrics. 2013;132(5):1–9.
15. de Muinck Keizer-Schrama SMPF, Mul D. Trends in pubertal development in Europe. Hum Reprod Update. 2001;7(3):287–91.
16. Aksglaede L, Sørensen K, Petersen JH, Skakkebaek NE, Juul A. Recent decline in age at breast development: the Copenhagen Puberty Study. Pediatrics. 2009;123(5):e932–9.
17. Zhai L, Liu J, Zhao J, Liu J, Bai Y, Jia L, et al. Association of obesity with onset of puberty and sex hormones in Chinese girls: a 4-year longitudinal study. PLoS One. 2015;10(8), e0134656.
18. Demerath EW, Towne B, Chumlea WC, Sun SS, Czerwinski SA, Remsberg KE, et al. Recent decline in age at menarche: the Fels Longitudinal Study. Am J Hum Biol. 2004;16:453–7.
19. Kaplowitz PB. Link between body fat and the timing of puberty. Pediatrics. 2008;121 Suppl 3:S208–17.
20. Rosenfeld RL, Lipton RB, Drum ML. Thelarche, pubarche, and menarche attainment in children with normal and elevated body mass index. Pediatrics. 2009;123(1):84–8. Erratum in: Pediatrics. 2009;123(4):1255.
21. Sørensen K, Juul A. BMI percentile-for-age overestimates adiposity in early compared with late maturing pubertal children. Eur J Endocrinol. 2015;173(2):227–35.
22. Boyne MS, Thame M, Osmond C, Fraser RA, Gabay L, Reid M, et al. Growth, body composition, and the onset of puberty: longitudinal observations in Afro-Caribbean children. J Clin Endocrinol Metab. 2010;95:3194–200.
23. Ong KK, Ahmed ML, Dunger DB. Lessons from large population studies on timing and tempo of puberty (secular trends and relation to body size): the European trend. Mol Cell Endocrinol. 2006;254–255:8–12.
24. Tomova A, Lalabonova C, Robeva RN, Kumanov PT. Timing of pubertal maturation according to the age at first conscious ejaculation. Andrologia. 2011;43:163–6.
25. Parent AS, Teilmann G, Jull A, Skakkebaek NE, Toppari J, Bourguignon JP. The timing of normal puberty and the age limits of sexual precocity: variation around the world, secular trend, and changes after migration. Endocr Rev. 2003;24:668–93.
26. Bau AM, Ernert A, Schenk L, Wiegand S, Martus P, Grutrs A, et al. Is there a further acceleration in the age at onset of menarche? A cross-sectional study in 1840 school children focusing on age and bodyweight at the onset of menarche. Eur J Endocrinol. 2009;160(1):107–13.
27. Hernandez MI, Unanue N, Gaete X, Cassorla F, Codner E. Age of menarche and its relationship with body mass index and socioeconomic status. Rev Med Chil. 2008;135(11):1429–36.
28. Dos Santos Silva I, De Stavola BL, Mann V, Kuh D, Hardy R, Wadsworth ME. Prenatal factors, childhood growth trajectories and age at menarche. Int J Epidemiol. 2002;31(2):405–12.
29. Dunger DB, Ahmed ML, Ong KK. Early and late weight gain and the timing of puberty. Mol Cell Endocrinol. 2006;254–255:140–5.
30. Tomova A, Makker K, Kirilov G, Agarwal A, Kumanov P. Disturbances in gonadal axis in women with anorexia nervosa. Eat Weight Disord. 2007;12(4):e92–7.
31. Tolle V, Kadem M, Bluet-Pajot MT, Frere D, Foulon C, Bossu C, et al. Balance in ghrelin and leptin plasma levels in anorexia nervosa patients and constitutionally thin women. J Clin Endocrinol Metab. 2003;88(1):109–16.

32. Karlberg J. Secular trends in pubertal development. Horm Res. 2002;57 Suppl 2:19–30.
33. Lee JM, Kaciroti N, Appugliese D, Corwyn RF, Bradley RH, Lumeng JC. Body mass index and timing of pubertal initiation in boys. Arch Pediatr Adolesc Med. 2010;164:139–44.
34. Herman-Giddens ME, Steffes J, Harris D, Slora E, Hussey M, Dowshen SA, et al. Secondary sexual characteristics in boys: data from the pediatric research in office settings network. Pediatrics. 2012;130:e1058–1068.
35. Vizmanos B, Martí-Henneberg C. Puberty begins with a characteristic subcutaneous body fat mass in each sex. Eur J Clin Nutr. 2000;54:203–8.
36. Tinggaard J, Aksglaede L, Sørensen K, Mouritsen A, Wohlfahrt-Veje C, Hagen CP, et al. The 2014 Danish references from birth to 20 years for height, weight and body mass index. Acta Paediatr. 2014;103:214–24.
37. Karpati AM, Rubin CH, Kieszak SM, Marcus M, Troiano RP. Stature and pubertal stage assessment in American boys: the 1988–1994 Third National Health and Nutrition Examination Survey. J Adolesc Health. 2002;30:205–12.
38. Ankarberg-Lindgren C, Norjavaara E. Changes of diurnal rhythm and levels of total and free testosterone secretion from pre to late puberty in boys: testis size of 3 ml is a transition stage to puberty. Eur J Endocrinol. 2004;151:747–57.
39. Palmert MR, Dunkel L. Delayed puberty. N Engl J Med. 2012;366:443–53.
40. Tinggaard J, Mieritz MG, Sørensen K, Mouritsen A, Hagen CP, Aksglaede L, et al. The physiology and timing of male puberty. Curr Opin Endocrinol Diabetes Obes. 2012;19:197–203.
41. Tanner JM, Whitehouse RH. Clinical longitudinal standards for height, weight, height velocity, weight velocity, and stages of puberty. Arch Dis Child. 1976;51:170–9.
42. Tomova A, Robeva R, Kumanov P. Influence of the body weight on the onset and progression of puberty in boys. J Pediatr Endocrinol Metab. 2015;28(7–8):859–65.
43. Juul A, Magnusdottirs S, Scheike T, Prytz S, Skakebaek NE. Age at voice break in Danish boys: effects of pre-pubertal body mass index and secular trend. Int J Androl. 2007;30(6):537–42.
44. Fu JF, Dong GP, Liang L, Jiang YJ, Chen LQ, Dayan C. Early activation of the inhibin B/FSH axis in obese Tanner stage G1PH1 boys. Clin Endocrinol (Oxf). 2006;65:327–32.
45. Sørensen K, Aksglaede L, Petersen JH, Juul A. Recent changes in pubertal timing in healthy Danish boys: association with body mass index. J Clin Endocrinol Metab. 2010;95:263–70.
46. Patton GC, Viner R. Pubertal transitions in health. Lancet. 2007;369:1130–39.
47. Ebling FJ. The neuroendocrine timing of puberty. Reproduction. 2005;129:675–83.
48. Styne D. Puberty. In: Gardner DG, Shoback D, editors. Greenspan's basic and clinical endocrinology. New York, Chicago, San Francisco: McGraw Hill; 2007. p. 611–40.
49. Araujo AB, Wittert GA. Endocrinology of the aging male. Best Pract Res Clin Endocrinol Metab. 2011;25(2):303–19.
50. Alwis G, Rosengren B, Stenevi-Lundgren S, Düppe H, Sernbo I, Karlsson MK. Normative dual energy X-ray absorptiometry data in Swedish children and adolescents. Acta Paediatr. 2010;99:1091–9.
51. Frisch RF, Revelle R. Height and weight at menarche and hypothesis of menarche. Arch Dis Child. 1971;46:695–701.
52. Baskin DG, Breininger JF, Schwartz MW. SOCS-3 expression in leptin-sensitive neurons of the hypothalamus of fed and fasted rats. Regul Pept. 2000;92(1–3):9–15.
53. Hill JW, Elmquist JK, Elias CF. Hypothalamic pathways linking energy balance and reproduction. Am J Physiol Endocrinol Metab. 2008;294:E827–32.
54. Biro FM, Greenspan LC, Galvezl MP. Puberty in girls of the 21st century. J Pediatr Adolesc Gynecol. 2012;25(5):289–94.
55. Fischer-Posovszky P, Wabitsch M, Hochberg Z. Endocrinology of adipose tissue: an update. Horm Metab Res. 2007;39:314–21.
56. Chehab FF. Leptin and reproduction: past milestones, present undertakings and future endeavors. J Endocrinol. 2014;223:T37–48.
57. Matkovic V, Ilich JZ, Skugor M, Badenhop NE, Goel P, Clairmont A, et al. Leptin is inversely related to age at menarche in human females. J Clin Endocrinol Metab. 1997;82(10):3239–45.

58. Rutters F, Nieuwenhuizen AG, Verhoef SP, Lemmens SG, Vogels N, Westerterp-Plantenga MS. The relationship between leptin, gonadotropic hormones, and body composition during puberty in a Dutch children cohort. Eur J Endocrinol. 2009;160(6):973–8.
59. Blum W, Englaro P, Hanitsch S, Juul A, Hertel NT, Muller G, et al. Plasma leptin levels in healthy children and adolescent: dependence on body mass index, body fat mass, gender, pubertal stage and testosterone. J Clin Endocrinol Metab. 1997;82(9):2904–10.
60. Singh R, Artaza JN, Taylor WE, Braga M, Yuan X, Gonzalez-Cadavid NF, et al. Testosterone inhibits adipogenic differentiation in 3T3 L1 cells: nuclear translocation of androgen receptor complex with β-catenin and T-cell factor 4 may bypass canonical Wnt signalling to down-regulate adipogenic transcription factors. Endocrinology. 2006;147:141–54.
61. Cornish J, Callon KE, Bava U, Lin C, Naot D, Hill BL, et al. Leptin directly regulates bone cell function in vitro and reduces bone fragility in vivo. J Endocrinol. 2002;175(2):405–15.
62. Turner RT, Kalra SP, Wong CP, Philbrick KA, Lindenmaier LB, Boghossian S, et al. Peripheral leptin regulates bone formation. J Bone Miner Res. 2013;28(1):22–34.
63. Shahab M, Mastronardi C, Seminara S, Crowley WF, Ojeda SR, Plant TM. Increased hypothalamic GPR54 signaling: a potential mechanism for initiation of puberty in primates. Proc Natl Acad Sci U S A. 2005;102(6):2129–34.
64. Plant T. The role of KISS-1 in the regulation of puberty in higher primates. Eur J Endocrinol. 2006;155:S11–6.
65. Zhang C, Bosch MA, Rønnekleiv OK, Kelly MJ. Gamma-aminobutyric acid B receptor mediated inhibition of gonadotropin-releasing hormone neurons is suppressed by kisspeptin-G protein-coupled receptor 54 signaling. Endocrinology. 2009;150(5):2388–94.
66. Ahmed ML, Ong KK, Dunger D. Childhood obesity and the timing of puberty. Trends Endocrinol Metab. 2009;20(5):237–42.
67. Lawrence C, Fraley GS. Galanin-like peptide (GALP) is a hypothalamic regulator of energy homeostasis and reproduction. Front Neuroendocrinol. 2011;32(1):1–9.
68. Rosen MP, Cedars MI. Female reproductive endocrinology and infertility. In: Gardner DG, Shoback D, editors. Greenspan's basic and clinical endocrinology. New York, Chicago, San Francisco etc: McGraw Hill comp; 2007. p. 502–61.
69. Moran A, Jacobs DR, Steinberger J, Hong CP, Prineas R, Luepker R, et al. Insulin resistance during puberty: results from clamp studies in 357 children. Diabetes. 1999;48(10):2039–44.
70. Marcovecchio ML, Chiarelli F. Obesity and growth during childhood and puberty. World Rev Nutr Diet. 2013;106:135–41.
71. Hounsgaard ML, Håkonsen LB, Vested A, Thulstrup AM, Olsen J, Bonde JP, et al. Maternal pre-pregnancy body mass index and pubertal development among sons. Andrology. 2014;2:198–204.
72. Novotny R, Daida YG, Grove JS, Acharya S, Vogt TM. Formula feeding in infancy is associated with adolescent body fat and earlier menarche. Cell Mol Biol (Noisy-le-grand). 2003;49(8):1289–93.
73. Den Hond E, Schoeters G. Endocrine disrupters and human puberty. Int J Androl. 2006;29:264–71.
74. Djurovic M, Pekic S, Petakov M, Damjanovic S, Doknic M, Dieguez C, et al. Gonadotropin response to clomiphene and plasma leptin levels in weight recovered but amenorrhoeic patients with anorexia nervosa. J Endocrinol Invest. 2004;27(6):523–7.
75. Tomova A, Kumanov P, Kirilov G. Factors related to sex hormone binding globulin concentrations in women with anorexia nervosa. Horm Metab Res. 1995;27(11):508–10.
76. True C, Grove KL, Smith MS. Beyond leptin: emerging candidates for the integration of metabolic and reproductive function during negative energy balance. Front Endocrinol. 2011;2:1–12.
77. He Q, Karlberg J. BMI in childhood and its association with height gain, timing of puberty, and final height. Pediatr Res. 2001;49:244–51.

Chapter 8
The Environmental Factors and Epigenetics of Gametogenesis in Puberty

Sezgin Gunes and Mehmet Alper Arslan

Introduction

Puberty is initiated by secretion of gonadotropin-releasing hormone (GnRH) and reactivation of hypothalamic-pituitary-gonadal (HPG) axis. The age of onset of puberty varies greatly from one person to another and between the genders [1, 2]. This variability can be determined by both genetics and environmental exposure of individuals. Twin studies indicated alterations in pubertal timing of even monozygotic twins though it is much more common in dizygotic twins [3]. This finding demonstrated the role of environmental factors in the timing of puberty, including nutrition and chemicals [1].

Environmental factors can involve a large variety of exposures, such as occupational exposures (workplace exposures), environmental exposures (ultraviolet light, radon gas, infectious agents, pesticides, traffic pollution), and exposures resulting from lifestyle choices (nutrition, smoking, cosmetics, physical activity) or medical treatments (radiation and medicines including chemotherapy, hormone drugs, drugs that suppress the immune system) [4]. Dioxin-like chemicals, metals, phytoestrogens, polychlorinated biphenyls, polycyclic aromatic hydrocarbons, phthalates, and several classes of pesticides are certain types of environmental pollutants that may interact with epigenetic mechanisms [5]. There is common belief that exposure to

S. Gunes (✉)
Department of Medical Biology, Faculty of Medicine, Ondokuz Mayis University, Samsun, Turkey

Department of Multidisciplinary Molecular Medicine, Health Sciences Institute, Ondokuz Mayis University, Samsun, Turkey
e-mail: sgunes@omu.edu.tr

M.A. Arslan
Department of Medical Biology, Faculty of Medicine, Health Sciences Institute, Samsun, Turkey

Department of Multidisciplinary Molecular Medicine, Health Sciences Institute, Ondokuz Mayis University, Samsun, Turkey

P. Kumanov, A. Agarwal (eds.), *Puberty*, DOI 10.1007/978-3-319-32122-6_8

environmental factors can impair development, onset of puberty, and gametogenesis (both spermatogenesis and oogenesis) in adults and reduce fertility.

Several studies have demonstrated detrimental effects of occupational exposures on gametogenesis. In a study, dibromochloropropane (DBCP), an active ingredient in nematicides, was shown to cause severe impairment of spermatogenesis and mostly irreversible fertility in highly exposed men [6, 7]. Persistent organic pollutants (POP) such as organic compounds including dichlorodiphenyltrichloroethane (DDT) and polychlorinated biphenyls (PCBs) are widely used around the world for industrial and agricultural processes and accumulate in adipose tissues. Bjerregaard and colleagues have found high PCB concentration in plasma lipid levels (67 %) of women at reproductive age and concluded that substantial portion of Greenlandic fetuses is prenatally exposed to harmful concentrations of PCBs [8]. However, other studies found no major link between occupational exposures and the impairment of gametogenesis [9, 10].

Endocrine-disrupting chemicals (EDC) are exogenous agents that interfere with the hormone action or aid in the elimination of hormones in the body that are responsible for the maintenance of development, behavior, and reproduction [11, 12]. Skincare products and basic toiletries contain some chemicals such as parabens and phthalates. In addition, phthalates and bisphenol A (BPA) are monomers of plastics. The EDCs and phthalates are antiandrogenic chemicals and therefore affect males greatly, compared to females. However, BPA and cadmium are estrogenic [13–15]. The potential adverse effects of parabens and phthalates on testosterone metabolism and spermatogenesis have been reported in a number of animal studies [16–18]. A few studies have found a significant relationship between urinary levels of monobutyl phthalates and poor semen parameters [19, 20].

Published studies on the reproductive toxicity of the pesticides and associated with semen parameter or oocyte quality are limited. Recent studies have demonstrated a link between impairment of gametogenesis and some environmental chemicals. Two studies have reported an association between nonpersistent insecticides and alterations in steroid hormone levels and sperm concentration, motility, and DNA integrity [21, 22]. Nevertheless, Swan and colleagues have shown a sufficiently significant correlation between urinary metabolite levels of the currently used pesticides (alachlor, atrazine, diazinon) and low sperm counts in males living in mid-Missouri, Colombia [23]. In this chapter, we have reviewed and discussed current evidence indicating that environmental factors may have a detrimental role in gametogenesis.

Epigenetics and Gametogenesis

Epigenetic modifications are heritable and reversible processes to regulate gene activity and expression, without any alteration of DNA sequences. These modifications include DNA methylation, histone tail modifications, and short noncoding RNAs and can be inherited through both mitotic and meiotic divisions. Epigenetic modifications can be altered by internal and external factors, including environmental chemicals, nutrition, and stress [24].

DNA Methylation

DNA methylation is the addition of a methyl group from *S*-adenosylmethionine to the fifth position of the cytosine ring (5meC) in the CpG islands (CGIs). CGIs are short interspersed C+G-rich DNA sequences and are localized in the promoters or regulatory regions of almost all housekeeping genes, developmental genes, and some tissue-specific genes [25, 26]. Methylation of these cytosines is correlated with inactivation or silencing of the associated promoter, whereas hypomethylation usually leads to activation of gene expression [26, 27]. Silencing of gene expression is either due to inhibition of transcription factor binding to methylated cytosines or repression mediated by methyl-CpG-binding proteins [26, 28].

DNA methylation is catalyzed by maintenance DNA methyltransferases (DNMTs) (DNMT1) and de novo DNMTs (DNMT3A, DNMT3B, DNMT3L) [29]. DNMT1 is responsible for maintenance of DNA methylation during DNA replication and termed as maintenance methyltransferase. DNMT3A, DNMT3B, and DNMT3L mediate de novo methylation of genomic DNA during early phase of embryonic development specifically in germ cells.

Sertoli cells proliferate in fetal life, postnatal/neonatal period, and prior to puberty. Sertoli cell number can be influenced by environmental factors during any of these periods. Sertoli cells can support only a limited number of mature germ cells; therefore, Sertoli cell proliferation during fetal life is critical for the number of sperms produced in adulthood. This proliferation is controlled by testosterone during fetal life and postnatal/neonatal period and by follicle-stimulating hormone (FSH) during puberty. Environmental factors may affect the proliferation of Sertoli cells during any one of these three periods, which may have an impact on sperm counts. Maternal lifestyle choices during pregnancy may be a determining factor for sperm count of the son during adulthood through the subsequent decrease in the number of Sertoli cells in testes [4, 30]. DNMT1 maintains DNA methylation patterns during mammalian oogenesis [31], and *DNMT1* gene homozygous mutations in mice cause severe genomic imprinting defects and X inactivation abnormalities [32].

Reprogramming of Non-imprinted Genes

The methylation marks of primordial germ cells (PGCs) are erased in a number of sequential reactions during the development of embryo between 8 and 13.5 days post coitum (dpc) in both sexes [33–35]. By 12.5 dpc, methylation marks of some single-copy genes including *alpha actin* and myosin light chain (*mylc*) are erased. Furthermore, some repetitive elements undergo substantial demethylation of their methylation marks, while other repetitive sequences are not completely erased [36, 37]. By 13.5 dpc, PGCs enter mitotic/meiotic arrest [34, 36]. The second demethylation mechanism removes methyl groups from CGIs within the inactive X chromosome, imprinted loci, and some genes expressed in germ cells [38]. After this demethylation process, a specific remethylation program starts to reestablish parental genomic imprints in germ cells. Remethylation program begins at around 15.5 dpc in spermatogonia and type I spermatocytes; hence, spermatozoa transmit the paternal imprint [39, 40]. In the mouse female germline, DNA remethylation takes place in oocytes that have entered meiosis and been arrested in diplotene of meiotic prophase I [37].

The methylation sequences of the oocyte and the sperm are both inside the genes and between the genes [38]. On the other hand, repeat methylation level in oocyte is lower than in spermatozoa and somatic cells [41].

Reprogramming of Imprinted Genes

Spermatozoa have unique DNA methylation patterns that are formed during early stages of development and are essential for proper sperm production and spermatogenesis [33]. Some genes are imprinted differentially by DNA methylation depending on which parent they are inherited from, which causes alterations in gene expression depending on the allele transmitted from the father or the mother [42]. *Igf2/H19*, *Rasgrf1*, *Dlk1-Gtl2*, and *Zdbf2* loci of sperm genome are methylated only in male germ cells [43]. Many imprinted genes are involved in the regulation of growth and development [44]. Several studies have demonstrated a significant association between methylation statuses of both maternally and paternally imprinted genes and sperm abnormalities [42, 45–51]. During mammalian oogenesis, the reprogramming process takes place for histone modification and short noncoding RNAs changed by both internal and external causes [52, 53]. DNA methylation pattern of imprinted genes in oocytes of mice and murine is altered by diabetes and obesity [54, 55]. Epigenetic alterations can occur at any time of life and can be transmitted to the future generations [56]. DNA methylation is the most common epigenetic aberration induced by environmental agents. These epimutations can be transgenerational or non-transgenerational in germline cells [57].

Environmental toxicants influence gene expression by epigenetic mechanisms and by directly binding to promoter regions of target genes. Additionally, in animal models, epigenetic modifications during oogenesis are effected by maternal diets [58].

Histone Modifications

Histones are basic proteins rich in lysine and arginine located in nucleus and are subject to posttranslational modifications on their N- and C-terminal tails via acetylation, methylation, phosphorylation, and ubiquitination [59]. These chemical modifications change binding capacity of regulatory factors to DNA and thus lead to alterations in gene activity and expression during development and in response to the environmental factors. Generally, acetylation of lysine (K) residues of histone 3

(H3) and histone 4 (H4) leads to active transcription by inducing open chromatin configuration and facilitating transcription factor binding in spermatogonial stem cells [60, 61]. On the contrary, deacetylation causes inactivation of transcription and generally correlates with methylation of histones [62].

During spermatogenesis, methylation of H3K and H4K histone tails is regulated by histone methyltransferases (HTM) and histone demethylases (HDM) [63, 64]. Acetylation of H2A, H2B, H3, and H4 were shown to be high in mouse spermatogonia, and these histones were deacetylated throughout meiosis in round spermatids and reacetylated in elongating spermatids [61]. Hyperacetylation of H4K has been shown to be responsible for the conversion of histone to protamines in elongating spermatids [61]. Recently, a few studies have investigated the role of histone tail modification in spermatogenesis. La Spina and colleagues evaluated the methylation of H3K4Me, H3K4Me3, H3K9Me2, H3K79Me2, and H3K36Me3 and acetylation of H3K4Ac and H4K5Ac in normal and abnormal human sperm. They reported the presence of unexpected and unexplained heterogeneous histone modifications, and the presence of H3K4Me1, H3K9Me2, H3K4Me3, H3K79Me2, and H3K36Me3 marks in poorly functional human sperm [65]. Further studies are required to evaluate the impact of histone tail modifications induced by environmental exposures.

Protamination

Sperm chromatin packaging is a critical process that serves to accommodate enormous amounts of DNA into a small sperm cell. Fertilization requires many physiological events including movement of sperm cells along the entire female reproductive system, attachment to zona pellucida, and penetration into the oocyte. For accomplishment of all these phases, a regulatory mechanism controlling the replacement of 85–95 % of histones by protamines becomes effective [66]. Protamines are small proteins rich in arginine. They are located in sperm nucleus and synthesized during later stages of spermatogenesis. Protamination of sperm chromatin facilitates compaction of nucleus required for sperm motility and also protects sperm genome from oxidation and harmful molecules within the female reproductive system [66].

Replacement of histones by protamines involves translocation of histones by selected histone variants which are expressed during spermatogenesis. Hyperacetylation of histone tails causes the unwinding of chromatin structure and stimulates DNA strand breaks by topoisomerase enzyme that, in turn, facilitates separation of histones and replacement by transition proteins (TPs) [67, 68]. TP1 and TP2 bind to DNA and are completely replaced by protamines. Transition proteins play a critical role in separation of histones and facilitate the condensation of sperm DNA by protamines at later stages [68]. Despite controversial publications, it is abundantly clear that deviations in protamine ratio might be associated with various phenotypic features including decreased sperm counts and function and poor embryonic quality [69, 70].

The Role of miRNAs in Gametogenesis

Spermatogenesis is a complex differentiation process that consists of at least three major phases starting with diploid spermatogonial stem cells and ending with haploid mature spermatozoa. The process requires prompt and timely transitions between mitotic, meiotic, and postmeiotic stages, which, as expected, are tightly regulated at both transcriptional and posttranscriptional levels [71]. Growing evidence has indicated that a specialized group of short noncoding RNAs termed microRNAs (miRNAs) exert an essential posttranscriptional control on each step of male germ cell differentiation [72].

miRNAs are 21–25 nucleotide long, endogenous noncoding RNAs that inhibit gene expression by binding to their target mRNAs, leading to either mRNA cleavage/degradation or translational repression. The biogenesis of miRNAs is a multistep process starting with RNA polymerase II-driven transcription of large precursor RNA molecules called pri-miRNAs [73]. Pri-miRNAs are processed in the nucleus by a type III RNase termed Drosha and its cofactor Pasha/DGCR8 to become pre-miRNAs. Pre-miRNAs are then exported from the nucleus into the cytoplasm by exportin 5. In the cytoplasm, cleavage of pre-miRNAs by another type III RNase called Dicer results in the generation of mature duplex miRNA molecules [74]. Either strand of the duplex may be incorporated into the so-called RNA-induced silencing complex (RISC) to downregulate its target mRNA via complementary base pairing at its 3′ untranslated region (3′UTR). The degree of miRNA-mRNA complementarity is considered to be the key factor in the choice of posttranscriptional mechanism employed by miRNAs [75]. Perfect base pairing results in mRNA cleavage and its subsequent degradation, whereas imperfect pairing leads to translational repression.

Recent studies have indicated that miRNAs are expressed in all phases of male germ cell differentiation and are required for spermatogenesis in mammalians [72]. The absolute requirement for miRNAs for spermatogenesis has been shown by two initial studies where *Dicer1* gene was knocked out in two different mouse models [76, 77]. Germ cell-specific deletion of Dicer1 in these models led to complete male infertility due to alterations in meiotic progression, increased spermatocyte apoptosis, and failure of haploid male germ cell differentiation. Since Dicer processes both miRNAs and endogenous siRNAs (endo-siRNAs) while Drosha is only limited to miRNA biogenesis, to dissect between the specific effects of miRNAs and endo-siRNAs, a following study has utilized *Drosha* and *Dicer* conditional knockout mouse models. In this study, it has been reported that both knockout males were infertile due to impaired spermatogenesis characterized by depletion of spermatocytes and spermatids leading to oligoteratozoospermia or azoospermia [78]. Interestingly, when compared to ones from *Dicer* knockouts, testes from *Drosha* knockouts were more severely disrupted in terms of spermatogenesis, which further highlights the significance of miRNAs for normal spermatogenesis and male fertility [78].

There have been several studies investigating the role of miRNAs in human spermatogenesis, and results have so far supported the abovementioned observations obtained from animal models. Next-generation sequencing analysis of short RNA transcriptome from three normal human testes has identified a total of 770 known and five novel human miRNAs, indicating the abundance and complexity of miRNAs in the human testis [79]. The most abundant miRNAs detected in this study were let-7 family members, miR-34c-5p, miR-103a-3p (meaning from the 3′arm), miR-202-5p, miR-508-3p, and miR-509-3-5p, which target gene transcripts involved in regulation of meiosis, spermatogenesis, germ cell apoptosis, testicular development, p53-related pathways, and homologous recombination pathways [79]. In a more recent study where the expression levels of 736 miRNAs were tested in spermatozoa from ten normozoospermic fertile men, 221 miRNAs were found to be consistently present in all individuals [80]. Potential targets of these miRNAs were found to be enriched in processes involved in development, morphogenesis, spermatogenesis, and embryogenesis. In the same study, three most stably expressed miRNAs, namely, miR-532-5p (meaning from the 5′arm), miR-374b-5p, and miR-564, have also been proposed by the authors to be used as fertility biomarkers [80].

Although cell stage-specific expression of miRNAs during spermatogenesis and their genuine and potential targets are relatively well defined in rodents, such studies are largely missing in humans [72, 74, 81]. Recently, one such study has isolated human spermatogenic cell populations from different stages of spermatogenesis and identified their miRNA expression profiles by microarray analysis [82]. A total of 559 miRNAs were found to be distinctively expressed by human spermatogonia, pachytene spermatocytes, and round spermatids. Comparative analyses revealed 32 miRNAs to be significantly upregulated and 78 miRNAs to be downregulated between human spermatogonia and pachytene spermatocytes, suggesting that these miRNAs have a role in meiotic and mitotic phases of spermatogenesis, respectively. In addition, 144 miRNAs were found to be upregulated, while 29 miRNAs were downregulated between pachytene spermatocytes and round spermatids, indicating a potential role for these miRNAs in the regulation of spermiogenesis [82]. Taken together, it has become more evident that in humans, as well as in rodents, miRNAs play essential roles in spatial and temporal control of gene expression, driving precise transitions between the major stages of spermatogenesis.

Finally, it is noteworthy to mention here the contribution of environmental factors to the epigenetic regulation of spermatogenesis. As is widely acknowledged, the male epigenome is subject to change due to certain environmental stressors, and these environmentally induced epigenetic changes can be transmitted to the next generations even though they are not exposed to the stressors themselves [83]. A miRNA microarray study performed with spermatozoa from adult men living in an environmentally polluted region in China has revealed 73 significantly upregulated and 109 downregulated miRNAs compared to the control group [84]. Since environmental pollution is one of the well-known factors accounting for decreased sperm quality in humans [4], these results suggest that differentially expressed miRNAs under such in men exposed to electronic waste pollution conditions might help explain the detrimental impact of environmental pollution on sperm quality and count [83].

Compared to spermatogenesis, investigating the connection between miRNA activity and oocyte development and oogenesis in humans has remained a poorly studied area. This may in part be due to the finding that despite their presence, gene regulation by miRNAs is kept in an inactive state in both mouse oocytes and early embryos [85, 86]. Although endo-siRNAs are thought to replace miRNAs in regulating gene expression and mRNA degradation at these stages [87], further studies are required to address the mechanism of action of endo-siRNAs and miRNAs in human oogenesis.

Conclusion

For several environmental exposures, it has been shown that these chemicals can alter the epigenetic profiles and subsequently lead to various diseases [57]. Epigenetic aberrations caused by environmental factors can be transmitted from oocyte and spermatozoan to the offspring. Germline cells undergo developmental epigenetic alterations during both spermatogenesis and oogenesis. Spermatogenesis does not start before puberty; however, the foundations of spermatogenesis begin during the fetal life, and abnormalities during this period may have subsequent effects on the quality of spermatogenesis in adulthood more than in adolescence period [3]. Environmentally induced germ cell differentiation and regulation in puberty is poorly understood. More work is necessary to understand the extent of epigenetic aberrations induced by environmental exposures during puberty. Epigenetic factors known to cause aberrant changes in epigenetic pathways are well documented; however, their exact mechanism in puberty has not been properly clarified. Further studies are required to elucidate the mechanisms relating to the origin of these alterations and to determine their significance and functional consequences for gametogenesis in puberty.

References

1. Rzeczkowska PA, et al. Epigenetics: a new player in the regulation of mammalian puberty. Neuroendocrinology. 2014;99(3–4):139–55.
2. Valeri C, Schteingart HF, Rey RA. The prepubertal testis: biomarkers and functions. Curr Opin Endocrinol Diabetes Obes. 2013;20(3):224–33.
3. Eaves L, et al. Genetic and environmental influences on the relative timing of pubertal change. Twin Res. 2004;7(5):471–81.
4. Sharpe RM. Environmental/lifestyle effects on spermatogenesis. Philos Trans R Soc Lond B Biol Sci. 2010;365(1546):1697–712.
5. Bollati V, Baccarelli A. Environmental epigenetics. Heredity (Edinb). 2010;105(1):105–12.
6. Whorton D, et al. Testicular function in DBCP exposed pesticide workers. J Occup Med. 1979;21(3):161–6.
7. Whorton D, Foliart D. DBCP: eleven years later. Reprod Toxicol. 1988;2(3–4):155–61.
8. Bjerregaard P, et al. Exposure of Inuit in Greenland to organochlorines through the marine diet. J Toxicol Environ Health A. 2001;62(2):69–81.
9. Bonde JP, Storgaard L. How work-place conditions, environmental toxicants and lifestyle affect male reproductive function. Int J Androl. 2002;25(5):262–8.
10. Larsen SB, et al. Semen quality and sex hormones among organic and traditional Danish farmers. ASCLEPIOS Study Group. Occup Environ Med. 1999;56(2):139–44.

11. Wan HT, et al. Targeting testis-specific proteins to inhibit spermatogenesis: lesson from endocrine disrupting chemicals. Expert Opin Ther Targets. 2013;17(7):839–55.
12. Euling SY, et al. Role of environmental factors in the timing of puberty. Pediatrics. 2008;121 Suppl 3:S167–71.
13. Taylor JA, et al. Estrogenic environmental chemicals and drugs: mechanisms for effects on the developing male urogenital system. J Steroid Biochem Mol Biol. 2011;127(1–2):83–95.
14. Kortenkamp A, Faust M. Combined exposures to anti-androgenic chemicals: steps towards cumulative risk assessment. Int J Androl. 2010;33(2):463–74.
15. Safe S. Cadmium's disguise dupes the estrogen receptor. Nat Med. 2003;9(8):1000–1.
16. David RM, et al. Chronic toxicity of di(2-ethylhexyl)phthalate in mice. Toxicol Sci. 2000;58(2):377–85.
17. Ishihara M, et al. Spermatogenic disturbance induced by di-(2-ethylhexyl) phthalate is significantly prevented by treatment with antioxidant vitamins in the rat. Int J Androl. 2000;23(2):85–94.
18. Oishi S. Effects of butylparaben on the male reproductive system in rats. Toxicol Ind Health. 2001;17(1):31–9.
19. Duty SM, et al. Phthalate exposure and human semen parameters. Epidemiology. 2003;14(3):269–77.
20. Hauser R, et al. The relationship between human semen parameters and environmental exposure to polychlorinated biphenyls and p, p'-DDE. Environ Health Perspect. 2003;111(12):1505–11.
21. Meeker JD, Calafat AM, Hauser R. Urinary metabolites of di(2-ethylhexyl) phthalate are associated with decreased steroid hormone levels in adult men. J Androl. 2009;30(3):287–97.
22. Meeker JD, Barr DB, Hauser R. Human semen quality and sperm DNA damage in relation to urinary metabolites of pyrethroid insecticides. Hum Reprod. 2008;23(8):1932–40.
23. Swan SH, et al. Semen quality in relation to biomarkers of pesticide exposure. Environ Health Perspect. 2003;111(12):1478–84.
24. Bird A. Perceptions of epigenetics. Nature. 2007;447(7143):396–8.
25. Zhu J, et al. On the nature of human housekeeping genes. Trends Genet. 2008;24(10):481–4.
26. Deaton AM, Bird A. CpG islands and the regulation of transcription. Genes Dev. 2011;25(10):1010–22.
27. Jones PA. Functions of DNA methylation: islands, start sites, gene bodies and beyond. Nat Rev Genet. 2012;13(7):484–92.
28. Klose RJ, Bird AP. Genomic DNA methylation: the mark and its mediators. Trends Biochem Sci. 2006;31(2):89–97.
29. Eden S, Cedar H. Role of DNA methylation in the regulation of transcription. Curr Opin Genet Dev. 1994;4(2):255–9.
30. Sharpe RM, et al. Proliferation and functional maturation of Sertoli cells, and their relevance to disorders of testis function in adulthood. Reproduction. 2003;125(6):769–84.
31. Mertineit C, et al. Sex-specific exons control DNA methyltransferase in mammalian germ cells. Development. 1998;125(5):889–97.
32. Panning B, Jaenisch R. DNA hypomethylation can activate Xist expression and silence X-linked genes. Genes Dev. 1996;10(16):1991–2002.
33. Santos F, Dean W. Epigenetic reprogramming during early development in mammals. Reproduction. 2004;127(6):643–51.
34. Hajkova P, et al. Epigenetic reprogramming in mouse primordial germ cells. Mech Dev. 2002;117(1–2):15–23.
35. Li E. Chromatin modification and epigenetic reprogramming in mammalian development. Nat Rev Genet. 2002;3(9):662–73.
36. Kagiwada S, et al. Replication-coupled passive DNA demethylation for the erasure of genome imprints in mice. EMBO J. 2013;32(3):340–53.
37. Tomizawa S, Nowacka-Woszuk J, Kelsey G. DNA methylation establishment during oocyte growth: mechanisms and significance. Int J Dev Biol. 2012;56(10–12):867–75.
38. Clarke HJ, Vieux KF. Epigenetic inheritance through the female germ-line: the known, the unknown, and the possible. Semin Cell Dev Biol. 2015;43:106–16

39. Davis TL, et al. The H19 methylation imprint is erased and re-established differentially on the parental alleles during male germ cell development. Hum Mol Genet. 2000;9(19):2885–94.
40. Boissonnas CC, Jouannet P, Jammes H. Epigenetic disorders and male subfertility. Fertil Steril. 2013;99(3):624–31.
41. Allegrucci C, et al. Epigenetics and the germline. Reproduction. 2005;129(2):137–49.
42. Camprubi C, et al. Semen samples showing an increased rate of spermatozoa with imprinting errors have a negligible effect in the outcome of assisted reproduction techniques. Epigenetics. 2012;7(10):1115–24.
43. Arnaud P. Genomic imprinting in germ cells: imprints are under control. Reproduction. 2010;140(3):411–23.
44. Horsthemke B. In brief: genomic imprinting and imprinting diseases. J Pathol. 2014;232(5):485–7.
45. Kobayashi H, et al. Aberrant DNA methylation of imprinted loci in sperm from oligospermic patients. Hum Mol Genet. 2007;16(21):2542–51.
46. Marques CJ, et al. Genomic imprinting in disruptive spermatogenesis. Lancet. 2004;363(9422):1700–2.
47. Marques CJ, et al. Abnormal methylation of imprinted genes in human sperm is associated with oligozoospermia. Mol Hum Reprod. 2008;14(2):67–74.
48. Marques CJ, et al. Methylation defects of imprinted genes in human testicular spermatozoa. Fertil Steril. 2010;94(2):585–94.
49. El Hajj N, et al. Methylation status of imprinted genes and repetitive elements in sperm DNA from infertile males. Sex Dev. 2011;5(2):60–9.
50. Minor A, Chow V, Ma S. Aberrant DNA methylation at imprinted genes in testicular sperm retrieved from men with obstructive azoospermia and undergoing vasectomy reversal. Reproduction. 2011;141(6):749–57.
51. Rotondo JC, et al. Methylation loss at H19 imprinted gene correlates with methylenetetrahydrofolate reductase gene promoter hypermethylation in semen samples from infertile males. Epigenetics. 2013;8(9):990–7.
52. Gu L, Wang Q, Sun QY. Histone modifications during mammalian oocyte maturation: dynamics, regulation and functions. Cell Cycle. 2010;9(10):1942–50.
53. Hales BF, et al. Epigenetic programming: from gametes to blastocyst. Birth Defects Res A Clin Mol Teratol. 2011;91(8):652–65.
54. Ge ZJ, et al. Maternal diabetes causes alterations of DNA methylation statuses of some imprinted genes in murine oocytes. Biol Reprod. 2013;88(5):117.
55. Ge ZJ, et al. Diabetic uterus environment may play a key role in alterations of DNA methylation of several imprinted genes at mid-gestation in mice. Reprod Biol Endocrinol. 2013;11:119.
56. Ryu HW, et al. Influence of toxicologically relevant metals on human epigenetic regulation. Toxicol Res. 2015;31(1):1–9.
57. Ruiz-Hernandez A, et al. Environmental chemicals and DNA methylation in adults: a systematic review of the epidemiologic evidence. Clin Epigenetics. 2015;7(1):55.
58. Steegers-Theunissen RP, et al. The periconceptional period, reproduction and long-term health of offspring: the importance of one-carbon metabolism. Hum Reprod Update. 2013;19(6):640–55.
59. Campos EI, Reinberg D. Histones: annotating chromatin. Annu Rev Genet. 2009;43:559–99.
60. Cairns BR. The logic of chromatin architecture and remodelling at promoters. Nature. 2009;461(7261):193–8.
61. Hazzouri M, et al. Regulated hyperacetylation of core histones during mouse spermatogenesis: involvement of histone deacetylases. Eur J Cell Biol. 2000;79(12):950–60.
62. Peng L, Seto E. Deacetylation of nonhistone proteins by HDACs and the implications in cancer. Handb Exp Pharmacol. 2011;206:39–56.
63. Lachner M, Jenuwein T. The many faces of histone lysine methylation. Curr Opin Cell Biol. 2002;14(3):286–98.
64. Carrell DT, Emery BR, Hammoud S. The aetiology of sperm protamine abnormalities and their potential impact on the sperm epigenome. Int J Androl. 2008;31(6):537–45.
65. La Spina FA, et al. Heterogeneous distribution of histone methylation in mature human sperm. J Assist Reprod Genet. 2014;31(1):45–9.

66. Torregrosa N, et al. Protamine 2 precursors, protamine 1/protamine 2 ratio, DNA integrity and other sperm parameters in infertile patients. Hum Reprod. 2006;21(8):2084–9.
67. Rousseaux S, et al. Molecular models for post-meiotic male genome reprogramming. Syst Biol Reprod Med. 2011;57(1–2):50–3.
68. Meistrich ML, et al. Roles of transition nuclear proteins in spermiogenesis. Chromosoma. 2003;111(8):483–8.
69. Nasr-Esfahani MH, et al. Effect of protamine-2 deficiency on ICSI outcome. Reprod Biomed Online. 2004;9(6):652–8.
70. de Mateo S, et al. Protamine 2 precursors (Pre-P2), protamine 1 to protamine 2 ratio (P1/P2), and assisted reproduction outcome. Fertil Steril. 2009;91(3):715–22.
71. Kotaja N. MicroRNAs and spermatogenesis. Fertil Steril. 2014;101(6):1552–62.
72. Yao C, et al. MicroRNAs and DNA methylation as epigenetic regulators of mitosis, meiosis and spermiogenesis. Reproduction. 2015;150(1):R25–34.
73. He Z, et al. Small RNA molecules in the regulation of spermatogenesis. Reproduction. 2009;137(6):901–11.
74. Hale BJ, et al. Small RNAs: their possible roles in reproductive failure. Adv Exp Med Biol. 2015;868:49–79.
75. Krol J, Loedige I, Filipowicz W. The widespread regulation of microRNA biogenesis, function and decay. Nat Rev Genet. 2010;11(9):597–610.
76. Korhonen HM, et al. Dicer is required for haploid male germ cell differentiation in mice. PLoS One. 2011;6(9), e24821.
77. Romero Y, et al. Dicer1 depletion in male germ cells leads to infertility due to cumulative meiotic and spermiogenic defects. PLoS One. 2011;6(10), e25241.
78. Wu Q, et al. The RNase III enzyme DROSHA is essential for microRNA production and spermatogenesis. J Biol Chem. 2012;287(30):25173–90.
79. Yang Q, et al. MicroRNA and piRNA profiles in normal human testis detected by next generation sequencing. PLoS One. 2013;8(6):e66809.
80. Salas-Huetos A, et al. New insights into the expression profile and function of micro-ribonucleic acid in human spermatozoa. Fertil Steril. 2014;102(1):213–222.e4.
81. Wang L, Xu C. Role of microRNAs in mammalian spermatogenesis and testicular germ cell tumors. Reproduction. 2015;149(3):R127–37.
82. Liu Y, et al. Fractionation of human spermatogenic cells using STA-PUT gravity sedimentation and their miRNA profiling. Sci Rep. 2015;5:8084.
83. O'Doherty AM, McGettigan PA. Epigenetic processes in the male germline. 2014. Reprod Fertil Dev.
84. Li Y, et al. A microarray for microRNA profiling in spermatozoa from adult men living in an environmentally polluted site. Bull Environ Contam Toxicol. 2012;89(6):1111–4.
85. Ma J, et al. MicroRNA activity is suppressed in mouse oocytes. Curr Biol. 2010;20(3):265–70.
86. Suh N, et al. MicroRNA function is globally suppressed in mouse oocytes and early embryos. Curr Biol. 2010;20(3):271–7.
87. Barckmann B, Simonelig M. Control of maternal mRNA stability in germ cells and early embryos. Biochim Biophys Acta. 2013;1829(6–7):714–24.

Chapter 9
Timing of Puberty and Secular Trend in Human Maturation

Anastasios Papadimitriou

Introduction

Puberty is a milestone in the transition from the immature child to the mature and capable for reproduction adult. Puberty refers to the physical changes that occur as a result of the reactivation of the hypothalamic-pituitary-gonadal (HPG) axis resulting in gonadal estradiol and testosterone secretion, whereas adolescence refers not only to somatic but the psychological changes that occur as a consequence of the HPG axis activation. The HPG axis is transiently activated during early infancy followed by a long period of relative quiescence. The process of puberty lasts for 3–5 years, and adolescence may last 10 years or more.

The timing of pubertal onset has been related to public health issues, e.g., early onset of puberty has been related to metabolic syndrome, hence increased cardiovascular risk, breast cancer in women, all-cause mortality, and testicular cancer in men [1–4], whereas delayed puberty has been linked to osteoporosis [5]. Therefore, there is a continuous interest on the timing of pubertal onset in the various populations and whether the age that puberty begins is decreasing.

Definitions

Onset of puberty is defined in girls as the first appearance of breast tissue (breast budding) and in boys as the attainment of a testicular volume more than 3 mL. Breast development must be determined by palpation, to avoid misclassification of fat (lipomastia) as breast, when the examination is only visual. Testicular volume (TV)

A. Papadimitriou (✉)
Third Department of Pediatrics, 'Attikon' University Hospital,
1 Rimini Street, Haidari, Athens 12462, Greece
e-mail: anpapad@med.uoa.gr

P. Kumanov, A. Agarwal (eds.), *Puberty*, DOI 10.1007/978-3-319-32122-6_9

is reliably determined by the Prader orchidometer, a graded series of ellipsoid beads on a string [6], in experienced hands. Nevertheless, the more accurate method of determining TV is by ultrasonography (US), because, in the measurements by US, scrotal skin and epididymis are not included [7].

Menarche is a girl's first menstrual bleeding, and *spermarche* is the boy's first conscious ejaculation, which is more appropriate to be called *ejacularche* that often occurs during sleep, i.e., nocturnal emission. Spermarche, i.e., the onset of sperm production, precedes ejacularche and is usually detected as spermatozoa in a morning urine specimen (spermaturia) [8].

Factors Influencing the Timing of Puberty

The various factors that are influencing the onset of puberty are covered in detail in other chapters of the book.

Here, within the limited space of this review, I refer briefly to the role of genetic and epigenetic, ethnic/racial, and environmental factors. Table 9.1 shows some of the main factors that influence the timing of puberty.

Genetic and Epigenetic

Although almost half of the variance in the age at menarche has been attributed to heritability [9, 10], knowledge of the specific factors regulating the onset of puberty is limited. Rare mutations have been identified as the cause of disordered pubertal timing, e.g., *ESR1*, *KISS1*, *KISSR1*, and *MKRN3*; however, these genes do not seem to determine the timing of puberty in the population. Genome Wide Association Studies (GWAS) examining genetic variations using large numbers of data explain only about 15% of the variance in menarcheal age [11]. It is notable that for a single nucleotide polymorphism rs314276 in intron 2 of *LIN28B* on chromosome 6, each major allele was associated with 0.12 years earlier menarche. In girls there was also association of this allele with earlier breast development and in boys with earlier voice breaking, suggesting earlier pubertal maturation. In line with early timing of puberty were the associations of *LIN28B* with a faster tempo of growth and shorter adult height in both sexes [12]. In a recent large-scale meta-analysis of 57 GWAS including data from 182.416 women, the authors found robust evidence for 123 signals at 106 genomic loci associated with age at menarche. Moreover, menarche signals were enriched in imprinted regions, with three loci (*DLK1/WDR25*, *MKRN3/MAGEL2*, and *KCNK9*) demonstrating parent-of-origin specific associations concordant with known parental expression patterns [11]. Further analysis implicated retinoic acid and gamma-aminobutyric acid-B2 receptor signaling pathways as novel mechanisms regulating pubertal timing in humans.

Table 9.1 Factors influencing the onset of puberty

	Effect	
Genetic and epigenetic	Boys	Girls
Mutations of ESR1	Normal puberty	Delayed puberty
KISS1 and KISSR1	Hypogonadotropic hypogonadism	Hypogonadotropic hypogonadism
MKRN3	Precocious puberty	Precocious puberty
SNP rs314276 of *LIN28B*	Earlier onset of puberty	Earlier onset of puberty/ menarche
Polymorphism of *FSHR*-29AA	–	Later onset of puberty
Epigenetic changes in polycomb group proteins (*Cbx7 and Eed*)	Signal pubertal onset	
Ethnic/racial differences		
Black race	Early puberty/no effect	Early puberty/menarche
Environmental factors		
Low socioeconomic status	Uncertain	Late menarche
Higher parental education	Uncertain	Early puberty
Absence of biological father	Uncertain	Early puberty
Urban environment	Uncertain	Early puberty
Adoption of Third World children	Inconsistent	Early puberty
Chronic stress (e.g., illness, wars)	Delayed puberty	Delayed puberty
Endocrine disruptors		
Phthalates	Uncertain	Early puberty/no effect
Bisphenol A	Uncertain	Early puberty/no effect
Pesticides (DDT, DDE)	Uncertain	Early puberty/no effect

The stronger genetic influence on pubertal onset in girls, so far, has been a polymorphism related to follicle-stimulating hormone receptor (FSHR) [13]. In girls homozygous for *FSHR*-29AA (reduced FSH receptor expression) pubertal onset occurred 7.4 months later than those with the common genotype variants *FSHR*-29GG+GA. Furthermore when *FSHR*-29GG+GA was combined with *FSHB*-211G>T (reduced FSH production), the age at pubertal onset increased with the number of minor alleles across the genotypes.

The role of epigenetic modification of genes in the control of pubertal onset has only recently been unraveled. Lomnizci et al. [14] demonstrated that increased promoter methylation and decreased expression of two polycomb group proteins (*Cbx7 and Eed*) leads to disinhibition of *kiss1* expression signaling pubertal onset. In the same study administration of 5-azacytidine, a pharmacological inhibitor of DNA methylation, prevented the increase of *Kiss1* expression that occurs prior to pubertal onset, resulting in pubertal delay.

Ethnic/Racial Influences

Several studies have shown the existence of ethnic/racial differences in the timing of pubertal maturation or menarche. Most of these studies refer to children in the USA and have been performed mostly in girls.

In a longitudinal 10-year study, which begun in 1986–1987 [15], black or white girls were examined annually. Mean onset of puberty in the white girls was 10.2 and in the black girls was 9.6 years. In the same study the age at menarche was 12.6 and 12.0 years, for the white and black girls, respectively.

In the Bogalusa Heart Study, black girls experienced menarche, on average, at the age of 12.3 years, 3 months earlier than did white girls experiencing menarche at 12.6 years [16]. Anthropometric differences, such as weight and height, which could be a confounding factor were controlled for; however, menarche remained significantly earlier among black girls, suggesting that race is an independent factor of pubertal development and timing of menarche. Black girls present higher insulin response to a glucose challenge and also have increased IGF1 levels compared to white girls [17]. Probably these biological differences have a genetic basis and are related with the more advanced skeletal and sexual maturation of the black compared to the white girls.

Contrary to the girls, only a few studies evaluated the existence of ethnic differences in the timing of puberty in boys. In the NHANES III study, conducted by the National Center for Health Statistics between 1988 and 1994, the median age at onset of pubertal maturation was approximately 9.2 years for black boys, 10.0 years for white boys, and 10.3 years for Mexican American boys, suggesting that, as African American girls do, African American boys enter puberty earlier than their peers of other origins [18].

However, in another US study, two hundred and twelve practitioners across the USA, in 144 well-child care pediatric offices, collected, cross-sectionally, Tanner stage and TV data on 4131 boys [19]. The data were collected between 2005 and 2010. Mean ages for attainment of TVs of ≥3 mL were reported to be 9.95 years for white, 9.71 years for African American, and 9.63 years for Hispanic boys and for ≥4 mL were 11.46, 11.75, and 11.29 years, respectively. Therefore, the latter data do not support the suggestion that African American boys mature earlier than European American boys. In line with this is an older observation in American children in which no difference was found at a testicular volume of 3 mL that usually heralds the onset of puberty (indeed most boys had attained a testicular volume of 4 mL within the next 6 months) between black and white children [20].

Environmental Factors

Environmental factors that impose a health hazard to the human are numerous and include air, water and food quality, waste disposal, hazardous substances, unsafe public space, and conditions within the house, e.g., stressful family environment.

Environmental factors that have been related to the timing of puberty include socioeconomic factors, place of residence, and endocrine-disrupting chemicals. More studies refer to females, and furthermore the results on boys are inconsistent or do not show a clear impact of the environmental factors to pubertal timing. Girls from families of low socioeconomic status experience menarche later than girls from affluent families [21, 22]. Parental education has been associated with the timing of puberty, higher education related to earlier onset of puberty. The absence of biological father, especially in the first 5 years of life, is also related to earlier puberty, and the association becomes stronger when the absence of biological father is combined with the presence of a stepfather and a stressful family environment [23, 24]. The place of residence during childhood is also important for the timing of puberty, urban girls experiencing menarche earlier than rural girls [25, 26].

Adoption of Third World children in Western Europe has been related to early puberty, especially in girls. The early sexual maturation may be triggered by the catch-up growth that is the usual growth pattern of these children after undernutrion [27] or recovery from psychosocial deprivation [28].

On the other hand, chronic illnesses, conditions of war [29], and in general conditions related to chronic stress result in suppression of HPG axis and delay in pubertal onset.

Endocrine Disruptors

Endocrine disruptors or endocrine-disrupting chemicals (EDCs) are mainly man-made, exogenous compounds (chemicals) that can interfere with the activity of endogenous hormones or disturb hormone signaling systems. EDCs mimic or block hormone signaling through the relevant hormonal receptor or modulate the synthesis, metabolism, and binding or elimination of natural hormones. EDCs are mainly used in industry, as solvents/lubricants [polychlorinated biphenyls (PCBs), polybrominated biphenyls (PBBs), dioxins], plastics [bisphenol A (BPA)], plasticizers (phthalates), pesticides [methoxychlor, chlorpyrifos, dichlorodiphenyltrichloroethane (DDT)], fungicides (vinclozolin), and also as pharmaceutical agents [diethylstilbestrol (DES)] [30]. EDCs may also be made by nature, e.g., phytoestrogens that interfere with endogenous endocrine function are produced by plants.

EDCs may affect the reproductive system via peripheral actions. Endocrine disruptors may have estrogenic activity, e.g., BPA; thus, their action is exerted through estrogen receptor; others, e.g., vinclozolin, interact with the androgen receptor, while other EDCs, e.g., fadrozole and ketoconazole, inhibit aromatase or steroidogenesis, respectively. On the other hand EDCs may affect puberty via CNS regulation. Atrazine delays puberty, reducing circulating LH and prolactin, in Sprague-Dawley (SD) and Long-Evans hooded (LE) rats [31]; phthalates and PCBs have been associated with earlier breast development and menarche, respectively [32].

The most commonly used and studied endocrine-disrupting chemicals are phthalates, bisphenol A, and pesticides.

Human exposure to phthalates is extremely prevalent and may occur through oral, inhaled, and topical routes. In a study on 129 Danish children and adolescents, the authors determined the concentrations of 11 phthalate metabolites of five different phthalate diesters on 24 h urine samples [33]. They found that phthalate metabolites were detectable in the urine of almost all children; younger children and boys were more exposed than older children and girls. The effect of phthalate exposure on the timing of puberty is controversial. In Puerto Rico high phthalate levels have been linked to premature thelarche [34]. In a study of 725 healthy Danish schoolgirls, it was demonstrated that high phthalate excretion in urine was associated with delayed pubarche, but not thelarche, which suggests antiandrogenic actions of phthalate [35]. Similar results were obtained in a study of US girls [36]. Some studies report early or precocious puberty, whereas others do not find such an association [37]. Moreover, in a study performed in China, elevated levels of phthalates were associated with constitutional delay of growth and puberty [38]. Therefore more studies are warranted to explore the effect of phthalate exposure on pubertal timing.

BPA is found in plastics (e.g., bottles, food cans, Tupperware, etc.), humans being exposed mainly through food contamination from plastic packaging. BPA is the most commonly found estrogen-like endocrine disruptor in the environment. Although it has been shown, in experimental animals, that BPA advances puberty [39], results on humans are inconsistent. In a study of 1151 girls, BPA had no influence on breast development [40]; however, in a Turkish study idiopathic central precocious puberty was associated with higher levels of BPA than control girls [41]. Thus, more studies are needed to clarify the existence of an association between BPA and pubertal maturation.

Pesticides are classified in various classes, e.g., insecticides are used for killing insects, and herbicides and fungicides are used against unwanted plants and fungi, respectively. Pesticides enter the human body through water, air, and food, and also, they can pass from the mother to the fetus via placenta and to the infant through mother's milk. Most of these substances cannot be broken down by the body, are lipophilic, and accumulate in adipose tissue, where they remain for long periods of time. The most widely studied pesticide compounds are DDT and its metabolite dichlorodiethyl dichloroethane (DDE). Although the agricultural use of DDT has been banned worldwide, in some developing countries, it is still used against the mosquitoes, as vectors of malaria.

Vasiliu et al. reported decrease in menarcheal age to girls exposed in utero to DDE [42]. However, when weight at menarche was controlled for, the significance of the association disappeared. In a Danish study of mothers who worked in greenhouses in the first trimester of pregnancy, the mothers were prenatally categorized as exposed or unexposed to pesticides. The female offspring of the exposed greenhouse workers had a significantly decreased age at onset of breast development at 8.9 years, compared with 10.4 years in the unexposed, and 10.0 years in a Danish reference population [43]. In a study examining the prenatal DDT exposure in relation to anthropometric and pubertal measures in adolescent males, no associations between prenatal exposure to any of the DDT compounds and any pubertal measures were noted [44]. Adopted or immigrant girls in Belgium, who presented central precocious puberty (CPP), had increased plasma levels of pesticides (DDE); thus, the authors suggested that CPP could be attributed to pesticide exposure [45]. However, other studies did not find an association between DDE levels and timing of menarche [46]. Also, in inner-city girls DDE, Pb, and dietary intakes of phytoestrogens were not significantly associated with breast stage [47].

The inconsistency of the results of the various studies examining the association of pesticides with onset of puberty makes imperative that more studies on the subject are needed.

Secular Trend in Human Maturation

Historical Data

One of the oldest inscriptions relating to age at menarche was from India, mainly by legislators, and they usually referred to upper-class girls. It is remarkable that from 500 BC until 500 AD, the age at menarche was reported to be 12 years [48].

At about the same time, the Greek philosopher and biologist Aristotle (384–322 BC) in his writings "Historia Animalium" reported the age at menarche to occur at 14 years and that at the same age ejacularche occurred in boys. Other physicians of the Greek-Roman era, i.e., Soranus of Ephesus (second half of first century AD), Galen (129–199 AD), and Oribasius (325 ca 400 AD), the personal physician of Julian the Apostate, also reported that in the majority of girls, menarche occurred at 14 years. However, these writings should be considered with care, since the age at menarche of 14 years may be related to the traditional mystical number 7.

For Chinese female, life is dominated by the number 7, first teeth erupting at 7 months of age and puberty, as marked by menarche, at 14 years. For boys the dominant number was 8, teeth erupting at 8 months and puberty, presumably ejacularche, occurring at 16 years [49].

In the medieval years, the age at menarche is generally reported to be similar to the classical years, i.e., 14 years, with a range from 12–15 years [50].

The age at menarche started to delay at the beginning of the modern era, especially after the industrial revolution, due to deterioration of hygiene and increasing population density that resulted in the spread of diseases. From available data it is estimated that in the second half of the eighteenth century, menarche occurred at 15–16 years of age. By mid-nineteenth century, the age at menarche in France was 15 years, whereas in Scandinavia was 17 years, suggesting the existence of a north to south gradient in pubertal maturation [51, 52].

Girls

Onset of Puberty in Girls

In the twentieth century the improvement of the socioeconomic conditions and the hygiene of the population resulted in increased somatic growth and earlier pubertal maturation of the children. The latter was most clearly evident in the age at menarche, which decreased substantially during the previous century. Although there is an abundance of studies on menarche and its secular trend in many countries, the studies that report on the timing of onset of puberty, i.e., breast development-B2 (thelarche), are much fewer. As far as pubic hair development is concerned, most experts believe that the onset of pubic hair development (PH2) is highly variable, depending on the individual, ethnicity, and race; therefore, the data are insufficient to establish a secular trend for PH2 [53].

Most studies on the secular trends of the onset of puberty refer to American or European girls.

In a developed country like Denmark, in a study performed in Copenhagen, onset of puberty, i.e., B2, occurred significantly earlier in the year 2006 (estimated mean age 9.86 years) compared to 1991 (estimated mean age 10.88 years), the difference remaining significant after adjustment for BMI [54]. In the Netherlands in a study examining the secular trend in three time points, i.e., in 1965, 1980, and 1997, it was shown that there was a decrease in the age of B2 between 1965 and 1980, but afterward the trend tended to stabilize, and median B2 was 11.0 years in 1965, 10.54 in 1980, and 10.7 years in 1997 [55]. In Krakow, Poland, age of thelarche declined between 1983 and 2010 from 10.9 to 10.3 years, respectively, that may be related to the socioeconomic changes that took place in Poland in the late twentieth century [56]. In Istanbul, Turkey, in a transitional society, i.e., a society undergoing large socioeconomic changes, the age at B2 decreased from 10 years in 1973 to 9.65 in 2009 [57]. In Athens, Greece, our group, in the 1990s, performed two studies, one cross-sectional and one longitudinal, examining the age of onset of female puberty [58]. In the cross-sectional study in 1995, we reported mean age at B2 to occur at 10.3 years, and in the longitudinal study, from 1990 to 1997, median age of onset of puberty was 10.0 years, and mean age was 9.9 years. In a study of Athenian girls in 1979, breast development occurred at 10.6 years [59]. These studies suggest a secular trend toward earlier onset of puberty between 1979 and 1995.

In 1997 in the USA, Herman-Giddens et al. [60] published a study performed by the Pediatric Research in Office Settings (PROS) network aiming to determine, by inspection, Tanner stages for breast and pubic hair development in 3-year-old to 12-year-old girls. The authors collected data on more than 17,000 girls (90 % white and 10 % black). The main finding of the study was that the mean age of onset of B2 was 10.0 years in white and 8.9 years in black girls, with a similar trend for pubic hair appearance that was 10.5 years for white and 8.8 years for black girls. All these estimates were earlier than those of previous studies. In the small longitudinal study of Nicolson and Hanley [61], children born in Berkeley, California, in 1928 and 1929, were followed yearly and when 8 years old half yearly until they reached the age of 18 years. Mean age of breast development in this sample was at 10.6 years and of pubic hair 11.6 years. In the Bogalusa Heart Study (9/1973-5/1974) mean age (±2 SE) of breast development in white girls was 10.37 (0.21) years and in black girls 10.22 (0.25) [61].

Table 9.2 Secular changes in the age at menarche (AAM)

	Time period	AAM (years)	Time period	AAM (years)	References
Decreasing AAM					
Canada	Year of birth <1933	13.2	Year of birth 1986–1990	12.5	[62]
China	Year of birth 1955–1960	15.7	Year of birth 1981–1985	14.7	[63]
India	Year of birth 1955–1964	13.8	Year of birth 1985–1989	13.6	[64]
Denmark	Year of study 1991	13.4	Year of study 2006	13.1	[54]
Israel	Year of birth 1969	13.4	Year of birth 1995	12.8	[65]
Korea	Year of birth 1920	16.8	Year of birth 1986	12.7	[66]
S. Africa (blacks)	Year of birth 1956	14.9	Year of birth 1990	12.4	[67]
UK	Year of birth 1945–1949	12.6	Year of birth 1990–1993	12.3	[69]
Slowing down or leveling off in AAM					
USA	Year of birth 1980	12.3	Year of birth 1993	12.3	[72]
France	Year of study 1994	12.6	Year of study 2009–2010	12.5	[75]
Greece	Year of study 1996	12.27	Year of study 2006	12.29	[77]
Netherlands	Year of study 1997	13.15	Year of study 2009	13.05	[78]

Age at Menarche

The studies examining the secular trend of age at menarche in various populations are numerous. Some of these studies are shown in Table 9.2. In general, for the most part of the twentieth century and the beginning of the twenty-first century, there is a trend for earlier ages at menarche. A secular change for earlier menarche is still occurring in developing and also in developed countries, e.g., Canada [62], China [63], Denmark [54], India [64], Israel [65], Korea [66], South Africa [67], Spain [68], and the UK [69].

In the USA, the mean age at menarche was more than 14 years in the nineteenth century [70], and in the NHANES III, in the late twentieth century (between 1988 and 1994) [71], it decreased to 12.43 years. The Fels Longitudinal Study of girls born in 1980 showed that menarche was at a slightly younger age at 12.34 years [72]. Comparing the data of NHANES III to those of NHES II/III [73], there was a decrease in menarcheal age of 4 months from 1963–1970 to 1988–1994. In the latest report on age at menarche in US girls [74], it was shown that girls born in 1993 had menarche at 12.3 years of age, at is similar to those born in 1980.

As in the latest report from the USA, and in some other countries, this trend is slowing down or has stabilized, e.g., France [75], Germany [76], Greece [77], and the Netherlands [78].

Furthermore, it is noteworthy that in Israel [65] and the UK [69], there is a recent decline in the age at menarche after decades of stabilization.

Menarche is often used as a proxy for the onset of puberty. However, studies from the USA and Denmark have shown that the decrease in onset of puberty (B2) is not accompanied by an analogous decrease in age at menarche. This discrepancy may be due to maturational tempo differences.

Maturational Tempo Differences and Age at Menarche

Early studies on the correlation between menarche and onset of puberty, in women born between 1920 and the 1960s, showed high correlations (0.64–0.86), whereas data from women born between 1977 and 1979 showed only a moderate correlation (0.37–0.38) [15]. An explanation of this may be a change in maturational tempo in girls born in the last part of the twentieth century. Several studies performed during the last two decades showed early-maturing girls to present a compensatory delay in pubertal progression [79–81] that is associated with greater pubertal height gain and a longer period of pubertal growth, thus explaining the moderate correlation between onset of puberty and age at menarche.

Boys

Onset of Puberty in Boys

The studies referring to the onset of puberty of boys are much fewer than those referring to girls. This may be due to refusal of the boys to be examined in the genital area or because of less interest in male puberty reflecting less cultural awareness for male pubertal maturation compared with girls [53]. Therefore, the secular trend of pubertal onset is less well studied in boys. In general, whereas the secular trend for earlier maturation is well established in girls, that is not the case for boys.

A substantial number of studies do not show secular trends in male pubertal onset. In the Netherlands in a study on pubertal maturation between 1965 and 1997, the authors did not detect a secular trend after 1980, attainment of TV of 4 mL being at 11.5 years [55]. In Istanbul, Turkey, in a longitudinal study from 1989 to 1999, TV of 4 mL was attained at a mean age of 11.6 years, whereas pubic hair development was at 12.3 years [82]. In an older Turkish study of boys born between 1955 and 1960, pubic hair was reported to develop at 11.8 years (no TV was measured), indirectly suggesting no secular trend [83]. In Athens, Greece, we did not find a significant change in the attainment of genital stage 2 (G2) between 1996 and 2007–2009, mean ages of G2 being 11.4 and 11.3 years, respectively [84]. In the USA, an expert panel that examined in 2005 possible secular trends in boys' puberty had the unanimous opinion that the data are insufficient to suggest or establish a trend for earlier puberty. This opinion was based on the lack of data quality, quantity, and marker reliability [53]. Many studies did not assess the more meaningful measure of pubertal onset, i.e., TV >3 mL. In 2012 the PROS network published their findings on male pubertal onset. The attainment of a TV of ≥4 mL was 11.46 for white, 11.75 for African American, and 11.29 for Hispanic boys and for PH2 was 11.47, 10.25, and 11.43 years, respectively. The authors concluded that testicular growth and pubic hair development were 6 months to 2 years earlier than in the past [19]. A secular trend for earlier onset of puberty was observed also in Copenhagen, Demark [85]. Between 2006–2008 and 1991–1993, mean onset of puberty decreased by 3 months, i.e., from 11.92 to the older to 11.66 years to the latest study.

Spermarche (Ejacularche)

If the data on pubertal onset in boys are relatively few, the age of the first conscious ejaculation (ejacularche) is scarcely examined. In boys, ejacularche may be considered analogous to menarche in girls. The term spermarche, in some studies, defines the first appearance of spermatozoa in urine samples (spermaturia), whereas other studies by spermarche define the first conscious ejaculation; however, the latter is best defined by the term ejacularche. Tanner in "Normal Growth and Growth assessment" [86] reports that ejacularche occurs about a year after the acceleration of penile growth, based on the work of Laron [87]. In their study Laron et al. found that despite a wide variation in the chronological age, the first ejaculation occurred, bone age, i.e., biological age, was 13.5 (±0.5) years, even in boys with delayed puberty.

In a longitudinal study, about 30 years ago, in Denmark [88], spermaturia occurred at a median age of 13.4 years (range 11.7–15.3 years), median TV being 11.5 mL (range 4.7–19.6 mL). In most boys spermaturia preceded peak height velocity. In a Mexican cross-sectional study, published in 1992, median age at spermaturia was 13.4 years, spermaturia occurring at a genital stage 2 [89], whereas in another Mexican study of teenagers and young adults (10–25 years of age) interviewed in 1987, the average age of ejacularche was 14 years [90]. In a Bulgarian study conducted in the 1990s, mean age of ejacularche was reported to occur at 13.27 (±1.08) [91]. In that study the authors reported a clear secular trend when their data were compared to studies of the year 1914, ejacularche occurring at 17 years, and of 1953, when ejacularche occurred at 15 years of age. In a Chinese study conducted in the year 1995, schoolchildren were interviewed about ejacularche. In urban males median age of ejacularche was 13.8 and in rural males 14.24 years [92]. In a study of urban Chinese boys conducted between 2003 and 2005, ejacularche was reported to occur at a median age of 14.05 years [93]. In 2004 it was reported that boys in Estonia presented ejacularche at a mean age of 13.35 (±0.99) years [94].

Therefore, from the limited available studies, it can be deduced that ejacularche in European boys occurs at around the age of 13.5 years. It is of historical interest that Aristotle wrote that, in Athenian boys in the fourth century BC, ejacularche occurred at 14 years of age!

References

1. Key TJ, Verkasalo PK, Banks E. Epidemiology of breast cancer. Lancet Oncol. 2001;2:133–40.
2. Velie EM, Nechuta S, Osuch JR. Lifetime reproductive and anthropometric risk factors for breast cancer in postmenopausal women. Breast Dis. 2005;24:17–35.
3. Lakshman R, Forouhi NG, Sharp SJ, Luben R, Bingham SA, Khaw KT, Wareham NJ, Ong KK. Early age at menarche associated with cardiovascular disease and mortality. J Clin Endocrinol Metab. 2009;94:4953–60.
4. Golub MS, Collman GW, Foster PM, Kimmel CA, Rajpert-De Meyts E, Reiter EO, Sharpe RM, Skakkebaek NE, Toppari J. Public health implications of altered puberty timing. Pediatrics. 2008;121 Suppl 3:S218–30.
5. Naves M, Diaz-Lopez JB, Gomez C, Rodriguez-Rebollar A, Cannata-Andia JB. Determinants of incidence of osteoporotic fractures in the female Spanish population older than 50. Osteoporos Int. 2005;16:2013–7.
6. Slora EJ, Bocian AB, Herman-Giddens ME, Harris DL, Pedlow SE, Dowshen SA, Wasserman RC. Assessing inter-rater reliability (IRR) of Tanner staging and orchidometer use with boys: a study from PROS. J Pediatr Endocrinol Metab. 2009;22(4):291–9.
7. Sotos JF, Tokar NJ. Testicular volumes revisited: a proposal for a simple clinical method that can closely match the volumes obtained by ultrasound and its clinical application. Int J Pediatric Endocrinol 2012;2012:17.
8. Laron Z. Age at first ejaculation (spermarche)--the overlooked milestone in male development. Pediatr Endocrinol Rev. 2010;7(3):256–7.
9. Sørensen K, Juul A, Christensen K, Skytthe A, Scheike T, Kold JT. Birth size and age at menarche: a twin perspective. Hum Reprod. 2013;28(10):2865–71.
10. Morris DH, Jones ME, Schoemaker MJ, Ashworth A, Swerdlow AJ. Familial concordance for age at menarche: analyses from the breakthrough generations study. Paediatr Perinat Epidemiol. 2011;25(3):306–11.
11. Perry JR, Day F, Elks CE, Sulem P, Thompson DJ, Ferreira T, et al. Parent-of-origin-specific allelic associations among 106 genomic loci for age at menarche. Nature. 2014;514(7520):92–7.
12. Ong KK, Elks CE, Li S, Zhao JH, Luan J, Andersen LB, et al. Genetic variation in LIN28B is associated with the timing of puberty. Nat Genet. 2009;41(6):729–33.
13. Hagen CP, Sørensen K, Aksglaede L, Mouritsen A, Mieritz MG, Tinggaard J, Wohlfart-Veje C, Petersen JH, Main KM, Rajpert-De Meyts E, Almstrup K, Juul A. Pubertal onset in girls is strongly influenced by genetic variation affecting FSH action. Sci Rep. 2014;4:6412.
14. Lomniczi A, Loche A, Castellano JM, Ronnekleiv OK, Bosch M, Kaidar G, Knoll JG, Wright H, Pfeifer GP, Ojeda SR. Epigenetic control of female puberty. Nat Neurosci. 2013;16:281–9.
15. Biro FM, Huang B, Crawford PB, Lucky AW, Striegel-Moore R, Barton BA, Daniels S. Pubertal correlates in black and white girls. J Pediatr. 2006;148:234–40.
16. Freedman DS, Khan LK, Serdula MK, Dietz WH, Srinivasan SR, Berenson GS. Relation to age at menarche to race, time period, and anthropometric dimensions: the Bogalusa heart study. Pediatrics. 2002;110, e43.
17. Higgins PB, Fernandez JR, Goran MI, Gower BA. Early ethnic difference in insulin-like growth factor-1 is associated with African genetic admixture. Pediatr Res. 2005;58:850–4.
18. Sun SS, Schubert CM, Chumlea WC, Roche AF, Kulin HE, Lee PA, Himes JH, Ryan AS. National estimates of the timing of sexual maturation and racial differences among US children. Pediatrics. 2002;110(5):911–9.
19. Herman-Giddens ME, Steffes J, Harris D, Slora E, Hussey M, Dowshen SA, Wasserman R, Serwint JR, Smitherman L, Reiter EO. Secondary sexual characteristics in boys: data from the Pediatric Research in Office Settings Network. Pediatrics. 2012;130(5):e1058–68.
20. Biro FM, Lucky AW, Huster GA, Morrison JA. Pubertal staging in boys. J Pediatr. 1995;127:100–2.
21. Wronka I, Pawlinska-Chmara R. Menarcheal age and socioeconomic factors in Poland. Ann Hum Biol. 2005;32:630–8.

22. Deardorff J, Ekwaru JP, Kushi LH, Ellis BJ, Greenspan LC, Mirabedi A, Landaverde EG, Hiatt RA. Father absence, body mass index, and pubertal timing in girls: differential effects by family income and ethnicity. J Adolesc Health. 2011;48:441–7.
23. Ellis BJ, Garber J. Psychosocial antecedents of variation in girls' pubertal timing: maternal depression, stepfather presence, and marital and family stress. Child Dev. 2000;71:485–501.
24. Culpin I, Heron J, Araya R, Joinson C. Early childhood father absence and depressive symptoms in adolescent girls from a UK Cohort: the mediating role of early menarche. J Abnorm Child Psychol. 2014;20. epub ahead of print.
25. Padez C. Social background and age of menarche in Portuguese university students: a note on the secular changes in Portugal. Am J Hum Biol. 2003;15:415–27.
26. Szwed A, John A, Czapla Z, Kosińska M. Influence of socioeconomic factors on age at menarche of Polish girls. Anthropol Anz. 2013;70(4):455–70.
27. Proos L, Gustafsson J. Is early puberty triggered by catch-up growth following undernutrition? Int J Environ Res Public Health. 2012;9:1791–809.
28. Dominé F, Parent AS, Rasier G, Lebrethon MC, Bourguignon JP. Assessment and mechanism of variations in pubertal timing in internationally adopted children: a developmental hypothesis. Eur J Endocrinol. 2006;155:S17–25.
29. Tahirović HF. Menarchal age and the stress of war: an example from Bosnia. Eur J Pediatr. 1998;157:978–80.
30. Diamanti-Kandarakis E, Bourguignon JP, Guidice LC, Hauser R, Prins GS, Soto AM, Zoeller RT, Gore AC. Endocrine disrupting- chemicals: an endocrine society scientific statement. Endocr Rev. 2009;30:293–342.
31. Cooper RL, Stoker TE, Tyrey L, Goldman JM, Mc Elroy WK. Atrazine disrupts the hypothalamic control of pituitary ovarian function. Toxicol Sci. 2000;53:297–307.
32. Jacobson-Dickman E, Lee MM. The influence of endocrine disruptors on pubertal timing. Curr Opin Endocrinol Diabetes Obes. 2009;16:25–30.
33. Frederiksen H, Aksglaede L, Sorensen K, Skakkebaek NE, Juul A, Andersson AM. Urinary excretion of phthalate metabolites in 129 healthy Danish children and adolescents: estimation of daily phthalate intake. Environ Res. 2011;111:656–63.
34. Colon I, Caro D, Bourdony CJ, Rosario O. Identification of phthalate esters in the serum of young Puerto Rican girls with premature breast development. Environ Health Perspect. 2000;108:895–900.
35. Frederiksen H, Sørensen K, Mouritsen A, Aksglaede L, Hagen CP, Petersen JH, Skakkebaek NE, Andersson AM, Juul A. High urinary phthalate concentration associated with delayed pubarche in girls. Int J Androl. 2012;35:216–26.
36. Wolff MS, Teitelbaum SL, McGovern K, Windham GC, Pinney SM, Galvez M, Calafat AM, Kushi LH, Biro FM, Breast Cancer and Environment Research Program. Phthalate exposure and pubertal development in a longitudinal study of US girls. Hum Reprod. 2014;29(7):1558–66.
37. Lomenick JP, Calafat AM, Melguizo Castro MS, Mier R, Stenger P, Foster MB, et al. Phthalate exposure and precocious puberty in females. J Pediatr. 2010;156:221–5.
38. Xie C, Zhao Y, Gao L, Chen J, Cai D, Zhang Y. Elevated phthalates' exposure in children with constitutional delay of growth and puberty. Mol Cell Endocrinol. 2015;407:67–73.
39. Howdeshell KL, Hotchkiss AK, Thayer KA, Vandenbergh JG, vom Saal FS. Exposure to bisphenol a advances puberty. Nature. 1999;401:763–4.
40. Wolff MS, Teitelbaum SL, Pinney SM, Windham G, Liao L, Biro F, Kushi LH, Erdmann C, Hiatt RA, Rybak ME, Calafat AM, Breast Cancer and Environment Research Centers. Investigation of relationships between urinary biomarkers of phytoestrogens, phthalates, and phenols and pubertal stages in girls. Environ Health Perspect. 2010;118:1039–46.
41. Durmaz E, et al. Urinary bisphenol a levels in girls with idiopathic central precocious puberty. J Clin Res Pediatr Endocrinol 2014;6:16–21.
42. Vasiliu O, Muttineni J, Karmaus W. In utero exposure to organochlorines and age at menarche. Hum Reprod. 2004;19:1506–12.

43. Wohlfahrt-Veje C, Andersen H, Schmidt I, Aksglaede L, Sørensen K, Juul A, Jensen T, Grandjean P, Skakkebaek N, Main K. Early breast development in girls after prenatal exposure to non-persistent pesticides. Int J Androl 2012;35:273–82.
44. Gladen BC, Klebanoff MA, Hediger ML, Katz SH, Barr DB, Davis MD, Longnecker MP. Prenatal DDT exposure in relation to anthropometric and pubertal measures in adolescent males. Environ Health Perspect. 2004;112:1761–7.
45. Krstevska-Konstantinova M, Charlier C, Craen M, Du Caju M, Heinrichs C, de Beaufort C, Plomteux G, Bourguignon JP. Sexual precocity after immigration from developing countries to Belgium: evidence of previous exposure to organochlorine pesticides. Hum Reprod. 2001;16:1020–6.
46. Denham M, Schell LM, Deane G, Gallo MV, Ravenscroft J, DeCaprio AP, Akwesasne Task Force on the Environment. Relationship of lead, mercury, mirex, dichlorodiphenyl dichloroethylene, hexachlorobenzene, and polychlorinated biphenyls to timing of menarche among Akwesasne Mohawk girls. Pediatrics. 2005;115:e127–34.
47. Wolff MS, Britton JA, Boguski L, Hochman S, Maloney N, Serra N, Liu Z, Berkowitz G, Larson S, Forman J. Environmental exposures and puberty in inner-city girls. Environ Res. 2008;107:393–400.
48. Datta B, Gupta D. The age at menarche in classical India. Ann Hum Biol. 1981;8:351–9.
49. Medvei VC. The ancient Chinese. In: A history of endocrinology. MTP Press Limited, Lancaster, England; 1982. p. 15–18.
50. Amundsen DW, Diers CJ. The age of menarche in medieval Europe. Hum Biol. 1973;45:363–9.
51. Ducros A, Pasquet P. Evolution de l'âge d'apparition des premières règles (ménarche) en France. Biometrie Humaine. 1978;13:35–43.
52. Eveleth PB. Population differences in growth: environmental and genetic factors. In: Falkner F, Tanner JM, editors. Human growth. New York: Plenum Press; 1978. p. 373–94.
53. Euling SY, Herman-Giddens ME, Lee PA, Selevan SG, Juul A, Sørensen TI, Dunkel L, Himes JH, Teilmann G, Swan SH. Examination of US puberty-timing data from 1940 to 1994 for secular trends: panel findings. Pediatrics. 2008;121(Suppl 3):S172–91.
54. Aksglaede L, Sørensen K, Petersen JH, Skakkebaek NE, Juul A. Recent decline in age at breast development: the Copenhagen Puberty Study. Pediatrics. 2009;123:e932–9.
55. Mul D, Fredriks AM, van Buuren S, Oostdijk W, Verloove-Vanhorick SP, Wit JM. Pubertal development in The Netherlands 1965–1997. Pediatr Res. 2001;50:479–86.
56. Woronkowicz A, Cichocka BA, Kowal M, Kryst L, Sobiecki J. Physical development of girls from Krakow in the aspect of socioeconomical changes in Poland (1938–2010). Am J Hum Biol. 2012;24:626–32.
57. Atay Z, Turan S, Guran T, Furman A, Bereket A. Puberty and influencing factors in schoolgirls living in Istanbul: end of the secular trend? Pediatrics. 2011;128:e40–5.
58. Papadimitriou A, Pantsiotou S, Douros K, Papadimitriou DT, Nicolaidou P, Fretzayas A. Timing of pubertal onset in girls: evidence for non-Gaussian distribution. J Clin Endocrinol Metab. 2008;93:4422–5.
59. Dacou-Voutetakis C, Klontza D, Lagos P, Tzonou A, Katsarou E, Antoniadis S, Papazisis G, Papadopoulos G, Matsaniotis N. Age of pubertal stages including menarche in Greek girls. Ann Hum Biol. 1983;10:557–63.
60. Herman-Giddens ME, Slora EJ, Wasserman RC, et al. Secondary sexual characteristics and menses in young girls seen in office practice: a study from the Pediatrics Research in Office Settings Network. Pediatrics. 1997;99:505–12.
61. Nicolson AB, Hanley C. Indices of physiological maturity: derivation and interrelationships. Child Dev. 1953;24:3–38.
62. Harris MA, Prior JC, Koehoorn M. Age at menarche in the Canadian population: secular trends and relationship to adulthood BMI. J Adolesc Health. 2008;43(6):548–54.
63. Lyu Y, Mirea L, Yang J, Warre R, Zhang J, Lee SK, Li Z. Secular trends in age at menarche among women born between 1955 and 1985 in Southeastern China. BMC Womens Health. 2014;14:155.

64. Pathak PK, Tripathi N, Subramanian SV. Secular trends in menarcheal age in India-evidence from the Indian human development survey. PLoS One. 2014;9(11), e111027.
65. Flash-Luzzatti S, Weil C, Shalev V, Oron T, Chodick G. Long-term secular trends in the age at menarche in Israel: a systematic literature review and pooled analysis. Horm Res Paediatr. 2014;81(4):266–71.
66. Hwang JY, Shin C, Frongillo EA, Shin KR, Jo I. Secular trend in age at menarche for South Korean women born between 1920 and 1986: the Ansan Study. Ann Hum Biol. 2003;30(4):434–42.
67. Jones LL, Griffiths PL, Norris SA, Pettifor JM, Cameron N. Age at menarche and the evidence for a positive secular trend in urban South Africa. Am J Hum Biol. 2009;21(1):130–2.
68. Soriano Guillén L, Blanco Rodríguez M, Cortés Martín M, Martínez MC. Secular trend of menarcheal age in Spanish adolescents. Med Clin (Barc). 2008;131(9):355–6.
69. Morris DH, Jones ME, Schoemaker MJ, Ashworth A, Swerdlow AJ. Secular trends in age at menarche in women in the UK born 1908–93: results from the Breakthrough Generations Study. Paediatr Perinat Epidemiol. 2011;25(4):394–400.
70. Wyshak G, Frisch RE. Evidence for a secular trend in age of menarche. N Engl J Med. 1982;306:1033–5.
71. Chumlea WC, Schubert CM, Roche AF, Kulin HE, Lee PA, Himes JH, Sun SS. Age at menarche and racial comparisons in US girls. Pediatrics. 2003;111:110–3.
72. Demerath EW, Towne B, Chumlea WC, Sun SS, Czerwinski SA, Remsberg KE, Siervogel RM. Recent decline in age at menarche: the Fels Longitudinal Study. Am J Hum Biol. 2004;16:453–7.
73. MacMahon B. Age at menarche. Rockville, MD: National Center for Health Statistics; 1973. DHEW publication (HRA) 74–1615.
74. Finer LB, Philbin JM. Trends in ages at key reproductive transitions in the United States, 1951–2010. Womens Health Issues. 2014;24(3):e271–9.
75. Lalys L, Pineau JC. Age at menarche in a group of French schoolgirls. Pediatr Int. 2014;56(4):601–4.
76. Gohlke B, Woelfle J. Growth and puberty in German children: is there still a positive secular trend? Dtsch Arztebl Int. 2009;106(23):377–82.
77. Papadimitriou A, Fytanidis G, Douros K, Bakoula C, Nicolaidou P, Fretzayas A. Age at menarche in contemporary Greek girls: evidence for levelling-off of the secular trend. Acta Paediatr. 2008;97(6):812–5.
78. Talma H, Schönbeck Y, van Dommelen P, Bakker B, van Buuren S, Hirasing RA. Trends in menarcheal age between 1955 and 2009 in the Netherlands. PLoS One. 2013;8(4), e60056.
79. Marti- Henneberg C, Vizmanos B. The duration of puberty in girls is related to the timing of its onset. J Pediatr. 1997;131:618–21.
80. Biro FM, McMahon RP, Striegel-Moore R, Crawford P, Obarzanek E, Barton BA, Falkner F. Impact of timing of pubertal maturation on growth in black and white female adolescents the NHLBI Growth and Health Study. J Pediatr. 2001;138:636–43.
81. Pantsiotou S, Papadimitriou A, Douros K, Priftis K, Nicolaidou P, Fretzayas A. Maturational tempo differences in relation to the timing of the onset of puberty in girls. Acta Paediatr. 2008;97:217–20.
82. Bundak R, et al. Analysis of puberty and pubertal growth in healthy boys. Eur J Pediatr. 2007;166(6):595–600.
83. Neyzi O, Alp H, Yalçindag A, Yakacikli S, Orphon A. Sexual maturation in Turkish boys. Ann Hum Biol. 1975;2:251–9.
84. Papadimitriou A, Douros K, Kleanthous K, et al. Pubertal maturation of contemporary Greek boys: no evidence of a secular trend. J Adolesc Health. 2011;49:434–6.
85. Sørensen K, Aksglaede L, Petersen JH, Juul A. Recent changes in pubertal timing in healthy Danish boys: associations with body mass index. J Clin Endocrinol Metab. 2010;95(1):263–70.
86. Tanner JM. Normal growth and techniques of growth assessment. Clin Endocrinol Metab. 1986;15(3):411–51.

87. Laron Z, Arad J, Gurewitz R, Grunebaum M, Dickerman Z. Age at first conscious ejaculation: a milestone in male puberty. Helv Paediatr Acta 1980;35(1):13–20.
88. Nielsen CT, Skakkebaek NE, Richardson DW, Darling JA, Hunter WM, Jørgensen M, Nielsen A, Ingerslev O, Keiding N, Müller J. Onset of the release of spermatozoa (spermarche) in boys in relation to age, testicular growth, pubic hair, and height. J Clin Endocrinol Metab. 1986;62(3):532–5.
89. Guízar-Vázquez JJ, Rosales-López A, Ortiz-Jalomo R, Nava-Delgado SE, Salamanca-Gómez F. Age of onset of spermaturia (spermache) in 669 Mexican children and its relation to secondary sexual characteristics and height. Bol Med Hosp Infant Mex. 1992;49(1):12–7.
90. García-Baltazar J, Figueroa-Perea JG, Reyes-Zapata H, Brindis C, Pérez-Palacios G. The reproductive characteristics of adolescents and young adults in Mexico City. Salud Publica Mex. 1993;35(6):682–91.
91. Tomova A, Lalabonova C, Robeva RN, Kumanov PT. Timing of pubertal maturation according to the age at first conscious ejaculation. Andrologia. 2011;43(3):163–6.
92. Yan H, Dibley MJ, D'Este K, Hou R. The national survey on the constitution and health of chinese students in 1995: nutritional status of school students aged 10–17 years in Shaanxi, China. Asia Pac J Clin Nutr. 1999;8(2):121–8.
93. Ma HM, Chen SK, Chen RM, Zhu C, Xiong F, Li T, Wang W, Liu GL, Luo XP, Liu L, Du ML, Pubertal Study Group of the Society of Pediatric Endocrinology and Genetic Disease, Chinese Medical Association. Pubertal development timing in urban Chinese boys. Int J Androl. 2011;34(5 Pt 2):e435–45.
94. Veldre G, Jürimäe T. Anthropometric parameters and sexual maturation in 12- to 15-year-old Estonian boys. Anthropol Anz. 2004;62(2):203–15.

Chapter 10
Precocious Puberty

Juliane Léger and Jean-Claude Carel

Introduction

Precocious puberty is defined as the onset of clinical signs of puberty before the age of 8 years in girls and 9.5 years in boys. However, the onset of puberty may be subject to the effects of environmental (secular trends, adoption, absence of the father, and possible exposure to estrogenic endocrine-disrupting chemicals), nutritional (body mass index), and constitutional (genetics, ethnicity) factors [1–4], with implications for the definition of precocious puberty.

PP may be caused by central or peripheral mechanisms [1]. Precocious puberty leads to the progressive development of secondary sexual characteristics including breast development in girls and testicular enlargement in boys, together with the development of pubic hair, and an acceleration of growth velocity and bone maturation, resulting in premature fusion of the growth plates, potentially responsible for adult height deficit [1].

Premature sexual maturation is a frequent cause for referral. Clinical evaluation is generally sufficient to reassure the patients and their families, but premature sexual maturation may reveal severe conditions, and thorough evaluation is therefore required to identify its cause and potential for progression, so that appropriate treatment can be proposed.

The clinical expression of precocious puberty is polymorphic. In addition to progressive central PP, with a progressive deterioration of adult height prognosis in the absence of treatment, there are very slowly progressive forms which do not modify predicted final height. It is not always straightforward to recognize these different clinical forms at the initial evaluation. Nevertheless, their correct identification is

J. Léger (✉) • J.-C. Carel
Department of Paediatric Endocrinology and Diabetology, INSERM UMR 1141,
DHU PROTECT, Reference Center for Rare Endocrine Growth Diseases,
Denis Diderot Paris 7 University, Hôpital Robert Debré, 75019 Paris, France
e-mail: juliane.leger@aphp.fr

P. Kumanov, A. Agarwal (eds.), *Puberty*, DOI 10.1007/978-3-319-32122-6_10

very important, because the indicated treatments differ [5–7]. The heterogeneity of precocious puberty, in terms of its clinical presentation and definition, can be explained by the gradual nature of the transition to puberty. Indeed, the pulsatile secretion of LH begins before the onset of clinical signs of puberty, and an increase in the amplitude of the LH peaks is the key biological sign of pubertal maturation of the gonadotropic pituitary axis. GnRH stimulation tests indirectly reveal pulsatile endogenous GnRH secretion, as this secretion determines the response to exogenous GnRH. The available data indicate that there is no clear boundary between prepubertal and pubertal status, accounting for the frequency of "marginal" forms of precocious puberty.

Etiologies and Mechanisms Underlying Premature Sexual Development

Central precocious puberty (CPP), which is much more common in girls than in boys [8], results from premature reactivation of the hypothalamic–pituitary–gonadal axis and pulsatile GnRH secretion, with a hormonal pattern similar to that of normal puberty. Premature sexual development results from the action of sex steroids or compounds with sex steroid activity on target organs. CPP may be due to hypothalamic lesions, but is idiopathic in most cases, particularly in girls (Table 10.1) [1]. Recent studies have implicated the inactivation of makorin ring finger 3 (*MKRN3*) genes in "idiopathic" CPP [9, 10]. *MKRN3* is an imprinted gene located on the long arm of chromosome 15, with a potentially inhibitory effect on GnRH secretion. *MKRN3* gene defects have been identified as a cause of paternally transmitted familial CPP, but such defects do not underlie maternally transmitted CPP and are rarely involved in sporadic forms [11].

Peripheral or gonadotropin-independent precious puberty is due to the production of sex steroids by gonadal or adrenal tissue, independently of gonadotropins which are generally suppressed. Peripheral precocious puberty can result from gonadal, adrenal, or hCG-producing tumors, activating mutations in the gonadotropic pathway, and exposure to exogenous sex steroids (Table 10.2). Peripheral precocious puberty can rarely lead to activation of pulsatile GnRH secretion and to central precocious puberty (Table 10.1).

Exposure to exogenous sex steroids or to compounds with steroidal activity can also result in premature sexual development.

It is also important to recognize that most cases of premature sexual maturation correspond to benign variants of normal development that can occur throughout childhood. They can mimic precocious puberty but do not lead to long-term consequences and are usually benign. This is particularly true in girls below the age of 2–3 where the condition is known as premature thelarche. Similarly in older girls, at least 50 % of cases of premature sexual maturation will regress or stop progressing and no treatment is necessary [5, 6]. Although the mechanism underlying these

Table 10.1 Clinical characteristics of the various forms of central precocious puberty

Cause	Symptoms and signs	Evaluation
Due to a CNS lesion		
Hypothalamic hamartoma	May be associated with gelastic (laughing attacks), focal, or tonic–clonic seizures	MRI: mass in the floor of the third ventricle iso-intense to normal tissue without contrast enhancement
Or other hypothalamic tumors: • Glioma involving the hypothalamus and/or the optic chiasm • Astrocytoma • Ependymoma • Pinealoma • Germ cell tumors	May include headache, visual changes, cognitive changes, symptoms/signs of anterior or posterior pituitary deficiency (e.g., decreased growth velocity, polyuria–polydipsia), fatigue, visual field defects If CNS tumor (glioma) associated with neurofibromatosis may have other features of neurofibromatosis (cutaneous neurofibromas, café au lait spots, Lisch nodules, etc.)	MRI: contrast-enhanced mass that may involve the optic pathways (chiasm, nerve, tract) or the hypothalamus (astrocytoma, glioma) or that may involve the hypothalamus and pituitary stalk (germ cell tumor), may have evidence of intracranial hypertension, may have signs of anterior or posterior pituitary deficiency (e.g., hypernatremia) If germ cell tumor: βhCG detectable in blood or CSF
Cerebral malformations involving the hypothalamus: • Suprasellar arachnoid cyst • Hydrocephalus • Septooptic dysplasia • Myelomeningocele • Ectopic neurohypophysis	May have neurodevelopmental deficits, macrocrania, visual impairment, nystagmus, obesity, polyuria–polydipsia, decreased growth velocity	May have signs of anterior or posterior pituitary deficiency (e.g., hypernatremia) or hyperprolactinemia
Acquired injury: • Cranial irradiation • Head trauma • Infections • Perinatal insults	Relevant history Symptoms and signs of anterior or posterior pituitary deficiency may be present	MRI may reveal condition-specific sequelae or may be normal
Idiopathic—No CNS lesion	≈92 % of girls and ≈ 50 % of boys History of familial precocious puberty or adoption may be present	No hypothalamic abnormality on the head MRI. The anterior pituitary may be enlarged MKRN 3 gene evaluation if paternally transmitted
Secondary to early exposure to sex steroids		
After cure of any cause of gonadotropin-independent precocious puberty	Relevant history	

cases of nonprogressive precocious puberty is unknown, the gonadotropic axis is not activated. Premature thelarche probably represents an exaggerated form of the physiological early gonadotropin surge that is delayed in girls relatively to boys.

Table 10.2 Clinical characteristics of the various forms of peripheral precocious puberty

Disorder	Characteristic symptoms and signs	Test results
Autonomous gonadal activation		
McCune–Albright syndrome and recurrent autonomous ovarian cysts due to somatic activating mutation of the GNAS gene resulting in increased signal transduction in the Gs pathway	Mostly in girls. Typically rapid progression of breast development and early occurrence of vaginal bleeding (before or within a few months of breast development) Precocious puberty may be isolated or associated with café au lait pigmented skin lesions or bone pain due to polyostotic fibrous dysplasia. More rarely other signs of endocrine hyperfunction (e.g., hypercortisolism, hyperthyroidism), liver cholestasis, or cardiac rhythm abnormalities	Typically large ovarian cyst or cysts on pelvic ultrasound examination Bone lesions of fibrous dysplasia May have laboratory evidence of hypercortisolism, hyperthyroidism, increased GH secretion, hypophosphatemia, liver cholestasis
Familial male-limited precocious puberty due to germinal activating mutations of the LH receptor gene	A familial history of dominant precocious puberty limited to boys (but transmitted by mothers) may be present but some cases are sporadic	Activating mutation of the LH receptor gene
Germ line mutations of GNAS gene resulting in dual loss and gain of function (rare)	Single case report of a boy with concomitant pseudohypoparathyroidism and gonadotropin-independent precocious puberty	
Tumors		
Granulosa cell tumors of the ovary	Rapid progression of breast development; abdominal pain may occur. The tumor may be palpable on abdominal examination	Tumor detection on ultrasound or CT scan
Androgen producing ovarian tumors	Progressive virilization	Tumor detection on ultrasound or CT scan
Testicular Leydig cell tumors	Progressive virilization; testicular asymmetry (the tumor itself is rarely palpable)	Tumor detection on testicular ultrasound
hCG-producing tumors	Tumors can originate in the liver or mediastinum. Pubertal symptoms in boys only. May be associated with Klinefelter syndrome	Elevated serum hCG
Adrenal disorders	Manifest with signs of androgen exposure	
Congenital adrenal hyperplasia	Increased androgen production leading to virilization in boys and girls	Increased adrenal steroid precursors in serum, mainly 17-OH-progesterone (basal or after an ACTH stimulation test)
Adrenal tumor	Increased androgen production leading to virilization in boys and girls. Very rarely, estrogen-producing adrenal tumor	Tumor on abdominal ultrasound or CT scan Elevated DHEAS, or adrenal steroid precursors

(continued)

Table 10.2 (continued)

Disorder	Characteristic symptoms and signs	Test results
Generalized glucocorticoid resistance	Symptoms and signs of mineralocorticoid excess, such as hypertension and hypokalemic alkalosis	Elevated free urinary cortisol and plasma cortisol
Environmental agents		
Exogenous sex steroids	Manifestations vary with the type of preparation (androgenic or estrogenic); most commonly described after topical exposure to androgens; tracing the source of exposure may be difficult	Endocrine evaluation can be misleading due to widely variable serum levels of sex steroids with time
Exposure to estrogenic endocrine-disrupting chemicals	May play a role in precocious puberty in adopted children (by modulating the timing of pubertal gonadotropic axis activation) although this remains unproven	No validated biochemical test
Severe untreated primary hypothyroidism	Signs of hypothyroidism. No increase of growth velocity Manifest mostly with increased testicular volume in the absence of virilization. Due to a cross-reactivity of elevated TSH to the FSH receptor	Elevated serum TSH levels, low free T4 level. No bone age advancement

Consequences of Precocious Puberty

Progressive premature sexual maturation can have consequences on growth and psychosocial development. Growth velocity is accelerated as compared to normal values for age, and bone age is advanced in most cases. The acceleration of bone maturation can lead to premature fusion of the growth plate and short stature. Several studies have assessed adult height in individuals with a history of precocious puberty. In older published series of untreated patients, mean heights ranged from 151 to 156 cm in boys and 150 to 154 cm in girls, corresponding to a loss of about 20 cm in boys and 12 cm in girls relative to normal adult height [12]. However, these numbers correspond to historical series of patients with severe early onset precocious puberty which are not representative of the majority of patients seen in the clinic today. Height loss due to precocious puberty is inversely correlated with the age at pubertal onset, and currently treated patients tend to have later onset of puberty than those in historical series [12].

Parents often seek treatment in girls because they fear early menarche [13]. However, there is little data to predict the age of menarche following early onset of puberty [14]. In the general population, the time from breast development to menarche is longer for children with an earlier onset of puberty, ranging from a mean of 2.8 years when breast development begins at age 9–1.4 years when breast development begins at age 12 [15].

In the general population, early puberty timing has been shown to be associated with several health outcomes in adult life with higher risks for cardiovascular disease and type 2 diabetes in both women and men [16]. However, there is no long-term data on these aspects in case of precocious puberty.

Adverse psychosocial outcomes are also a concern, but the available data specific to patients with precocious puberty have serious limitations [17]. In the general population, a higher proportion of early-maturing adolescents engage in exploratory behaviors (sexual intercourse, legal and illegal substance use) and at an earlier age than adolescents maturing within the normal age range or later [18, 19]. In addition, the risk for sexual abuse seems to be higher in girls or women with early sexual maturation [20]. However, the relevance of these findings to precocious puberty is unclear, and they should not be used to justify intervention.

Evaluation of the Child with Premature Sexual Development

The evaluation of patients with premature sexual development should address several questions: (1) Is sexual development really occurring outside the normal temporal range? (2) What is the underlying mechanism and is it associated with a risk of a serious condition, such as an intracranial lesion? (3) Is pubertal development likely to progress, and (4) would this impair the child's normal physical and psychosocial development?

Clinical Diagnosis

Precocious puberty manifests as the progressive appearance of secondary sexual characteristics—breast development, pubic hair, and menarche in girls and enlargement of testicular volume (testicular volume greater than 4 ml or testicular length greater than 25 mm) and penis and pubic hair development in boys [21, 22] Fig 10.1—together with an acceleration of height velocity and bone maturation, which is frequently very advanced (by more than 2 years relative to chronological age). However, a single sign may remain the only sign for long periods, making diagnosis difficult, particularly in girls, in which isolated breast development may precede the appearance of pubic hair or the increase in growth velocity and bone maturation by several months. However, in some children, the increase in height velocity precedes the appearance of secondary sexual characteristics [23].

The clinical evaluation should guide the diagnosis and discussions about the most appropriate management (Table 10.3).

The interview is used to specify the age at onset and rate of progression of pubertal signs, to investigate neonatal parameters (gestational age, birth measurements) and whether the child was adopted, together with any evidence suggesting a possible central nervous disorder, such as headache, visual disturbances, or neurological

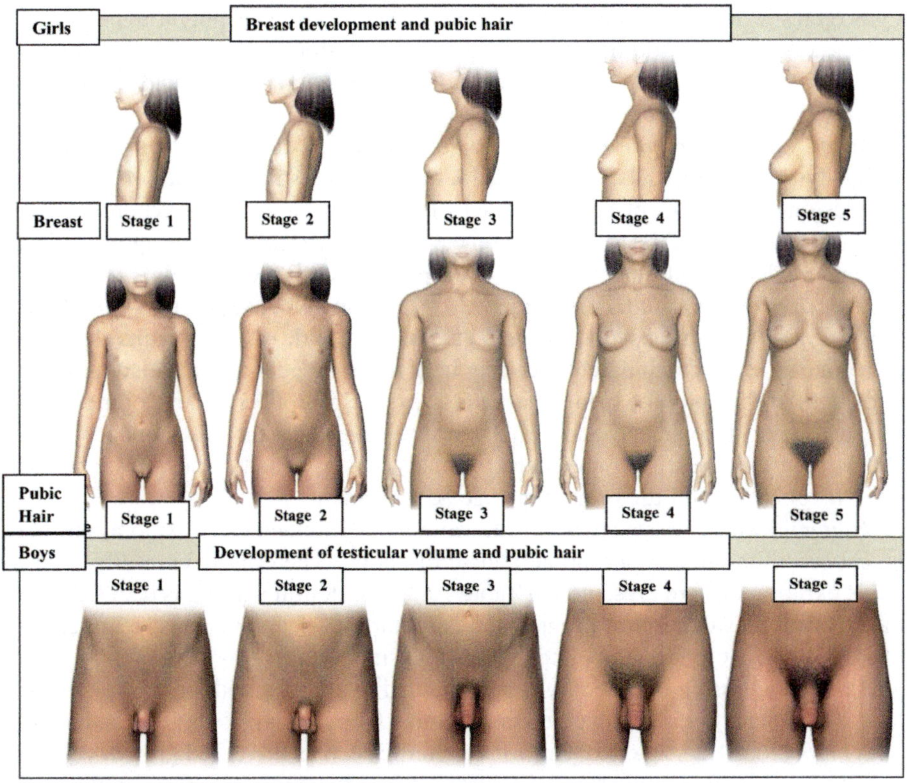

Fig. 10.1 Pubertal stage as a function of Tanner stage: figure adapted from ref. [1]

Table 10.3 When should suspected precocious puberty be explored?

Girls	Boys
Breast development before the age of 8 years	Increase in testicular volume before the age of 9.5 years
Pubic hair before the age of 8 years	Pubic hair before the age of 9.5 years
Breast development between the ages of 8 and 9 years. Exploration only if: • Onset of pubertal development before 8 years • Growth velocity >6 cm/year, adult height prognosis below target height • Rapid progression of pubertal development (transition from one stage to another in less than 6 months) • Clinical evidence for a neurogenic etiology • Clinical evidence of peripheral precocious puberty	Pubertal development seen around 10 years. Exploration only if: • Onset of pubertal development before 9.5 years • Growth velocity >6 cm/year, adult height prognosis below target height • Rapid progression of pubertal development (transition from one stage to another in less than 6 months) • Clinical evidence of a neurogenic etiology. Clinical evidence of peripheral precocious puberty
Menarche before the age of 10 years	

signs (gelastic attacks), or pituitary deficiency, such as asthenia, polyuria–polydipsia, and the existence of a known chronic disease or history of cerebral radiotherapy. The evaluation also includes the height and pubertal age of parents and siblings and family history of early or advanced puberty.

The physical examination assesses height, height velocity (growth curve), weight and body mass index, pubertal stage, and, in girls, the estrogenization of the vulva, skin lesions suggestive of neurofibromatosis or McCune–Albright syndrome, neurological signs (large head circumference with macrocephaly, nystagmus, visual change or visual field defects, neurodevelopmental deficit), symptoms or signs of anterior or posterior pituitary deficiency (low growth velocity, polyuria–polydipsia, fatigue), and the neuropsychological status of the child, which remains the major concern of the child and parents seeking help for early puberty. It is also important to recognize clinically the benign variants of precocious pubertal development, usually involving the isolated and nonprogressive development of secondary sexual characteristics (breasts or pubic hair), normal growth velocity or slight increase in growth velocity, and little or no bone age advancement.

Following this assessment, watchful waiting or complementary explorations may be chosen as the most appropriate course of action. The criteria currently used to guide explorations are presented in Table 10.3. If watchful waiting is decided upon, then careful reevaluation of progression is required 3–6 months later, to assess the rate of progression of puberty and any changes in growth.

Additional testing is generally recommended in all boys with precocious pubertal development, in girls with precocious Tanner 3 breast stage or higher, and in girls with precocious B2 stage and additional criteria, such as increased growth velocity, or symptoms or signs suggestive of central nervous system dysfunction or of peripheral precocious puberty.

These tests include the assessment of bone age (which is usually advanced in patients with progressive precocious puberty), hormonal determinations, pelvic or testicular (if peripheral PP is suspected) ultrasound scans, and brain magnetic resonance imaging (MRI).

Biological Diagnosis

The biological diagnosis of precocious puberty is based on the evaluation of sex steroid secretion and its mechanisms. The diagnosis of central precocious puberty is based on pubertal serum gonadotropin concentrations, with the demonstration of an activation of gonadotropin secretion [24].

Sex Steroid Determinations

In boys, testosterone is a good marker of testicular maturation, provided it is assessed with a sensitive method. RIA is generally used in practice. In girls, estradiol determination is uninformative, because half the girls displaying central precocious puberty have estradiol levels within the normal range of values in prepubescent girls. Very sensitive methods are required, and only RIA methods meet this requirement. The increase in estradiol concentration is also highly variable, due to the fluctuation, and sometimes intermittent secretion of this hormone. Very high estradiol levels are generally indicative of ovarian disease (peripheral PP due to cysts or tumors). Estrogenic impregnation is best assessed by pelvic ultrasound scans, on which the estrogenization of the uterus and ovaries may be visible [25].

Gonadotropin Determinations

Basal gonadotropin levels are informative and are generally significantly higher in children with PP than in prepubertal children [26]. However, basal serum LH concentration is much more sensitive than basal FSH concentration and is the key to diagnosis. Ultrasensitive assays should be used to determine serum LH concentration. Prepubertal LH concentrations are <0.1 IU/l, so LH assays should have a detection limit close to 0.1 IU/l [27–29].

The response to GnRH stimulation is considered the gold standard for the diagnosis of central precocious puberty. Stimulation tests involving a single injection of GnRH analogs can also be used [30, 31]. The major problem is defining the decision threshold. In both sexes, a central cause of precocious puberty is demonstrated an increase in pituitary gonadotropin levels. Indeed, the underlying mechanism of early central puberty is linked to premature activation of the hypothalamic–pituitary–gonadal axis, with the onset of pulsatile LH secretion and an increase in the secretion of pituitary gonadotropins both in basal conditions and after stimulation with GnRH. Before the onset of puberty, the FSH peak is greater than the LH surge. During and after puberty, the LH surge predominates. In cases of central precocious puberty, basal serum LH concentration usually is ≥0.3 IU/l and serum LH concentration after stimulation is ≥5 IU/l [1, 32]. FSH is less informative than LH, because FSH levels vary little during pubertal development. However, the stimulated LH/FSH ratio may make it easier to distinguish between progressive precocious puberty (with an LH/FSH ratio >0.66) and nonprogressive variants not requiring GnRH agonist therapy.

Place of Imaging in the Evaluation of Precocious Puberty

Pelvic ultrasound scans can be used to assess the degree of estrogenic impregnation of the internal genitalia in girls, through measurements of size and morphological criteria. A uterine length ≥35 mm is the first sign of estrogen exposure. Morphological features are also important, as the prepubertal state is marked by a tubular uterus, which becomes more pearl-like in shape during the course of puberty, with a bulging fundus. Measurements of uterine volume increase the reliability of the examination (prepubertal ≤2 ml). Endometrial thickening on an endometrial ultrasound scan

Table 10.4 Differentiation between true precocious puberty and slowly progressive forms

		Progressive precocious puberty	Slowly progressive precocious puberty
Clinical	Pubertal stage	Passage from one stage to another in 3–6 months	Spontaneous regression or stabilization of pubertal signs
	Growth velocity	Accelerated: >6 cm/year	Normal for age
	Bone age	Typically advanced, variable, at least 2 years	Variable, but usually within 1 year of chronological age
	Predicted adult height	Below-target height or decreasing on serial determinations	Within target height range
Pelvic ultrasound scan	Uterus	Length >34 mm or volume >2 ml	Length ≤34 mm or volume ≤2 ml
		Pearl-shaped uterus	Prepubertal, tubular uterus
		Endometrial thickening (endometrial ultrasound scan)	
	Ovaries	Not very informative	Not very informative
Hormonal evaluation	Estradiol (RIA ++)	Not very informative, usually measurable	Not detectable or close to the detection limit
	LH peak after stimulation with GnRH	In the pubertal zone ≥5 IU/l	In the prepubertal range
	Basal LH determination	Useful if value is high (≥3 IU/l) and frankly in the pubertal range	No definitive value

provides a second line of evidence. Ovary size and the number of follicles are not criteria for the assessment of pubertal development [25, 31, 33].

Testicular ultrasound should be performed if the testicles differ in volume or if peripheral precocious puberty is suspected, to facilitate the detection of Leydig cell tumors, which are generally not palpable.

Neuroimaging is essential in the etiological evaluation in progressive central precocious puberty. Magnetic resonance imaging (MRI) is the examination of choice in the study of the brain and of the hypothalamic–pituitary region, for the detection of hypothalamic lesions. The prevalence of such lesions is higher in boys (30–80 % of cases) than in girls (8–33 %) and is much lower when puberty starts after the age of 6 years in girls, this population accounting for the majority of cases. It has been suggested that an algorithm based on age and estradiol levels could replace MRI, but such an approach has not been clearly validated [34–36].

At the end of this analysis, the diagnostic approach should help to determine the progressive or nonprogressive nature of pubertal precocity (Table 10.4) and to differentiate between the etiologies of central or peripheral precocious puberty.

Indeed, many girls with idiopathic precocious puberty display very slowly progressive puberty, or even regressive puberty, with little change to predicted adult height and a normal final height close to their parental target height [5, 6]. Therapeutic abstention is the most appropriate approach in most of these cases, because puberty progresses slowly, with menarche occurring, on average, 5.5 years after the onset of clinical signs of puberty, and patient reaching a normal final height relative to parental target height. However, in some cases (about one third of subjects), predicted adult stature may decrease during the progression of puberty, in parallel with the emergence of evident biological signs of estrogenization and a highly progressive form of central PP. Thus, children for whom no treatment is justified at the initial assessment should undergo systematic clinical assessment, at least until the age of 9 years, to facilitate the identification of girls subsequently requiring treatment to block central precocious puberty.

Peripheral precocious puberty is completely independent of the hypothalamic–pituitary axis, with high serum estradiol levels in girls and high serum testosterone levels in boys, low basal and peak serum LH concentrations after GnRH stimulation, advanced bone age, and an estrogenized uterus on ultrasound scans for girls. The gonads or adrenal glands are responsible for excess steroid production, but they may also promote the activation of pubertal maturation of the gonadal axis, resulting in central precocious puberty [1].

The Normal Variants of Puberty

The distinction between early puberty and normal puberty is not clear-cut. There are several variants of normal puberty, which may pose problems for differential diagnosis, particularly as they have a high prevalence [37–39].

Isolated Premature Breast Development or Premature Thelarche

Premature thelarche is isolated breast development before the age of 8 years. There are two peaks in the frequency of premature thelarche: the neonatal period, which is marked by gonadotropin activation, this peak potentially lasting for 2 or 3 years, and the prepubertal period [33]. Premature thelarche differs from early puberty in the absence of any other aspect of sexual development, usually with a lack of scalability of breast development and no acceleration of height velocity or significant advance in bone maturation (≥2 years). Uterine ultrasound scans provide a simple means of checking that there is no change in the uterus. No further exploration or treatment is required, and the outcome is the persistence of moderate breast development (in two thirds of cases) or regression (one third of cases). However, isolated premature breast development may precede the onset of central precocious puberty, which should not be ignored if patients develop other pubertal signs and an acceleration of height velocity.

Premature Development of Pubic Hair or Premature Pubarche

Premature pubarche is the appearance of pubic hair before the age of 8 years in girls and 9 years in boys. It may be accompanied by clinical signs of hyperandrogenism: acne, axillary hair, accelerated growth rate. It corresponds to adrenal maturation (adrenarche) and is not a differential diagnosis for central precocious puberty. Possible differential diagnoses to be systematically excluded include adrenal tumors and congenital adrenal hyperplasia [40, 41].

Slow Progressive Forms of Precocious Puberty

Such forms present clinically as early puberty with the development of secondary sexual characteristics and a moderate advance in bone age. On ultrasound scans, the uterus may show very early estrogen impregnation. However, the response to GnRH is of the prepubertal type. The mechanism underlying these cases of nonprogressive precocious puberty is unknown, but the gonadotropic axis is not activated. Studies monitoring these benign variants of precocious puberty have shown that treatment with GnRH agonists is not appropriate because there tends to be either a total regression of pubertal signs or a slow progression toward puberty [5, 6]. Table 10.4 provides elements guiding differentiation between slowly progressive and progressive forms of central precocious puberty.

Psychosocial Aspects

Psychosocial aspects of early puberty are the major concern of patients and families seeking help for early puberty, whereas doctors generally focus on etiological aspects and height prognosis. Psychological assessment usually reveals a normal IQ. Patients tend to be rather solitary, with high scores for isolation, and a tendency to become depressed. They are mostly concerned about their appearance, whereas parents are generally worried about the onset of periods. Little is known about the long-term psychosocial consequences of early puberty or about the psychosocial integration of patients treated for precocious puberty [13, 42].

Management

Central Precocious Puberty

GnRH Agonists

GnRH agonists are generally indicated in progressive central precocious puberty, with the aim to restore genetic growth potential and to stabilize or regress pubertal symptoms. GnRH agonists continuously stimulate the pituitary gonadotrophs, leading to desensitization and decreases in LH release and, to a lesser extent, FSH release [43]. Several GnRH agonists are available in various depot forms and the approval for use of the various formulations varies with countries. Despite nearly 30 years of use of GnRH agonists in precocious puberty, there are still ongoing questions on their optimal use, and an international consensus statement has summarized the available information and the areas of uncertainty as of 2007 [17].

GnRH agonist treatments should be followed by experienced clinicians and result in the regression or stabilization of pubertal symptoms, decrease of growth velocity, and bone age advancement [17]. GnRHa-injection dates should be recorded and adherence with the dosing interval monitored. A suppressed LH response to the stimulation by GnRH, GnRH agonist, or after an injection of the depot preparation (which contains a fraction of free GnRH agonist) is indicative of biochemical efficacy of the treatment but is not recommended routinely. Progression of breast or testicular development usually indicates poor compliance, treatment failure, or incorrect diagnosis and requires further evaluation.

There are no randomized controlled trials assessing *long-term outcomes* of the treatment of central precocious puberty with GnRH agonists, and height outcome has been mostly evaluated. Among approximately 400 girls treated until a mean age of 11 years, the mean adult height was about 160 cm and mean gains over predicted height varied from 3 to 10 cm [12]. Individual height gains were very variable, but were calculated using predicted height, which is itself poorly reliable. Factors affecting height outcome include initial patient characteristics (lower height if bone age is markedly advanced and shorter predicted height at initiation of treatment) and, in some series, duration of treatment (higher height gains in patients starting treatment at a younger age and with longer durations of treatment). No height gain benefit has been shown in girls treated after the age of 9 years.

Other outcomes to consider include bone mineral density, risk of obesity and metabolic disorders, and psychosocial outcomes. Bone mineral density may decrease during GnRH agonist therapy. However, subsequent bone mass accrual is preserved, and peak bone mass does not seem to be negatively affected by treatment [17]. There has been concern that GnRH agonist use may affect BMI. However, childhood obesity is associated with earlier pubertal development in girls, and early sexual maturation is associated with increased prevalence of overweight and obesity. Altogether, the available data indicate that long-term GnRH agonist treatment does not seem to cause or aggravate obesity or have repercussions for body composition, bone mineral density, fertility, and metabolic or cancer comorbidities. General health status is not different as compared to women with normal puberty [44–46]. The development of polycystic ovarian syndrome remains controversial [47–50], and further studies are still required to assess the potential risk of premature ovarian dysfunction. Data concerning psychosocial outcomes are scarce, and there is little evidence to show whether treatment with GnRH agonists is associated with improved psychological outcome [13, 46]. Studies of this aspect are required.

Although *tolerance* to GnRH agonist treatment is generally considered good, it may be associated with headaches and menopausal symptoms such as hot flushes. Local complications (3–13 %) such as sterile abscesses may result in a loss of efficacy, and anaphylaxis has been described [51].

The optimal time to stop treatment has not been established, and factors that could influence the decision to stop GnRH agonists include aiming at maximizing height, synchronizing puberty with peers, ameliorating psychological distress, or facilitating care of the developmentally delayed child. However, data only permit analysis of factors that affect adult height. Several variables can be used to decide on when to stop treatment including chronological age, duration of therapy, bone age, height, target height, and growth velocity. However, these variables are closely interrelated and cannot be considered independently. In addition, retrospective analyses suggest that continuing treatment beyond the age of 11 years is associated with no further gains [52]. Therefore, it is reasonable to consider these parameters and informed parent and patient preferences, with the goal of menarche occurring near the population norms [17]. Pubertal manifestations generally reappear within months of GnRH agonist treatment being stopped, with a mean time to menarche of 16 months [53]. Long-term fertility has not been fully evaluated, but preliminary observations are reassuring [46, 53].

The addition of growth hormone [54] or oxandrolone [55] when growth velocity decreases or if height prognosis appears to be unsatisfactory has been proposed, but data are limited on the efficacy and safety of these drugs in children with precocious puberty.

Management of Causal Lesions

When precocious puberty is caused by a hypothalamic lesion (e.g., mass or malformation), management of the causal lesion generally has no effect on the course of pubertal development. Hypothalamic hamartomas should not be treated by surgery for the management of precocious puberty. Precocious puberty associated with the presence of a hypothalamic lesion may progress to gonadotropin deficiency.

Peripheral Precocious Puberty

Management of Causal Lesions

Surgery is indicated for gonadal tumors, and postoperative chemo- or radiotherapy should be discussed as part of a multidisciplinary team including surgeons and oncologists.

Large ovarian cysts (greater than 20 ml or 3.4 cm in diameter and typically more than 75 ml or 5.2 cm) should be managed very carefully given the risk of adnexal torsion [56]. In such cases, puncture possibly ultrasound guided should be considered and allows molecular analysis of the cystic fluid for activating GNAS mutation.

Removal of exogenous exposure to sex steroids is obvious but the search for occupational exposure is often very difficult and requires careful investigation.

Medications

There is no etiological treatment for peripheral causes of precocious puberty, and the rarity of the diseases renders evaluation of therapeutic strategies very difficult. In McCune–Albright syndrome and recurrent ovarian cysts, aromatase inhibitors [57] and SERMs [58] have been used to inhibit the production or action of estrogens, respectively [59]. These approaches are partly effective but no definitive strategy has emerged. In familial male precocious puberty due to LH receptor activating mutations, ketoconazole, an inhibitor of androgen biosynthesis, has been shown to be effective in the long term [60], and the combination of anti-androgens and aromatase inhibitors has been proposed. However, caution must be used with the use of ketoconazole given the risk of liver toxicity. Nonclassical forms of congenital adrenal hyperplasia should be managed with glucocorticoids.

Conclusion

A knowledge of the different clinical forms of precocious puberty is essential, to determine whether there is a tumor (intracranial, or in the gonads or adrenal glands) or other disease (neurofibromatosis, McCune–Albright syndrome, congenital adrenal hyperplasia) and the indications for treatment or an abstention from treatment. The psychological aspects of precocious puberty should also be evaluated during the treatment of these patients.

References

1. Carel JC, Leger J. Clinical practice. Precocious puberty. N Engl J Med. 2008;358(22):2366–77.
2. Kaplowitz PB, Slora EJ, Wasserman RC, Pedlow SE, Herman-Giddens ME. Earlier onset of puberty in girls: relation to increased body mass index and race. Pediatrics. 2001;108(2):347–53.
3. Biro FM, Galvez MP, Greenspan LC, Succop PA, Vangeepuram N, Pinney SM, et al. Pubertal assessment method and baseline characteristics in a mixed longitudinal study of girls. Pediatrics. 2010;126(3):e583–90.
4. Sorensen K, Mouritsen A, Aksglaede L, Hagen CP, Mogensen SS, Juul A. Recent secular trends in pubertal timing: implications for evaluation and diagnosis of precocious puberty. Horm Res Paediatr. 2012;77(3):137–45.
5. Palmert MR, Malin HV, Boepple PA. Unsustained or slowly progressive puberty in young girls: initial presentation and long-term follow-up of 20 untreated patients. J Clin Endocrinol Metab. 1999;84(2):415–23.
6. Leger J, Reynaud R, Czernichow P. Do all girls with apparent idiopathic precocious puberty require gonadotropin-releasing hormone agonist treatment? J Pediatr. 2000;137(6):819–25.
7. Prete G, Couto-Silva AC, Trivin C, Brauner R. Idiopathic central precocious puberty in girls: presentation factors. BMC Pediatr. 2008;8:27.
8. Teilmann G, Pedersen CB, Jensen TK, Skakkebaek NE, Juul A. Prevalence and incidence of precocious pubertal development in Denmark: an epidemiologic study based on national registries. Pediatrics. 2005;116(6):1323–8.
9. Abreu AP, Dauber A, Macedo DB, Noel SD, Brito VN, Gill JC, et al. Central precocious puberty caused by mutations in the imprinted gene MKRN3. N Engl J Med. 2013;368(26):2467–75.

10. Bulcao Macedo D, Nahime Brito V, Latronico AC. New causes of central precocious puberty: the role of genetic factors. Neuroendocrinology. 2014;100(1):1–8.
11. Macedo DB, Abreu AP, Reis AC, Montenegro LR, Dauber A, Beneduzzi D, et al. Central precocious puberty that appears to be sporadic caused by paternally inherited mutations in the imprinted gene makorin ring finger 3. J Clin Endocrinol Metab. 2014;99(6):E1097–103.
12. Carel JC, Lahlou N, Roger M, Chaussain JL. Precocious puberty and statural growth. Hum Reprod Update. 2004;10(2):135–47.
13. Xhrouet-Heinrichs D, Lagrou K, Heinrichs C, Craen M, Dooms L, Malvaux P, et al. Longitudinal study of behavioral and affective patterns in girls with central precocious puberty during long-acting triptorelin therapy. Acta Paediatr. 1997;86(8):808–15.
14. Giabicani E, Lemaire P, Brauner R. Models for predicting the adult height and age at first menstruation of girls with idiopathic central precocious puberty. PLoS One. 2015;10(3), e0120588.
15. Marti-Henneberg C, Vizmanos B. The duration of puberty in girls is related to the timing of its onset. J Pediatr. 1997;131(4):618–21.
16. Day FR, Elks CE, Murray A, Ong KK, Perry JR. Puberty timing associated with diabetes, cardiovascular disease and also diverse health outcomes in men and women: the UK Biobank study. Sci Rep. 2015;5:11208.
17. Carel JC, Eugster EA, Rogol A, Ghizzoni L, Palmert MR, Antoniazzi F, et al. Consensus statement on the use of gonadotropin-releasing hormone analogs in children. Pediatrics. 2009; 123(4):e752–62.
18. Michaud PA, Suris JC, Deppen A. Gender-related psychological and behavioural correlates of pubertal timing in a national sample of Swiss adolescents. Mol Cell Endocrinol. 2006;254–255:172–8.
19. Schoelwer MJ, Donahue KL, Bryk K, Didrick P, Berenbaum SA, Eugster EA. Psychological assessment of mothers and their daughters at the time of diagnosis of precocious puberty. Int J Pediatr Endocrinol. 2015;2015(1):5.
20. Wise LA, Palmer JR, Rothman EF, Rosenberg L. Childhood abuse and early menarche: findings from the black women's health study. Am J Public Health. 2009;99 Suppl 2:S460–6.
21. Marshall WA, Tanner JM. Variations in pattern of pubertal changes in girls. Arch Dis Child. 1969;44(235):291–303.
22. Marshall WA, Tanner JM. Variations in the pattern of pubertal changes in boys. Arch Dis Child. 1970;45(239):13–23.
23. Papadimitriou A, Beri D, Tsialla A, Fretzayas A, Psychou F, Nicolaidou P. Early growth acceleration in girls with idiopathic precocious puberty. J Pediatr. 2006;149(1):43–6.
24. Nathan BM, Palmert MR. Regulation and disorders of pubertal timing. Endocrinol Metab Clin North Am. 2005;34(3):617–41. ix.
25. de Vries L, Horev G, Schwartz M, Phillip M. Ultrasonographic and clinical parameters for early differentiation between precocious puberty and premature thelarche. Eur J Endocrinol. 2006;154(6):891–8.
26. Resende EA, Lara BH, Reis JD, Ferreira BP, Pereira GA, Borges MF. Assessment of basal and gonadotropin-releasing hormone-stimulated gonadotropins by immunochemiluminometric and immunofluorometric assays in normal children. J Clin Endocrinol Metab. 2007;92(4):1424–9.
27. Neely EK, Wilson DM, Lee PA, Stene M, Hintz RL. Spontaneous serum gonadotropin concentrations in the evaluation of precocious puberty. J Pediatr. 1995;127(1):47–52.
28. Pasternak Y, Friger M, Loewenthal N, Haim A, Hershkovitz E. The utility of basal serum LH in prediction of central precocious puberty in girls. Eur J Endocrinol. 2012;166(2):295–9.
29. Houk CP, Kunselman AR, Lee PA. Adequacy of a single unstimulated luteinizing hormone level to diagnose central precocious puberty in girls. Pediatrics. 2009;123(6):e1059–63.
30. Yazdani P, Lin Y, Raman V, Haymond M. A single sample GnRHa stimulation test in the diagnosis of precocious puberty. Int J Pediatr Endocrinol. 2012;2012(1):23.
31. Sathasivam A, Rosenberg HK, Shapiro S, Wang H, Rapaport R. Pelvic ultrasonography in the evaluation of central precocious puberty: comparison with leuprolide stimulation test. J Pediatr. 2011;159(3):490–5.

32. Fuqua JS. Treatment and outcomes of precocious puberty: an update. J Clin Endocrinol Metab. 2013;98(6):2198–207.
33. de Vries L, Guz-Mark A, Lazar L, Reches A, Phillip M. Premature thelarche: age at presentation affects clinical course but not clinical characteristics or risk to progress to precocious puberty. J Pediatr. 2010;156(3):466–71.
34. Chalumeau M, Hadjiathanasiou CG, Ng SM, Cassio A, Mul D, Cisternino M, et al. Selecting girls with precocious puberty for brain imaging: validation of European evidence-based diagnosis rule. J Pediatr. 2003;143(4):445–50.
35. Stanhope R. Gonadotrophin-dependent [correction of dependant] precocious puberty and occult intracranial tumors: which girls should have neuro-imaging? J Pediatr. 2003;143(4):426–7.
36. Pedicelli S, Alessio P, Scire G, Cappa M, Cianfarani S. Routine screening by brain magnetic resonance imaging is not indicated in every girl with onset of puberty between the ages of 6 and 8 years. J Clin Endocrinol Metab. 2014;99(12):4455–61.
37. Atay Z, Turan S, Guran T, Furman A, Bereket A. The prevalence and risk factors of premature thelarche and pubarche in 4- to 8-year-old girls. Acta Paediatr. 2012;101(2):e71–5.
38. Mogensen SS, Aksglaede L, Mouritsen A, Sorensen K, Main KM, Gideon P, et al. Diagnostic work-up of 449 consecutive girls who were referred to be evaluated for precocious puberty. J Clin Endocrinol Metab. 2011;96(5):1393–401.
39. Kaplowitz P. Clinical characteristics of 104 children referred for evaluation of precocious puberty. J Clin Endocrinol Metab. 2004;89(8):3644–50.
40. Oberfield SE, Sopher AB, Gerken AT. Approach to the girl with early onset of pubic hair. J Clin Endocrinol Metab. 2011;96(6):1610–22.
41. Ghizzoni L, Gasco V. Premature pubarche. Horm Res Paediatr. 2010;73(5):420–2.
42. Baumann DA, Landolt MA, Wetterwald R, Dubuis JM, Sizonenko PC, Werder EA. Psychological evaluation of young women after medical treatment for central precocious puberty. Horm Res. 2001;56(1–2):45–50.
43. Lahlou N, Carel JC, Chaussain JL, Roger M. Pharmacokinetics and pharmacodynamics of GnRH agonists: clinical implications in pediatrics. J Pediatr Endocrinol Metab. 2000;13 Suppl 1:723–37.
44. Thornton P, Silverman LA, Geffner ME, Neely EK, Gould E, Danoff TM. Review of outcomes after cessation of gonadotropin-releasing hormone agonist treatment of girls with precocious puberty. Pediatr Endocrinol Rev. 2014;11(3):306–17.
45. Lazar L, Meyerovitch J, de Vries L, Phillip M, Lebenthal Y. Treated and untreated women with idiopathic precocious puberty: long-term follow-up and reproductive outcome between the third and fifth decades. Clin Endocrinol (Oxf). 2014;80(4):570–6.
46. Lazar L, Lebenthal Y, Yackobovitch-Gavan M, Shalitin S, de Vries L, Phillip M, et al. Treated and untreated women with idiopathic precocious puberty: BMI evolution, metabolic outcome, and general health between third and fifth decades. J Clin Endocrinol Metab. 2015;100(4):1445–51.
47. Heger S, Partsch CJ, Sippell WG. Long-term outcome after depot gonadotropin-releasing hormone agonist treatment of central precocious puberty: final height, body proportions, body composition, bone mineral density, and reproductive function. J Clin Endocrinol Metab. 1999;84(12):4583–90.
48. Franceschi R, Gaudino R, Marcolongo A, Gallo MC, Rossi L, Antoniazzi F, et al. Prevalence of polycystic ovary syndrome in young women who had idiopathic central precocious puberty. Fertil Steril. 2010;93(4):1185–91.
49. Magiakou MA, Manousaki D, Papadaki M, Hadjidakis D, Levidou G, Vakaki M, et al. The efficacy and safety of gonadotropin-releasing hormone analog treatment in childhood and adolescence: a single center, long-term follow-up study. J Clin Endocrinol Metab. 2010;95(1):109–17.
50. Chiavaroli V, Liberati M, D'Antonio F, Masuccio F, Capanna R, Verrotti A, et al. GNRH analog therapy in girls with early puberty is associated with the achievement of predicted final

height but also with increased risk of polycystic ovary syndrome. Eur J Endocrinol. 2010;163(1):55–62.
51. Carel JC, Lahlou N, Jaramillo O, Montauban V, Teinturier C, Colle M, et al. Treatment of central precocious puberty by subcutaneous injections of leuprorelin 3-month depot (11.25 mg). J Clin Endocrinol Metab. 2002;87(9):4111–6.
52. Carel JC, Roger M, Ispas S, Tondu F, Lahlou N, Blumberg J, et al. Final height after long-term treatment with triptorelin slow-release for central precocious puberty: importance of statural growth after interruption of treatment. J Clin Endocrinol Metab. 1999;84:1973–8.
53. Heger S, Muller M, Ranke M, Schwarz HP, Waldhauser F, Partsch CJ, et al. Long-term GnRH agonist treatment for female central precocious puberty does not impair reproductive function. Mol Cell Endocrinol. 2006;254–255:217–20.
54. Pasquino AM, Pucarelli I, Segni M, Matrunola M, Cerroni F, Cerrone F. Adult height in girls with central precocious puberty treated with gonadotropin-releasing hormone analogues and growth hormone. J Clin Endocrinol Metab. 1999;84(2):449–52.
55. Vottero A, Pedori S, Verna M, Pagano B, Cappa M, Loche S, et al. Final height in girls with central idiopathic precocious puberty treated with gonadotropin-releasing hormone analog and oxandrolone. J Clin Endocrinol Metab. 2006;91(4):1284–7.
56. Linam LE, Darolia R, Naffaa LN, Breech LL, O'Hara SM, Hillard PJ, et al. US findings of adnexal torsion in children and adolescents: size really does matter. Pediatr Radiol. 2007;37(10):1013–9.
57. Shulman DI, Francis GL, Palmert MR, Eugster EA. Use of aromatase inhibitors in children and adolescents with disorders of growth and adolescent development. Pediatrics. 2008;121(4):e975–83.
58. Eugster EA, Rubin SD, Reiter EO, Plourde P, Jou HC, Pescovitz OH. Tamoxifen treatment for precocious puberty in McCune-Albright syndrome: a multicenter trial. J Pediatr. 2003;143(1):60–6.
59. Mieszczak J, Eugster EA. Treatment of precocious puberty in McCune-Albright syndrome. Pediatr Endocrinol Rev. 2007;4 Suppl 4:419–22.
60. Soriano-Guillen L, Lahlou N, Chauvet G, Roger M, Chaussain JL, Carel JC. Adult height after ketoconazole treatment in patients with familial male-limited precocious puberty. J Clin Endocrinol Metab. 2005;90(1):147–51.

Chapter 11
Constitutional Delayed Puberty

Peter A. Lee and Christopher P. Houk

Definition and Age of Puberty

Puberty is the period of human growth and development when sexual maturity and fertility are established. The timing and tempo of puberty is dependent upon a host of genetic and environmental factors. The physical changes of puberty progress in a predictable sequence within an expected time related to hormone stimulation. Onset of puberty is considered when breast development becomes apparent in girls (Tanner stage 2) or when testicular growth is documented in boys (length greater than 2.5 cm or volume greater than 3–4 mL). Progression through puberty typically occurs within 2.5–3 years; generally progression to the next Tanner stage is expected within 6–12 months. Progression may differ between breast or genital staging and pubic hair stage. The age range of pubertal development varies among racial-ethnic groups, appearing earlier among African-Americans, then Hispanics, followed by Caucasian and occurring on average somewhat later in studied Asian populations. However, precise data are not available for the age of completion of puberty, and generally it is considered that puberty is delayed if physical evidence of onset (breast development or testicular enlargement) is not present by 13 years among girls or by 14 years for boys [1]. Delayed puberty is much more common in boys and is usually benign; however, pubertal delay in girls represents pathology in the majority.

The onset of pubic hair growth does not signal the onset of puberty as this may be a consequence of adrenarche, the increase of adrenal androgen secretion that

P.A. Lee (✉)
Department of Pediatrics, Hershey Medical Center, Penn State College of Medicine,
500 University Drive, Hershey, PA 17033-0850, USA
e-mail: plee@psu.edu

C.P. Houk
Department of Pediatrics, Georgia Regents University,
1446 Harper Street, Augusta, GA 30912, USA
e-mail: chouk@gru.edu

P. Kumanov, A. Agarwal (eds.), *Puberty*, DOI 10.1007/978-3-319-32122-6_11

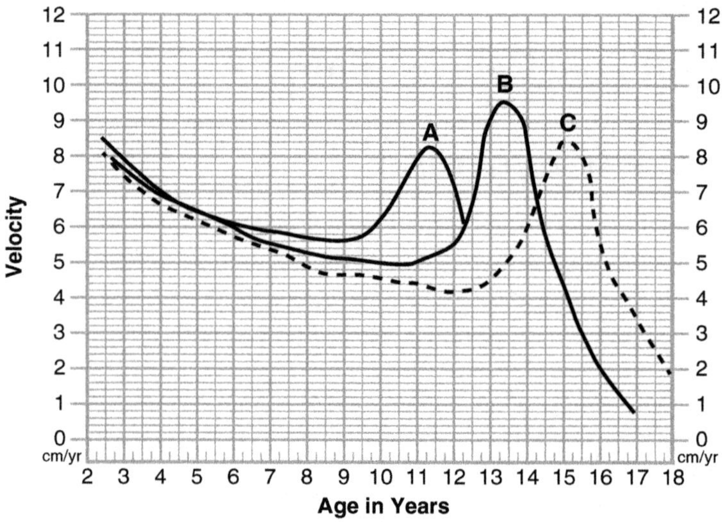

Fig. 11.1 Height velocity for age for a (**A**) girl and a (**B**) boy with normal puberty occurring at an average age and a (**C**) boy with CDP (based on charts developed by the National Center for Health Statistics)

begins during late childhood, and does not indicate onset of gonadal function. Further, a girl with minimal breast development and no progression of pubertal changes, particularly in those who are heavy, does not necessarily signal the onset of pubertal ovarian secretion as progression is an obligate feature of puberty. A growth spurt (Fig. 11.1) follows a nadir of growth rate just before pubertal onset. Among girls it occurs early, together with breast budding as the first signs of puberty. In boys, the growth spurt occurs in mid-to-late puberty.

Definition of Delayed Puberty

Delayed puberty represents the late onset or the delayed progression of physical puberty. Delayed puberty is defined as the onset of puberty beyond the mean age of onset by approximately 2–2.5 standard deviations (approximately 13 years in girls and 14 years in boys) [1]. Absence of menarche by age 15 is also evidence of lack of normal progression and is called primary amenorrhea.

Constitutionally delayed puberty (CDP), as the name implies, has traditionally been considered puberty that is temporarily delayed in onset or completion and has been considered as a normal variant [2]. It is felt to occur as a result of a delay in the onset of pubertal gonadotropin stimulation of the gonads or a lag in the progression of such secretion in an individual who ultimately attains normal adult gonadotropin secretion. Those with CDP are expected to complete puberty and attain adult height by 18 years of age [3]. CDP is distinct from other categories of delayed puberty that have an identifiable underlying pathology such as:

1. *Functional pubertal delay* as a consequence of a physiologic abnormality such as systemic disease and therapy which delays normal growth and maturation, can be considered a temporary hypogonadotropic hypogonadism.
2. *Hypothalamic-pituitary dysfunction* resulting in lack of gonadotropin secretion (hypogonadotropic hypogonadism, HH), traditionally considered to be a permanent defect.
3. *Gonadal failure* because of lack of functional gonadal tissue; characterized by elevated circulating levels of gonadotropins due to a lack of negative gonadal feedback (hypergonadotropic hypogonadism).

When puberty is delayed, constitutional delay and the first two pathologic categories above present with low gonadotropin levels and are usually difficult to differentiate one from another, in contrast to elevated gonadotropin levels in gonadal failure. Features at initial presentation help to categorize patients presenting with delayed puberty (Table 11.1), although the category needs to be subsequently confirmed in most instances.

CDP designation is typically, but is not always, synonymous with constitutional delay of growth and puberty (CDGP). The later involves delayed maturation including statural growth delay during prepubertal years [4, 5]. CDGP presents with short stature compared with expected height based on parents' heights, with a commensurate delay of skeletal age and low or borderline low growth rates. Their puberty can be expected to begin when skeletal age reaches 10–11 years for girls and 11.5–12.5 years for boys. CDGP is an inclusive term including those who did not have apparent delay of maturity during childhood, while CDGP occurs during adolescence.

Etiology

Historically our view of CDP has been that it represents the far end of the normal distribution of normal pubertal development. More recently, the identification of gene modifications that are associated with both transient CDP and permanent hypogonadotropic hypogonadism has suggested that our paradigm for understanding CDP is too simple.

The currently identified genes related to reproductive function have been recently summarized [6]. Because of the complexity of genetic and physiologic factors controlling both puberty and growth, it is reasonable to presume that multiple genetic/environmental factors impact both the age of onset and rate of progression of puberty. Thus, it is reasonable to hypothesize that the expression of gene variants results in a spectrum of diagnoses related to the resurgence of the hypothalamic-pituitary-gonadal axis that heralds the onset of puberty. This spectrum in pubertal onset/progression ranges from individuals who attain a normal adult height and adult gonadal function, to those with a foreshortened adult height or subfertility, to

Table 11.1 Approach to patients with delayed puberty

Girls	No or minimal breast development with no progression in previous 6 months		
Boys	Prepubertal genitalia with		
	Testicular volume	<4 mL	Likely early changes in CDP
		>4 mL	HH or CDP with no early changes
First-tier screening testing—LH, FSH (plus testosterone in males or estradiol in females), prolactin. CBC, CMP, skeletal age X-ray, olfaction testing; depending on linear growth-free T4, TSH, IGF1; karyotype based on clinical findings			
Gonadotropin levels mIU/mL (using third-generation assay)			
Random LH levels[a]			
<0.3—prepubertal or hypogonadotropic levels			
CDP (delayed but essentially normal puberty)			
Functional pubertal delay (consequence of a chronic disease or condition in a patient with a potential of normally functioning hypothalamic-pituitary-gonadal axis)			
Anorexia nervosa			
Chronic cardiac, pulmonary, and renal disease			
CNS tumors (prolactinoma, craniopharyngioma)			
Excessive exercise (e.g., gymnastics)			
Growth hormone deficiency			
Hypothyroidism			
Inflammatory bowel disease			
Hypercortisolism			
Malnutrition/eating disorder			
Multiple pituitary hormone deficiency			
Psychogenic or stress related			
Hypogonadotropic hypogonadism (permanent deficiency—some with anosmia)			
>0.9—pubertal levels indicating normal HPG axis			
CDP			
>9.0—elevated levels suggestive of gonadal failure			
Hypergonadotropic hypogonadism			
Turner syndrome			
Klinefelter syndrome			

[a]FSH less useful but may be confirmatory, levels >12 are consistent with hypergonadotropic hypogonadism

those who felt to have HH who unexpectedly develop normal gonadal function later in adult life [7]. This occurrence of endogenous reproductive hormone secretion in individuals diagnosed with permanent HH, some of whom carry a genetic mutation associated with permanent HH, suggests a spectrum of clinical severity extending to a portion of those patients previously classified as having constitutional delayed puberty, having relatively mild alterations in genes [8].

Evidence for incomplete or disordered pubertal development in patients with CDP includes failure to reach target height [9], lower adult bone mineral density (BMD) [10], and diminished adult fertility. These findings suggest that mild alterations of genes related to gonadotropin deficiency and genes related to growth and maturation may constitute distinct but often overlapping etiologies of CDP. This hypothesis supports by the identification of gene alterations that may delay puberty eventually results in attainment of normal function [11] and other genetic changes that delay puberty but show persistence of partial HH. Families in which multiple individuals share the same genetic mutation have been reported where some individuals manifest permanent HH, while others show CDP [12]. The increased incidence of CDP in kindreds with permanent idiopathic hypogonadotropic hypogonadism (IHH) (idiopathic to distinguish from forms of known etiology such as Kallmann syndrome) is indirect evidence that genetic alterations often show a variable clinical expression of differing severity involving secretion and action of gonadotropin-releasing hormone (GnRH) secretion [2].

HH genes have been evaluated in individuals comparing kindred with IHH with or without delayed puberty versus a kindred with no family history of IHH [11]. Potential variants were for a presumed neurodevelopmental gene involved in the initial fate specification of GnRH neurons (IL17RD) and the gene for neurokinin B (TAC 3). In the kindred with IHH, in those with pubertal delay, 53 % had a variant of the IHH gene compared to 12 % of the control family. Among those with delayed puberty with no family history, 14 % had a genetic variant and 5.6 % of controls did. These results are consistent with IHH gene variants being an etiology of CDP. Normal reproductive function among adults who have previously been diagnosed with IHH has been found to be associated with genetic variants of neurokinin B (TAC3) [13] and its receptor (TACR3) [7].

The gonadotropin-releasing hormone receptor (GNRHR) gene has also been studied using molecular analysis and in vitro experiments and correlated with phenotype in 74 male and 36 female patients with normosmic hypogonadotropic hypogonadism (IHH) and in 50 with CDP [14]. The phenotypic spectrum in patients with GNRHR mutations varied from complete GnRH deficiency to partial and reversible IHH, with evidence of genotype-phenotype correlation. However, no evidence was found that mutations in GNRHR were involved in the pathogenesis of CDP.

Associations of polymorphisms in the estrogen receptor α (ESR1) with CDP have been studied using three single nucleotide polymorphisms from intron 1 of ESR1 (rs3778609, rs12665044, and rs827421) as candidates [15]. The frequency of G/G genotype at rs827421 in intron 1 of ESR1 was increased in CDGP boys ($P=0.03$). This is consistent with genetic variation of ESR1 contributing to the etiologies of CDP.

To date, there is no evidence suggesting an association with CDP among loss-of-function mutations in the immunoglobulin superfamily member 1 (IGSF1). Such mutations result in an X-linked syndrome of central hypothyroidism, normal timing of testicular growth, but delayed rise of testosterone. Although the search found three novel variants among 30 patients with an apparent X-linked form of CDP, it did not provide evidence that IGSF1 mutations are also associated with CDP [16].

Significant linkage between the pericentromeric region of chromosome 2 and CDP among Finnish families has been recently reported [17], similar to a previous report [18]. However, the variation within the linked region that predisposes to delayed puberty has not been identified.

Natural History

As noted above, CDP is often identified at the age of puberty as a continuation of a delayed growth pattern described as constitutional delay of growth and puberty (CDGP). This may be identified earlier in childhood during evaluation of short stature. CDGP is characterized by short stature manifest early in childhood (Fig. 11.2) and borderline or low normal growth rates but without evidence of a pathologic cause of short stature. Skeletal maturity as judged by radiographic skeletal age is delayed for age and sex. It may be considered that the typical child with CDGP has a delay of "biologic age" compared with chronologic age. Whether or not delay is apparent during prepubertal years, patients with CDP have a delayed growth spurt (Fig. 11.1). This delayed growth acceleration may also not reach the maximum rate of typically puberty. Since patients continue to grow—albeit at a slow rate—until the growth spurt begins, it is often difficult to ascertain whether adult height has been compromised.

A positive family history of CDP is often present among same-sex relatives, i.e., fathers or uncles of boys and mothers or grandmothers of girls. Fifty to eighty percent of patients with CDGP have a positive family history [19, 20]. A recent assessment of families of 492 Finnish subjects [20] with CDGP (based upon delay of pubertal growth spurt) confirmed the heritability of CDGP but found only a slightly higher prevalence in male first-degree relatives over that seen in female relatives challenging the traditional view of a marked predominance of CDGP among males. Such clustering in families suggests a pattern consistent with autosomal dominant inheritance. While the onset and progression of puberty normally vary in a population over a number of years, the inclusion of CDGP as a variant of normal growth results in a significant skewing of the normal Gaussian distribution of puberty in males.

The numerous changes within the neural systems that regulate GnRH synthesis and puberty are impacted by metabolic factors related to body size and composition [21] and psychological, social, and other unknown factors. The relationship of obesity and puberty onset is unclear. When delayed puberty occurs in obese boys, the association of linear growth pattern is not that typically found in CDGP and tends to show a greater height for age, less delay of bone age, as well as taller stature for bone age [22]. Predicted heights are greater than midparental height in contrast to normal-weight boys with delayed puberty who typically have predicted adult heights within or below midparental height ranges. Hence, the relatively taller stature among obese boys is not associated with foreshortened adult height suggesting a different etiology of delayed puberty than the "typical" CDGP [23].

The diagnostic category of familial short stature (FSS) should be considered when assessing CDGP since findings also include diminishing height for age, slow growth rates, and skeletal age delay. While FSS involves adult family members with stature below the normal range, findings overlap at presentation of FSS and CDGP [24]. Among patients presenting with CDGP, 40 % have been reported to have short family members suggesting familial short stature [25]. Such is not surprising since both are descriptive categories with multiple etiologies related to numerous factors including multiple genes.

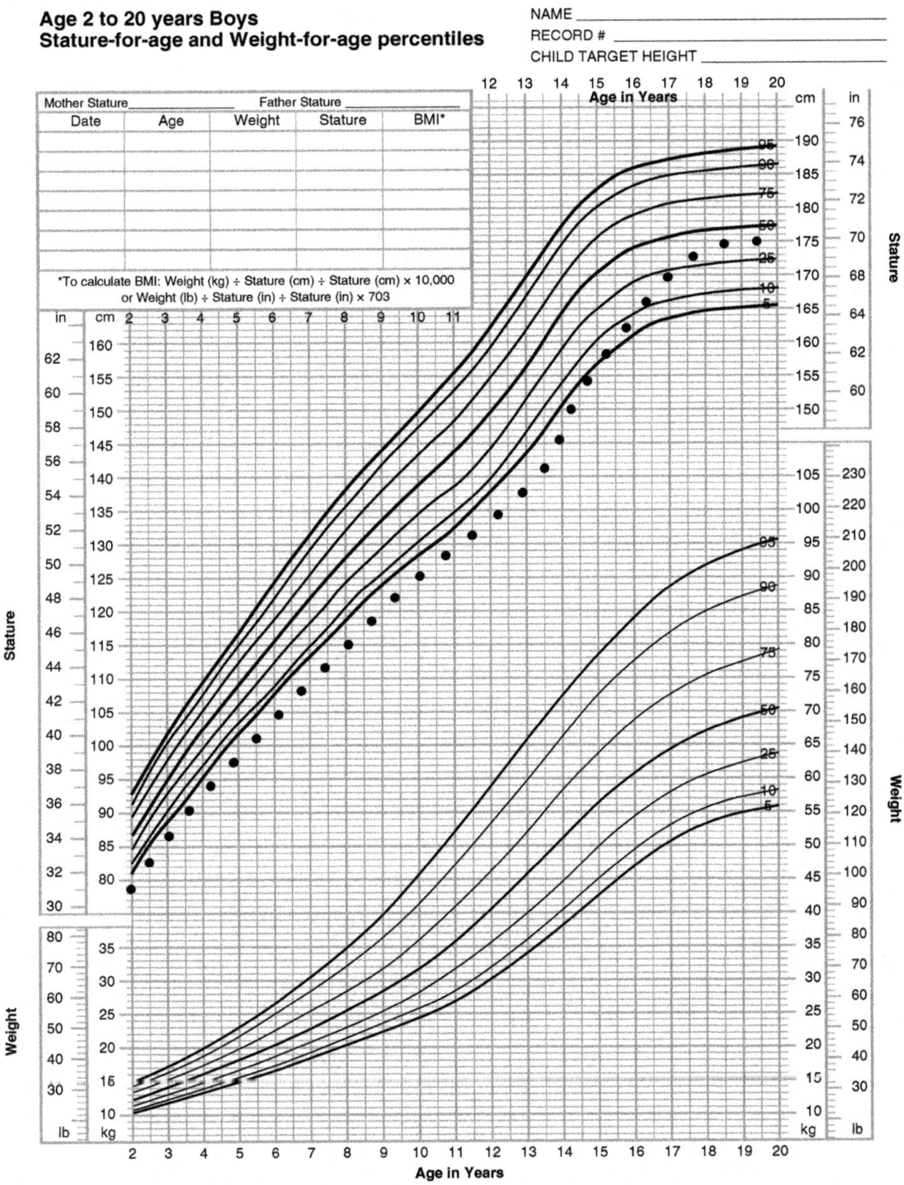

Fig. 11.2 Typical growth chart for a boy with CDGP showing low normal growth rates during childhood with deviation from the normal range at the typical age of puberty and later adolescent growth spurt of lesser magnitude than the average boy

Physical Observations

A common clinical criterion for the diagnosis of CDP among boys is the lack of evidence of the physical onset of puberty by age 14 years. The first evidence is an increase in testicular volume (greater than 4 mL. or a long axis greater than 2.5–3 cm.) in boys. Among girls, the first physical evidence is the onset of breast development (clear evidence of growth of mammary tissue); delay is commonly diagnosed if not present by 13 years of age. Onset should be followed by the timely attainment of pubertal milestones, including accelerated growth rates typical of sex. Growth rates for stage of puberty are informative, including the period of deceleration of growth rate in late childhood, since with CDP there may be a prolongation of this interval of slow growth rate. Upper-lower body proportions with relatively longer limbs, a finding characteristic of hypogonadal individuals, have been noted in CDGP; this suggests a prolonged duration of the childhood growth phase. In boys with CDP, the duration of the interval between the onset of puberty and the pubertal growth spurt is shortened as the duration of growth acceleration leading to an attenuation of the peak growth velocity. Those who have a height deficit early in childhood, typically described as CDGP, have a less favorable adult height prognosis than those who develop this deficit late in childhood [26].

Estimation of testicular volume when a boy presents with the complaint of delayed puberty is crucial. Testicular growth, as the first physical evidence of the onset of puberty in boys, is often evident at the time of presentation with the complaint of delayed puberty. Evidence of testicular growth suggests CDP rather than hypogonadism because this is an indication that puberty has begun. Among those with testicular volume at presentation of greater than 4 mL, at least 95 % have been found to have CDP, while among those with volume <4 mL, the likelihood of HH is much greater (40 % of series presenting with delayed puberty; all have been shown to have HH) [27].

A pubertal nomogram has recently been published for Danish boys classifying CDP using a puberty nomogram (genital stage < −2 SD for age) rather than the classical criteria (genital stage 1 at ≥ 14 years) [28]. In this study, results from 287 boys found that 78 (27 %) had delayed pubertal onset according to the classical criteria, whereas 173 (60 %) had impaired pubertal progression according to the puberty nomogram. These results suggest the CDP may be more even frequent when rates of progression are considered or that standards for progression are too narrow.

Laboratory Assessment

A reasonable approach to the boy presenting with pubertal delay would include determination of a random, preferably morning, testosterone level paired with an LH level. FSH often adds little additional information, except when abnormally high levels, indicative of gonadal failure, are noted. Anti-Müllerian hormone

(AMH) and inhibin B levels are higher among boys with CDP than HH. Values > 100 pmol/L and >35 pg/mL suggest CDP [29, 30]. While CDP among girls has not been studied extensively, a similar approach is appropriate, substituting a sensitive estradiol assay for testosterone. In addition, screening to rule out a functional cause of pubertal delay should be done based on history and physical findings. A skeletal age determination is also pertinent to determine biologic delay and estimate growth potential. Care for the patient with a tentative diagnosis of CDP involves follow-up to determine endogenous HPG axis function.

Virtually all presenting with the complaint of delayed puberty who have basal morning serum concentration of testosterone (T) of >1.7 nmol/L (48 ng/dL) have CDP, while if T is <1.7, 45 % had CDP with the rest having HH [26].

Over recent decades there have been reports of different endocrine tests to differentiate CDGP from HH at the time of presentation. A meta-analysis of publications concluded that basal and GnRH analog stimulated gonadotropin levels have limited diagnostic specificity because of overlap of values for these two diagnoses during adolescence [31]. Stimulation tests with GnRH agonists or hCG may have better discrimination, but they involve prolonged protocols, while an inhibin B level may provide good differentiation. A summary of differentiation criteria is discussed below comparing criteria for CDP vs. those of HH with some specificity and sensitivity data:

1. Testicular volume > vs. <4 mL [27]
2. Basal T > vs. <1.7 nmol/L (48 ng/dL) [27]
3. Basal LH <0.3 IU/L—*88 % specificity and 100 % sensitivity for HH* [32]
4. AMH > 110 vs. <110 pmol/L [30]
5. Inhibin B
   (a) >35 vs. <35 pg/mL [29]
   (b) <111 pg/mL—*92 % specificity and 100 % sensitivity for HH* [32]
6. Testosterone response to hCG
   (a) 1500 U ×3 every other day T > vs. <8 nmol/L (230 ng/dL) [33]
   (b) Three days of hCG T > vs. <9 nmol/L (260 ng/dL) [26]
   (c) Seven days post hCG every other day T > vs. <8 nmol/L [30]
   (d) 24 hours after IM dosage of 15 mg/kg T > vs. <6 nmol/L [34]
7. LH after GnRH
   (a) Nafarelin 0.1 mg/m^2—LH increment > 4.6 U/L vs. <increment < 2 U/L [35]
   (b) Three hour post triptorelin 0.1 mg/m^2 LH > vs. < 14 U/L [33]
   (c) Four hour post triptorelin 0.1 mg—*100% specificity and sensitivity for HH* [32]
   (d) Four hour post decapeptyl (0.1 mg/m^2 LH > vs. < 8 U/L [31]
   (e) Post low dose—10 mcg GnRH IV ++response vs. no response [36]
8. Combination of basal LH < 0.3 IU/L + inhibin B < 111 pg/mL—*specificity 98 % for HH* [32]

Because there is overlap of the prepubertal hypothalamic-pituitary-gonadal function in those with normal versus compromised hypothalamic-pituitary function, none of these tests clearly distinguish between CDP and HH. This may in part be explained by the current recent understanding that some instances of CDP may represent a partial gonadotropin deficiency in spite of later evidence of functioning HPG axis, albeit at a borderline or lower level.

Treatment

Short-term treatment of females with estrogen and males with testosterone may be diagnostic as well as therapeutic since not only should physical changes of puberty be stimulated, but also reassessment after a period of therapy may indicate that endogenous pubertal hormone secretion has begun. While there are more data for males, because of the higher frequency of CDP among boys, similar therapy among girls for whom other causes of pubertal delay have been ruled out is reasonable. It is pertinent that dosages of estrogen are low so that pubertal changes and particularly skeletal maturity is not stimulated to mature at a faster rate than concomitant statural growth. For CDP, treatment is given for short intervals, commonly of 3–6 months duration, followed by interruptions for at least 6–8 weeks so endogenous hormonal secretion, and testicular enlargement in males, can be assessed.

For girls, estrogen therapy is given using the lowest available dosages orally or transdermally. Some forms of patches can be cut and are used by some. Ethinyl estradiol should be avoided. For boys, treatment commonly involves depot T for several months. While it can be argued that the topical (transdermal) forms of testosterone therapy can be prescribed to more closely mimic the gradual rise of levels found in spontaneous puberty, such have generally not been popular among boys and offer no long-term advantage for those with CDP. However, adjusting dosages for those who require long-term therapy is a general practice. Depot testosterone injections are practical and effective, with the goal of therapy being to induce physical changes of puberty and accelerated growth without inappropriate advance of skeletal age. Overall, as long as initial dosages are low to moderate, results are satisfactory. Typically it is unnecessary to monitor T levels during therapy, but if levels are measured, it is important to realize that levels rise progressively over the first 5–7 days after injection and decline thereafter. A reasonable initial dosage would be 25–50 mg every month for the patient who has very low circulating testosterone levels (<30 ng/dL, 1 nmol/L), while 50–75 mg can be used for those whose pretreatment testosterone levels are somewhat higher. If a second course is needed, the dosage can be increased to 100–150 mg every 4 weeks. Since this therapy is a diagnostic and therapeutic trial, there is no need to develop a long-term plan with gradual increases of dosage unless there is evidence of permanent hypogonadism.

While the impact of short-term androgen in boys on inducing maturation of hypothalamic-pituitary axis is unclear [37], if endogenous testosterone 6 weeks later is within the pubertal range, interval maturation of the axis is suggested. During the same interval, testicular volume increase also confirms progression of endogenous secretion [38], since testosterone without gonadotropins (particularly FSH) has minimal impact on testicular growth. Some CDP patients require repeated short-term treatment courses before there is evidence of maturation of the HPG axis [39]. Ongoing monitoring is important.

Since eventual endogenous secretion is expected with CDP (as with the boy with early increase in testicular volume), the option of interval hormonal therapy should be discussed with the patient and parents. It should be made clear that normal but late development is expected, and the therapy is to avoid further delay in physical pubertal changes and growth. Because there is long-term experience with such therapy without long-term negative effects, it is reasonable to explain the presumed diagnosis to the patient and parents and give them treatment options to begin the changes, rather than wait until they happen. In the majority of such situations, patients chose therapy in order to begin growth and maturation.

Treatment is considered because delay may be prolonged with psychosocial problems, as well as a shorter adult height than target (sex-corrected midparental) heights and decreased BMD, and perhaps affect fertility. The psychosocial problems may involve feelings of incompetence, vulnerability, poor self-esteem, less participation in athletic activities, social isolation, impaired academic performance, substance abuse, and disruptive behavior [40].

If there is severe short stature or evidence of partial hypogonadism, other therapeutic regimens may be considered. Treatments that have been used include oxandrolone (which has primarily been used for the prepubertal-aged boys with short stature in an attempt to increase growth rate without inappropriate skeletal age advance), aromatase inhibitors (used concomitantly with testosterone therapy or alone for the older adolescent boys in an attempt to delay epiphyseal closure by lowering estradiol levels allowing for more time for growth), dihydrotestosterone levels (to stimulate pubertal changes since this is a substrate that is not aromatized to estradiol, so there is diminished stimulation of skeletal maturation), and growth hormone (GH) (used in an attempt to increase adult height, sometimes begun in the short prepubertal boy at the usual age of puberty before testosterone therapy).

It is, in fact, difficult to differentiate patients with CDP from those with mild GH deficiency based upon responses to GH stimulation testing. Because of the high variability seen in GH stimulation testing in normal patients and because patients presenting with CDP and mild GH deficiency frequently later demonstrate normal responses to GH stimulation after puberty, the diagnosis of mild GH deficiency in patients with CDP should be questioned. When GH stimulation testing is undertaken in pubertal aged children with CDP, it has been suggested that sex steroid priming be undertaken to improve the validity of testing by giving 25 mg testosterone 7–10 days before testing in boys or by using 1.25 mg of conjugated estrogen once daily for 3 days in girls. However, recent evidence fails to show that this method provides better evidence for the diagnosis of GH deficiency [41]. It is generally felt that consideration of GH therapy should be considered only for those patients whose heights are below –2.5 SD for age with predicted adult heights (based upon skeletal age) and height less than the normal adult range. If GH testing in such patients is consistent with GH deficiency, GH therapy can be initiated before or concomitant with sex steroid therapy with careful monitoring.

Summary

Constitutional delayed puberty continues to be a diagnosis of exclusion, requiring sufficient time for endogenous pubertal physiology to manifest itself. While traditionally viewed as a variant of normal growth, developing evidence suggests that a portion of this population may not achieve normal postpubertal status. Such evidence includes foreshortened adult height, diminished BMD, and adult reproductive function that may be less than the general population. While the later is difficult to document because of the wide range of variation of sexual function and fertility among adults, careful assessment suggests mild hypogonadism and subfertility in some patients previously diagnosed with CDP. Molecular genetic studies suggest that this may be related to genetic defects resulting in later or slower onset of puberty with outcome function at or below the range of normal. In the meantime, while further information is being learned, the diagnosis and treatment of these patients continues unchanged. This involves temporary androgen therapy as desired until onset of endogenous physiologic function with further assessment only if hormone levels are inadequate or infertility is apparent.

References

1. Palmert MR, Dunkel L. Clinical practice. Delayed puberty. N Engl J Med. 2012;366:443–53.
2. Yap F, Hogler W, Broidy J, Moore B, Howman-Giles R, Cowell CT. The skeletal phenotype of men with previous constitutional delay of puberty. J Clin Endocrinol Metab. 2004;89:4306–11.
3. Sykiotis GP, Pitteloud N, Seminara SB, Kaiser UB, Crowley WF, Jr. Deciphering genetic disease in the genomic era: the model of GnRH deficiency. Sci Transl Med. 2010;2:32rv32.
4. Arrigo T, Cisternino M, De Luca F, Saggese G, Messina MF, Pasquino AM, et al. Final height outcome in both untreated and testosterone-treated boys with constitutional delay of growth and puberty. J Pediatr Endocrinol Metab. 1996;9:511–7.
5. Sedlmeyer IL, Palmert MR. Delayed puberty: analysis of a large case series from an academic center. J Clin Endocrinol Metab. 2002;87:1613–20.
6. Valdes-Socin H, Rubio Almanza M, Tomé Fernández-Ladreda M, Debray FG, Bours V, Beckers A. Reproduction, smell, and neurodevelopmental disorders: genetic defects in different hypogonadotropic hypogonadal syndromes. Front Endocrinol (Lausanne). 2014;5:109. doi:10.3389/fendo.2014.00109. eCollection 2014.
7. Sidhoum VF, Chan Y-M, Lippincott MF, Balasubramanian R, Quiton R, Plummer L, et al. Reversal and relapse of hypogonadotropic hypogonadism: resilience and fragility of the reproductive neuroendocrine system. J Clin Endocrinol Metab. 2014;99:861–70.
8. Dunkel L, Quinton R. Transition in endocrinology: induction of puberty. Eur J Endocrinol. 2014;170:R229–39.
9. von Kalckreuth G, Haverkamp F, Kessler M. Constitutional delay of growth and puberty: do they really reach their target height? Horm Res. 1991;35:222–5.
10. Bertelloni S, Baroncelli GI, Ferdeghini M, Perri G, Saggese G. Normal volumetric bone mineral density and bone turnover in young men with histories of constitutional delay of puberty. J Clin Endocrinol Metab. 1998;83:4280–3.
11. Raivio T, Falardeau J, Dwyer A, Quinton R, Hayes FJ, Hughes VA, et al. Reversal of idiopathic hypogonadotropic hypogonadism. N Engl J Med. 2007;357:863–73.

12. Zhu J, Choa RE, Guo MH, Plummer L, Buck C, Palmert MR, et al. A shared genetic basis for self-limited delayed puberty and idiopathic hypogonadotropic hypogonadism. J Clin Endocrinol Metab. 2015;100(4):E646–54.
13. Gianetti E, Tusset C, Noel SD, Au MG, Dwyer AA, Hughes VA, Abreu AP, et al. *TAC3/TACR3* mutations reveal preferential activation of gonadotropin-releasing hormone release by neurokinin B in neonatal life followed by reversal in adulthood. J Clin Endocrinol Metab. 2010;95:2857–67.
14. Beneduzzi D, Trarbach EB, Min L, Jorge AA, Garmes HM, Renk AC, et al. Role of gonadotropin-releasing hormone receptor mutations in patients with a wide spectrum of pubertal delay. Fertil Steril. 2014;102(3):838–846.e2.
15. Kang BH, Kim SY, Park MS, Yoon KL, Shim KS. Estrogen receptor α polymorphism in boys with constitutional delay of growth and puberty. Ann Pediatr Endocrinol Metab. 2013;18:71–5.
16. Joustra SD, Wehkalampi K, Oostdijk W, Biermasz NR, Howard S, Silander TL, et al. IGSF1 variants in boys with familial delayed puberty. Eur J Pediatr. 2015;174:687–92.
17. Cousminer DL, Leinonen JT, Sarin AP, Chheda H, Surakka I, Wehkalampi K, et al. Targeted resequencing of the pericentromere of chromosome 2 linked to constitutional delay of growth and puberty. PLoS One. 2015;10(6), e0128524.
18. Wehkalampi K, Widen E, Laine T, Palotie A, Dunkel L. Association of the timing of puberty with a chromosome 2 locus. J Clin Endocrinol Metab. 2008;93:4833–9.
19. Sedlmeyer IL, Hirschhorn JN, Palmert MR. Pedigree analysis of constitutional delay of growth and maturation: determination of familial aggregation and inheritance patterns. J Clin Endocrinol Metab. 2002;87:5581–6.
20. Wehkalampi K, Widen E, Laine T, Palotie A, Dunkel L. Patterns of inheritance of constitutional delay of growth and puberty in families of adolescent girls and boys referred to specialist pediatric care. J Clin Endocrinol Metab. 2008;93:723–8.
21. Nathan BM, Sedlmeyer IL, Palmert MR. Impact of body mass index on growth in boys with delayed puberty. J Pediatr Endocrinol Metab. 2006;19:971–7.
22. Kaplowitz P. Delayed puberty in obese boys: comparison with constitutional delayed puberty and response to testosterone therapy. J Pediatr. 1998;133:745–9.
23. Wagner IV, Sabin MA, Pfäffle RW, Hiemisch A, Sergeyev E, Körner A, et al. Effects of obesity on human sexual development. Nat Rev Endocrinol. 2012;31:246–54.
24. Lanes R, Lee PA, Plotnick LP, Kowarski AA, Migeon CJ. Are constitutional delay of growth and familial short stature different conditions? Clin Pediatr. 1980;19:31–3.
25. Lindsay R, Feldkamp M, Harris D, Robertson J, Rallison M. Utah growth study: growths standards and the prevalence of growth hormone deficiency. J Pediatr. 1994;125:29–35.
26. Wehkalampia K, Vangonena K, Laines T, Dunkel L. Progressive reduction of relative height in childhood predicts adult stature below target height in boys with constitutional delay of growth and puberty. Horm Res. 2007;68:99–111.
27. Degros V, Cortet-Rudelli C, Soudan B, Dewailly D. The human chorionic gonadotropin test is more powerful than the gonadotropin-releasing hormone agonist test to discriminate male isolated hypogonadotropic hypogonadism from constitutional delayed puberty. Eur J Endocrinol. 2003;149:23–9.
28. Gerner Lawaetz J, Hagen CP, Grunnet Mieritz M, Blomberg Jensen M, Holm Petersen J, Juul A. Evaluation of 451 Danish boys with delayed puberty: diagnostic use of a new puberty nomogram and effects of oral testosterone therapy. J Clin Endocrinol Metab. 2015;100:1376–85.
29. Coutant R, Biette-Demeneix E, Bouvattier C, Bounours-Nouet N. Baseline inhibin B and anti-mullerian hormone measurements for diagnosis of hypogonadotropic hypogonadism in boys with delayed puberty. J Clin Endocrinol Metab. 2010;95:5225–32.
30. Hero M, Tommiska J, Varralahti K, Laitnen EM, Sipila I, Puhakka I, et al. Circulating anti-mullerian hormone levels in boys decline during early puberty and correlated with inhibin B. Fertil Steril. 2012;97:1242–7.
31. Harrington J, Palmert MR. Clinical review: distinguishing constitutional delay of growth and development from isolated hypogonadotropic hypogonadism: critical appraisal of available diagnostic tests. J Clin Endocrinol Metab. 2012;97:3056–67.

32. Binder G, Schweizer R, Blumenstock G, Braun R. Inhibin B plus LH vs GnRH agonist test for distinguishing constitutional delay of growth and puberty from isolated hypogonadotropic hypogonadism in boys. Clin Endocrinol (Oxf). 2015;82:100–5.
33. Kauschansky A, Dickerman Z, Phillip M, Weintrob N, Strich D. Use of GnRH agonist and human chorionic gonadotropin tests for differentiating constitutional delayed puberty from gonadotropin deficiency in boys. Clin Endocrinol (Oxf). 2002;56:603–7.
34. Martin MM, Martin AL. Constitutional delayed puberty in males and hypogonadotropic hypogonadism: a reliable and cost-effective approach to differential diagnosis. J Pediatr Endocrinol Metab. 2005;18:909–16.
35. Ghai K, Cara JF, Rosenfield RL. Gonadotropin releasing hormone agonist (nafarelin) test to differentiate gonadotropin deficiency from constitutionally delayed puberty in teen-age boys—a clinical research center study. J Clin Endocrinol Metab. 1995;80:2980–6.
36. Zevenhuijzen H, Kelnar CH, Crofton PM. Diagnostic utility of a low-dose gonadotropin-releasing hormone test in the context of puberty disorders. Horm Res. 2004;62:168–76.
37. De Luca F, Argente J, Cavallo L, Crowne E, Delemarre-Van de Wall HA, De Sanctis C, et al. Management of puberty in constitutional delay of growth and puberty. International workshop on management of puberty for optimal auxological results. J Pediatr Endocrinol Metab. 2001;14 Suppl 2:953–7.
38. Kaplowitz PB. Diagnostic value of testosterone therapy in boys with delayed puberty. Am J Dis Child. 1989;143:1001–2.
39. Kelly BP, Paterson WF, Donaldson MD. Final height outcome and value of height prediction in boys with constitutional delay in growth and adolescence treated with intramuscular testosterone 125 mg per month for 3 months. Clin Endocrinol (Oxf). 2003;58:267–72.
40. Poyrazoglu S, Gumoz H, Darendeliler F, Saka N, Bundak R, Bas F. Constitutional delay of growth and puberty: from presentation to final height. J Pediatr Endocrinol Metab. 2005;18:171–9.
41. Soliman A, Adel A, Sabt A, Elbukhari E, Ahmed H, De Sanctis V. Does priming with ex steroids improve the diagnosis of normal growth hormone secretion in short children? Indian J Endocrinol Metab. 2014;18 Suppl 1:S80–3.

Chapter 12
Pubertal Dysfunction: A Disorder of GnRH Pulsatility

Lauren C. Passby, Kavitha Rozario, and Jyothis T. George

Timely upregulation of gonadotropin-releasing hormone (GnRH) pulsatility is the fundamental neuroendocrine process underpinning puberty. GnRH is released from a population of approximately 1500 sparse and widely distributed hypothalamic neurons located predominantly in the median eminence of the hypothalamus. Input from rostral periventricular area of the third ventricle (RP3V) neurons controls GnRH secretion from nerve terminals into the hypophyseal portal circulation, which delivers the hormone to its cognate receptor located on the gonadotrope cells of the anterior pituitary. Binding of GnRH to its receptor stimulates the synthesis and release of luteinising hormone (LH) and follicle-stimulating hormone (FSH), which in turn regulate sex hormones from the gonads.

The 'Mini-Puberty'

In the first and second postnatal weeks, the GnRH pulse generator is disinhibited, resulting in the 'mini-puberty' of infancy. In males, this peaks between weeks 4–10 postnatally and is predominantly LH driven, before becoming quiescent by 6

L.C. Passby
Medical Sciences Division, University of Oxford, John Radcliffe Hospital,
43 Woodstock Road, Oxford OX2 6HG, Oxfordshire, UK
e-mail: laurenpassby@gmail.com

K. Rozario (✉)
Department of Paediatric Endocrinology, Oxford University Hospitals NHS Foundation Trust,
John Radcliffe Hospital, Headley Way, Oxford OX3 9DU, UK
e-mail: Kavitha.Rozario@ouh.nhs.uk

J.T. George
Royal Berkshire Hospital, Reading, UK

Boehringer Ingelheim, Bracknell, UK

P. Kumanov, A. Agarwal (eds.), *Puberty*, DOI 10.1007/978-3-319-32122-6_12

months. In females, this mini-puberty is longer, with GnRH secretion remaining active for up to 3 years.

In males, this mini-puberty is thought to facilitate expansion of the Sertoli cell population, with a subsequent increase in germ cell numbers. Exposure to sex steroids during this period potentially has important immediate and future developmental consequences, such as in phallic development and testicular descent—microphallus/micropenis and cryptorchidism are biological sequelae in which this brief window of gonadal axis activation is defective (as in isolated GnRH deficiency). Following the end of this mini-puberty, childhood is a period of reproductive quiescence, wherein there are very low amplitude secretions of GnRH, gonadotropins and sex steroids.

Puberty

The commencement of puberty is controlled by reactivation of the pulsatile release of GnRH. The onset of puberty is characterised in boys by testicular enlargement, penile growth and the development of pubic hair, typically occurring between the ages of 9 and 14. In girls, puberty usually takes place between the ages of 8 and 13 and begins with thelarche—breast bud development, pubic hair growth and menarche.

This reawakening of the hypothalamic-pituitary-gonadal (HPG) axis heralds the start of puberty, though the precise genetic basis of the onset of this pulsatile GnRH release remains one of human biology's greatest mysteries. The prismatic model of human GnRH deficiency presents an opportunity to unravel molecular mechanisms and to better understand the arousal of the GnRH pulse generator that signals puberty. The study of individuals with GnRH deficiency has made it possible to untangle some components of the neuroendocrine network, generating improved understanding of the ontogeny of GnRH-releasing hypothalamic neurons (Fig. 12.1).

GnRH deficiency has numerous genetic causes and, correspondingly, numerous possible phenotypes. Functionally, GnRH deficiency can be classified into three categories, which are discussed below.

Upstream Inhibition of GnRH Release

Mutations affecting the one or several of the upstream regulatory pathways of GnRH can result in hypogonadotropic hypogonadism.

Linkage analysis of consanguineous families facilitated the discovery of mutations in GPR54 [1] (now known as KISS1R), a G protein-coupled receptor, and its endogenous ligands: kisspeptins. Kisspeptins stimulate gonadotropin release from hypothalamic neurons, thereby functioning as upstream gatekeepers to GnRH release. Defects in this pathway can thus result in GnRH deficiency. A number of mutations in the *KISS1R* gene have been reported in individuals with normosmic idiopathic hypogonadotropic hypogonadism (nIHH) [2].

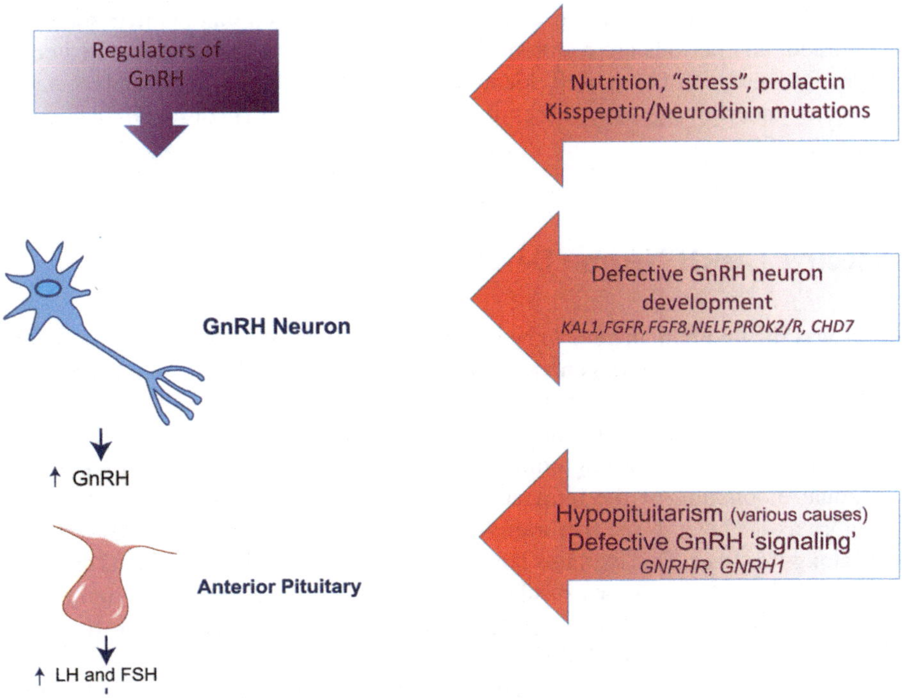

Fig. 12.1 Functional categorisation of defective pubertal development

Mutations in *KISS1* (the gene encoding kisspeptin) have been reported in individuals with a functional GnRH deficiency, though mutations have also been found in control populations in whom there is no evidence of pubertal failure (suggesting a role for other genes in contributing to the GnRH-deficient phenotype) [3]. *KISS1/KISS1R* mutations represent less than 5 % of cases of GnRH deficiency, possibly reflecting the evolutionary importance of this pathway in initiating reproductive capacity.

Further study of consanguineous families with nIHH led to the discovery of mutations in the gene encoding neurokinin B (*TAC3*) and its receptor (*TAC3R*) [4]. Male individuals with such mutations typically have a micropenis and fail to undergo puberty, implicating a role for neurokinin B signalling in the 'mini-puberty' of infancy as well as the initiation of puberty at adolescence. There is some evidence of HPG axis functional recovery during adulthood in nIHH patients with *TAC3/TAC3R* mutations [5], suggesting that the primary role for this pathway is during the neonatal period and puberty, with a reduced dependence upon this pathway in adulthood.

Adult-onset inhibition of GnRH secretion can also be seen in individuals with hypothalamic amenorrhoea (HA). This is a functionally reversible deficiency occurring in otherwise normal females, which is precipitated by stress, undernutrition and/or over-exercise in females. Upon removal of the precipitant, GnRH secretion is resumed, and periods are restored. Whilst the role of the above-mentioned environmental factors on HA is well documented, recent studies have also advocated a role for an underlying genetic susceptibility in this mildest form of functional GnRH deficiency [6].

Defective GnRH Neuron Development

KAL1 was the first human gene to be identified in patients with Kallmann syndrome (KS)—a syndrome of hypogonadotropic hypogonadism with anosmia [7, 8]. The *KAL1* gene comprises 14 exons, which produce glycoprotein anosmin-1. Anosmin-1 is required for the formation of the olfactory guidance platform that facilitates GnRH-secreting neuronal migration embryologically. Anosmin-1 plays a key role in axonal elongation of the intracerebral olfactory tract, as well as in attracting olfactory axons towards the forebrain. There is subsequent migration of GnRH neurons along this tract. This explains how a lack of Anosmin-1 in KS patients carrying *KAL1* deletions or mutations results in a loss of this trajectory and a failure for GnRH neurons to reach the hypothalamus. Deletions and mutations in *KAL1* account for 10–14 % of familial KS and 8–11 % of sporadic KS [9].

Some patients with KS and nIHH have been found to have loss-of-function mutations in fibroblast growth factor receptor 1 (*FGFR1* or *KAL2*) [10]. There is variation in the specific effects that different mutations have some impair expression of the receptor, whereas others impair the ligand-receptor interaction. Mutations in *FGFR1* account for up to 10 % of cases of both KS and nIHH.

Following identification of mutations in *FGFR1*, subsequent mutations in the ligands for this receptor have been found in patients with KS/nIHH. Fibroblast growth factor 8 (FGF8) binds FGFR1, and decreased FGF8 signalling has been shown to cause a deficiency of GnRH in humans and mice [11], with mutations in *FGF8* being found in patients with GnRH deficiency. FGFR1 is also known to be associated with anosmin-1, offering further evidence of the oligogenic nature of GnRH deficiency.

In mice, *NELF* (nasal embryonic LHRH factor) encodes a guidance molecule which has been shown to be associated with the guidance of olfactory and GnRH neuronal axons [12]. A unique rare sequence variant in *NELF* has been reported in human GnRH deficiency, though the biology of *NELF* remains unclear [13]. Given the role that this gene plays in mice, there is reason to believe that alterations in gene may contribute to GnRH deficiency in humans.

Another *gene PROK2* and its receptor PROKR2 are known regulators of the GnRH system, and loss-of-function mutations have been found in *PROK2* and *PROKR2* in individuals with KS/nIHH [14]. As with *FGF8/FGFR1* mutations, there is considerable phenotypic heterogeneity, and variable penetrance, further suggesting oligogenicity to underlie GnRH deficiency.

Defective GnRH Signalling

Mutations affecting GnRH signalling—either its production or its actions at its receptor—can also result in KS/nIHH.

GNRH1 is located on chromosome 8 and encodes the preprohormone that is sequentially processed to produce GnRH. The mouse hypogonadal (hpg) model carries a homozygous deletion of *GNRH1* and has hypogonadotropic hypogonadism. Supporting a role for pulsatile GnRH release in the 'mini-puberty' of early infancy, male patients with homozygous frameshift *GNRH1* mutations have microphallus [15]. Individuals carrying heterozygous mutations have also been reported, in whom there is phenotypic heterogeneity [16]. The presence of a GnRH-deficient phenotype in these individuals may be dependent upon the synergistic action of other rare variant alleles (oligogenicity) that, when present together, result in a hypogonadotropic hypogonadal phenotype.

Mutations in *GNRHR*, the gene encoding the receptor of GnRH, were first documented in patients with nIHH [17]. The effects of these mutations range from a reduction in ligand affinity to impairment of downstream signal transduction. *GNRHR* mutations account for up to 40 % of familial cases of nIHH and around 17 % of sporadic cases [18]. Reproductive symptoms are heterogeneous implicating oligogenicity underlying the pathology, as well as implicating a role for epigenetic changes in response to environmental factors.

Rationale for Genetic Underpinning of Puberty Timing

A Role for Genetics in Pubertal Timing

Timing of pubertal onset is a normally distributed trait. Other complex traits, such as height, show similar distributions and are known to be genetically influenced—which makes it likely that pubertal timing is heritable. Furthermore, several genes that play a role in puberty have been identified in individuals with pubertal disorders, suggesting that there is a strong genetic influence in determining pubertal timing.

Mothers and daughters tend to be of a similar age at time of menarche (which, whilst not the first indication of the onset of puberty, is a clear milestone in female development), despite there being a regression towards the mean in daughters (potentially due to the combined effects of genetics and important environmental influences).

Whilst the pedigrees of families carrying mutations that result in GnRH-deficient phenotypes are characteristically and expectedly small, studies of families situated at the other end of the pubertal-timing normal distribution curve—those with central precocious puberty (CPP)—have shown evidence for familial inheritance of the condition, thus a clear role for genetics in determining the precocious onset of puberty.

A Role for Environmental Factors in Pubertal Timing

Studies in migrant children have shown an increased incidence of CPP in girls migrating for foreign adoption in several Western European countries [19]. This mirrors a secular trend seen in the USA, where the age of menarche decreased from 17 in the mid-nineteenth century to less than 14 by the mid-twentieth century. This occurred in response to improved living conditions, smaller family sizes, decreased infectious disease and better nutrition and may offer the explanation to the observed phenomenon in migrant children.

Precocity in migrant children may be linked to improved nutrition and catch up growth priming maturation for puberty, though CPP is also seen in some non-deprived migrating children. Comparison of CPP in adopted migrating children and non-adopted migrating children (who migrated with their families) showed similar increased frequencies of precocity, suggesting that factors related to migration itself—such as removal of stressful former living conditions or nutritional changes—may be related to precocity. Geographical factors such as altitude, temperature, humidity and lighting levels are known to impact upon various neuronal networks and may similarly feed in to disrupt the neuroendocrine axis that triggers the initiation of puberty. A role for psychological factors also cannot be excluded, though it is difficult to quantify the effects of any of the stresses (both psychological and physical) encountered in these chronic situations.

Intrauterine growth retardation (IUGR) is known to have several effects on development throughout later life, so it is possible that this may also impact upon pubertal timing. Whilst it is convenient to postulate that many of the adopted children may have experienced IUGR due to being conceived in nutrient-deprived areas, there is a dearth of data to support such claims.

The study of migrant children permits for environmental and peripheral signals, which otherwise play minor modulatory roles in the timing of pubertal onset, to be studied in specific situations wherein their effects may play a crucial role in the onset of puberty. Though focused upon CPP, it is easy to see how nutrition and the environment can have important effects on the timing of puberty, alongside the actions of genes.

Conclusion

Studies into the timing of menarche, and twin studies, offer strong evidence for a genetic input into pubertal timing and provide further support for the claim that 50–80 % of the variation in pubertal onset can be attributed to genetic influence. At the same time, migration studies in populations in whom genetics remain unchanged have shown marked environmental effects upon the timing of puberty, which should not be underappreciated when investigating individuals with pubertal delay.

Genetics of Pubertal Delay

Pubertal delay arises when there is a delay in the reawakening of GnRH secretion. The most severe form of this is a total absence of GnRH secretion from the mini-puberty of infancy (resulting in micropenis/cryptorchidism) as well as a failure to spontaneously commence puberty. There is, however, a phenotypic spectrum of GnRH deficiency, resulting in heterogeneity in the signs and symptoms that individuals may present with. Baseline clinical presentations may vary in both sexes with respect to the presence or absence of anosmia; the degree, severity and timing of reproductive defects; patterns of endogenous GnRH secretion; and critical presence or absence of other, nonreproductive defects.

Constitutional delay of puberty (CDP) is the mildest defect in GnRH secretion and is defined as the failure to initiate puberty beyond 2SDs of the population mean age. Individuals spontaneously enter puberty eventually and characteristically remain reproductively normal thereafter. This phenotypic ‘recovery’ is in contrast to individuals with more complete forms of GnRH deficiency, in which there is a failure to initiate or complete puberty, resulting in either Kallmann syndrome (KS) or normosmic idiopathic hypogonadotropic hypogonadism (nIHH).

Kallmann syndrome describes isolated GnRH deficiency accompanied with anosmia (lack of sense of smell), whereas nIHH describes normosmic idiopathic hypogonadotropic hypogonadism, in which the sense of smell is preserved.

Adult-onset idiopathic hypogonadotropic hypogonadism describes a cessation of GnRH secretion following the completion of sexual development and puberty and typically responds to exogenous GnRH administration—demonstrating the hypothalamic nature of the defect. The defect in adult-onset idiopathic hypogonadotropic hypogonadism has been shown to be permanent, in contrast to the reversibility of hypothalamic amenorrhoea (HA).

HA represents a functional reversible deficiency that occurs in otherwise normal adult females and is the most common reproductive deficiency. Defects in GnRH secretion are precipitated by stress, undernutrition and/or over-exercise in females who otherwise underwent normal sexual and pubertal development, with complete recovery upon removal of the precipitant.

Nonreproductive features may also be present in patients presenting with pubertal delay or failure, which may serve to provide clues as to the underlying genetic defect. Well-described associations include:

- Craniofacial defects (cleft lip/palate, high arched palate, coloboma, choanal atresia)
- Renal agenesis, horseshoe kidney and GU duplications (e.g. bifid ureter)
- Skeletal defects
  - Digital anomalies (short fourth metacarpals, campylodactyly, syndactyly, clinodactyly)
  - Scoliosis
- Sensorineural deafness
- Dental agenesis

- Oculomotor abnormalities
- Bimanual synkinesis
- Cerebellar ataxia

The diversity in the nonreproductive features that may accompany GnRH deficiency is important to recognise, and detailed phenotyping of such patients is important in the targeting of genetic testing.

Given the diversity in the phenotypes seen in individuals with GnRH deficiency, it is clear that numerous genetic defects can contribute towards GnRH deficiency. Due to the variable degree of infertility that GnRH deficiency impacts upon individuals, most patients with GnRH deficiency present with sporadic genetic mutations. The genetic basis for 40–50 % of cases of GnRH deficiency is now known, though each of the genes identified individually account for a small percentage of cases. The genes found are involved in various functions and have been described above.

- Genes affecting GnRH development and migration (*KAL1, NELF)*
- Neuroendocrine genes (*GNRH1, GNRHR, KISS1, KISS1R, TAC3, TACR3*)
- Genes with neurodevelopment *and* neuroendocrine functions (*FGF8, FGFR1, PROK2, PROKR2*) (Fig. 12.2)

What remains unclear with the as yet-undiscovered genes is whether they will map on to already-known pathways of GnRH neuronal development and function or whether entirely novel pathways will be uncovered.

Making Use of Phenotypic Clues

Phenotypic clues can give hints to the specific underlying genetic mutations in conditions such as nIHH/KS. The incomplete penetrance of many of the identified genes involved in KS and nIHH emphasises the need to detect underlying genetic anomalies when offering genetic counselling to families, and use of specific phenotypic clues can be a cost-effective means of directing this process. When penetrant, there is a tendency for mutations in genes that are responsible for early embryonic development to manifest as KS (e.g. *KAL1*, *FGF8*, *FGFR1*, *NELF*, *CHD7*, *PROK2* and *PROKR2*), whereas genes controlling GnRH and its actions in puberty (e.g. *KISS1, KISS1R, GnRH1, GnRHR, TAC3,* and *TAC3R*) tend to present as nIHH. Furthermore, there are complex syndromic presentations of GnRH deficiency that are associated with particularly genes, such as *LEP/LEPR* (leptin and leptin receptor, respectively, giving nIHH associated with severe obesity) and *CHD7* (chromodomain-helicase-DNA-binding protein 7, associated with CHARGE syndrome), highlighting how the genetic heterogeneity underlying GnRH deficiency manifests in a similar heterogeneous fashion.

Leptin (*LEP*) and signalling through its receptor (*LEPR*) are known to play a key role in stimulating GnRH release from the hypothalamus. Leptin is a hormone produced by adipose tissue that influences the HPA axis and its downstream effects on satiety and energy expenditure. Mutations in the leptin gene result in early obesity,

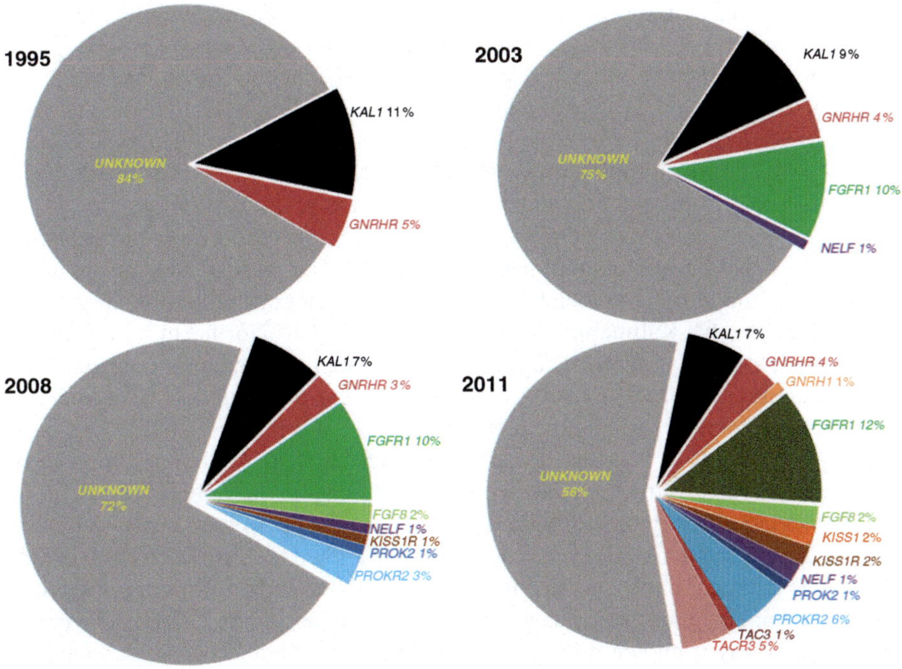

Fig. 12.2 Genetic causes of isolated GnRH deficiency: a historical perspective. Genetic aetiology of isolated GnRH deficiency with relative percentage contribution from each identified gene to the heritability of the syndrome from 1995 to 2011. From only two genes that were known in 1995, the number of genes discovered in subjects with isolated GnRH deficiency has steadily increased through 1995–2011. In 2011, the genetic cause of a nearly half of the subjects is known, whilst in the remaining half, the genes are yet to be identified (Data from the Harvard Reproductive Endocrine Sciences Center, Massachusetts General Hospital, Boston, MA) (Reprinted from Balasubramanian R, Crowley WF. Isolated GnRH deficiency: A disease model serving as a unique prism into the systems biology of the GnRH neuronal network. Molecular and Cellular Endocrinology 2011; 346(1–2): 4–12. With permission from Elsevier)

whilst individuals with mutations in the leptin receptor exhibit this early onset obesity as well as a failure of pubertal development [20]. This reflects a widespread reduction in pituitary function, which extends to reduced growth hormone and thyrotropin secretion, generating a distinct clinical picture for this cause of nIHH.

Mutations in *DAX1* have been found in patients with X-linked adrenal hypoplasia congenital (AHC) and nIHH [21]. *DAX1* encodes an orphan nuclear receptor that is expressed in the adrenal cortex, gonads, hypothalamus and anterior pituitary. Whilst the adrenal failure is clinically apparent at or shortly after birth, the hypogonadotropic hypogonadism of this X-linked form of AHC is often not recognised until the expected time of puberty. Mouse studies and case reports have further indicated that *DAX1* plays a role in spermatogenesis, adding further clues that can be investigated when trying to determine the genetic basis of a case of nIHH.

SOX10 is a transcription factor in which mutations are associated with Waardenburg syndrome (WS). WS is a rare disorder characterised by pigmentation and deafness, though may also include olfactory agenesis. Loss-of-function mutations of SOX10 have been found in approximately one third of individuals with Kallmann syndrome with deafness, indicating a clear role for this gene in this particular phenotype [22]. In patients presenting with Kallmann syndrome and deafness, there is thus the rationale to look for genetic mutations on and around the region of the *SOX10* gene.

A relationship between *FGFR1* mutations and split hand/foot malformation (SHFM) has also been in a small patient sample [23]. A particular mutation in the receptor was found to be associated with GnRH deficiency and SHFM in patients with CHH both Kallmann Syndrome (KS) and Normosmic Idiopathic Hypogonadotropic Hypogonadism (niHH) seven out of eight patients described carried a mutation in *FGFR1*. *FGFR1* mutations account for around 10 % of all cases of CHH, though in the patients sampled in this study, this increased to 88 % of cases of CHH where SHFM was also seen, suggesting that this phenotypic clue can be informative in identifying the underlying genetic cause of the CHH.

PROK2 and its receptor PROKR2 are known regulators of the GnRH system, as discussed above, and mutations in these genes are known to result in KS [14]. Study of families carrying mutations in PROK2 or PROKR2 show intriguing pedigrees, with some homozygous individuals having KS and others having nIHH. The prokineticin 2 pathway is known to play a role in olfactory bulb neurogenesis, so the KS phenotype is expected. The nIHH phenotype, however, indicates a further role for this pathway in regulation of either GnRH synthesis, secretion and/or action. Family members carrying identical mutations can, however, show a wide spectrum of reproductive and nonreproductive phenotypes, suggesting a role for oligogenicity in the manifestation of their condition. These individuals highlight the potential pitfalls of relying upon phenotypic clues to direct the search for a genetic diagnosis.

Monogenicity vs. Oligogenicity

Some of the genes identified as playing a role in GnRH deficiency are thought to be dominant, and pedigrees show full penetration of the reproductive and olfactory phenotypes (e.g. in males with *KAL1* mutations). Likewise, individuals with homozygous mutations in several genes known to play a role in GnRH deficiency have a concordance of reproductive and nonreproductive phenotypes (e.g. in *GNRH1, RnRHR, TAC3, TAC3R, PROK2, PROKR2, KISS1R* mutations).

In documented pedigrees where the mutation is heterozygous, however, there is often considerable phenotypic variability amongst family members in whom the mutant allele is identical (seen in *FGFR1, FGF8, PROK2, PROKR2* and *GNRHR* mutations). Oligogenicity is the phenomenon in which two individually rare genetic variants synergise, or act in a concerted fashion, resulting in the pathogenic phenotype. So, in the case of GnRH deficiency and phenotypic variability, some family members inherit the mutated gene associated with GnRH deficiency, as well as mutated forms of as-yet unidentified genes, which synergise to give the GnRH deficiency phenotype.

Other family members will inherit only one of the genes required to act in synergism to produce the phenotype, thus will be phenotypically normal. Large studies of 400 GnRH-deficient families have shown that digenicity occurs in almost a quarter of all those in whom rare sequence variants could be identified [9]. The prevalence of oligogenicity in patients with GnRH deficiency is known to be at least 15 %, and this is likely to increase when the genetic causes of GnRH deficiency are better understood (currently only 40–50 % of genetic causes are known). Oligogenicity explains the hitherto unexplained phenotypic variability seen in GnRH deficiency, which flouts the laws of strict Mendelian inheritance.

Clinical Utility of Genetic Diagnosis

The majority of the genetic causes of GnRH deficiency have yet to be identified. As there is this considerable phenotypic heterogeneity, enabling individuals to receive a specific genetic diagnosis could facilitate better management of other phenotype features seen in their particular instance of GnRH deficiency. In young adults, it might also be necessary to distinguish a permanent failure of GnRH release, from a constitutional delay, allowing for better management of the physical and psychological sequelae of either outcome.

Differentiation from Constitutional Pubertal Delay

Investigating the genetic cause underlying an individual's failure to spontaneously enter puberty potentially allows for the distinction to be made between a constitutional delay of puberty (CDP) and a failure of puberty. CDP is the mildest form of GnRH deficiency, and individuals typically spontaneously enter puberty without any intervention being required. In contrast, a failure to enter puberty altogether will require medical management, and providing an early genetic diagnosis permits for earlier recognition of this.

Identifying Pubertal Prognosis

If a defect in a pathway known to be involved in regulating puberty is identified, a pubertal prognosis can be generated. It is unclear whether patients presenting with a pubertal delay will eventually enter into puberty (CDP), or whether there is a complete failure to enter puberty (KS/nIHH). When even the mildest manifestation of GnRH deficiency—the constitutional delay of puberty—can result in a psychologically challenging phenotype, there is a great need to identify the specific genetic diagnosis such that appropriate counselling and treatment options can be provided, dependent upon the pubertal prognosis.

Differing manifestations of GnRH deficiency have different pubertal prognoses. Individuals with CDP eventually enter puberty spontaneously and characteristically remain reproductively normal thereafter. This contrasts with the pubertal prognoses for individuals in whom the deficiency of GnRH is more complete (in which there is a failure to initiate or complete puberty, resulting in either KS or nIHH).

Allelic heterogeneity further complicates the phenotype of individuals with GnRH deficiency—different family members carrying the same disease mutations may have different phenotypes as a result of oligogenicity. Along with oligogenicity, there is also a role for epigenetic modifications in contributing to the phenotypic heterogeneity of GnRH deficiency.

Future Directions

Whilst work in recent decades has identified several genes involved in GnRH deficiency, those discovered are responsible for a few per cent of cases each and represent the rare causes of GnRH deficiency. These historic efforts to targeted candidate-gene searching have not been very successful, given our limited understanding of the physiological neuroendocrine networks being perturbed. This may be overcome with exome or genome sequencing, and with the costs of these ever decreasing, the wealth of data that can be gathered from individuals with GnRH deficiency has never been greater. As with all big data endeavours, however, limitations lie within the development and proper use of bioinformatic platforms with which to interpret the data. Challenges also lie within understanding the functional significance of each datum gathered from each individual, for which large collaborative efforts will be required to untangle. To better facilitate this, the COST research consortium—Cooperation on Science and Technology organisation—funded formation of a European-wide research consortium in 2011, with the aims of promoting international collaboration.

References

1. Seminara SB, et al. The GPR54 gene as a regulator of puberty. N Engl J Med. 2003;349:1614–27.
2. De Roux N, et al. Hypogonadotropic hypogonadism due to loss of function of the KiSS1-derived peptide receptor GPR54. Proc Natl Acad Sci U S A. 2003;100:10972–6.
3. Chan Y-M, et al. GnRH-deficient phenotypes in humans and mice with heterozygous variants in KISS1/Kiss1. J Clin Endocrinol Metab. 2011;96:E1771–81.
4. Topaloglu AK, et al. TAC3 and TACR3 mutations in familial hypogonadotropic hypogonadism reveal a key role for Neurokinin B in the central control of reproduction. Nat Genet. 2009;41:354–8.
5. Gianetti E, et al. TAC3/TACR3 mutations reveal preferential activation of gonadotropin-releasing hormone release by neurokinin B in neonatal life followed by reversal in adulthood. J Clin Endocrinol Metab. 2010;95:2857–67.

6. Caronia LM, et al. A genetic basis for functional hypothalamic amenorrhea. N Engl J Med. 2011;364:215–25.
7. Legouis R, et al. The candidate gene for the X-linked Kallmann syndrome encodes a protein related to adhesion molecules. Cell. 1991;67:423–35.
8. Franco B, et al. A gene deleted in Kallmann's syndrome shares homology with neural cell adhesion and axonal path-finding molecules. Nature. 1991;353:529–36.
9. Sykiotis GP, et al. Oligogenic basis of isolated gonadotropin-releasing hormone deficiency. Proc Natl Acad Sci U S A. 2010;107:15140–4.
10. Pitteloud N, et al. Mutations in fibroblast growth factor receptor 1 cause both Kallmann syndrome and normosmic idiopathic hypogonadotropic hypogonadism. Proc Natl Acad Sci U S A. 2006;103:6281–6.
11. Falardeau J, et al. Decreased FGF8 signaling causes deficiency of gonadotropin-releasing hormone in humans and mice. J Clin Invest. 2008;118:2822–31.
12. Kramer PR, Wray S. Novel gene expressed in nasal region influences outgrowth of olfactory axons and migration of luteinizing hormone-releasing hormone (LHRH) neurons. Genes Dev. 2000;14:1824–34.
13. Miura K, Acierno JS, Seminara SB. Characterization of the human nasal embryonic LHRH factor gene, NELF, and a mutation screening among 65 patients with idiopathic hypogonadotropic hypogonadism (IHH). J Hum Genet. 2004;49:265–8.
14. Martin C, et al. The role of the prokineticin 2 pathway in human reproduction: evidence from the study of human and murine gene mutations. Endocr Rev. 2011;32:225–46.
15. Chan Y-M, et al. GNRH1 mutations in patients with idiopathic hypogonadotropic hypogonadism. Proc Natl Acad Sci U S A. 2009;106:11703–8.
16. Chesover A, Kim S, Ahlquist J, Bouloux P. Identification of a novel compound heterozygous mutation in the gonadotrophin releasing hormone receptor in two siblings with isolated hypogonadotrophic hypogonadism. 2008. http://www.endocrine-abstracts.org/ea/0015/ea0015oc11.htm
17. De Roux N, et al. A family with hypogonadotropic hypogonadism and mutations in the gonadotropin-releasing hormone receptor. N Engl J Med. 1997;337:1597–602.
18. Genç DB, Özkan MA, Büyükgebiz A. McCune-Albright syndrome mimicking malignancy: an endocrine disease from oncologist's perspective. J Clin Res Pediatr Endocrinol. 2012;4:160–3.
19. Parent A-S, et al. The timing of normal puberty and the age limits of sexual precocity: variations around the world, secular trends, and changes after migration. Endocr Rev. 2003;24:668–93.
20. Clément K, et al. A mutation in the human leptin receptor gene causes obesity and pituitary dysfunction. Nature. 1998;392:398–401.
21. Seminara SB, Achermann JC, Genel M, Jameson JL, Crowley WF. X-linked adrenal hypoplasia congenita: a mutation in DAX1 expands the phenotypic spectrum in males and females. J Clin Endocrinol Metab. 1999;84:4501–9.
22. Pingault V, et al. Loss-of-function mutations in SOX10 cause Kallmann syndrome with deafness. Am J Hum Genet. 2013;92:707–24.
23. Villanueva C, et al. Congenital hypogonadotropic hypogonadism with split hand/foot malformation: a clinical entity with a high frequency of FGFR1 mutations. Genet Med. 2014. doi:10.1038/gim.2014.166.

Chapter 13
Pubertal Gynecomastia

Philip Kumanov

Introduction

Gynecomastia is a benign enlargement of the male breast due to the proliferation of mammary glandular tissues. In contrast, pseudogynecomastia (adipomastia or lipomastia) represents increase of subareolar fat without proliferation of the breast glandular component [1, 2]. Gynecomastia occurs in males of all ages. The term, derived from the Greek words γυνη gyne (female) and μαστοζ mastos (breast), was first introduced by Galen in the second century AD [2].

Enlargement of the breast in males is not a disease. It is a sign of an underlying disturbance in hormonal physiology, mainly that of steroids [3].

In three periods of life, male breast enlargement may be regarded as a normal developmental variant rather than a pathologic finding. These three forms are neonatal, pubertal (adolescent), and involutional gynecomastia and they occur shortly after birth, during puberty, and in old age, respectively [4]. They correspond to times of hormonal changes [2] and are generally united under the name physiologic gynecomastia [4, 5]. Although not so adequate this term is used to underline their transient character and that not a strong pathologic process is the cause for these forms of gynecomastia.

Gynecomastia should be regarded as unusual in prepubertal children and men of reproductive age [6].

P. Kumanov (✉)
Clinical Center of Endocrinology, Medical Faculty, Medical University of Sofia, 2, Zdrawe Street, Sofia 1431, Bulgaria
e-mail: phkumanov@lycos.com

P. Kumanov, A. Agarwal (eds.), *Puberty*, DOI 10.1007/978-3-319-32122-6_13

Normal Breast Development

In human embryo, bilateral mammary lines develop from the ectoderm during the first trimester and give rise to a single pair of placodes [7]. Due to the epithelial/mesenchymal interactions [5], the placodes descent into the underlying mesenchyme and produce the ductal structure of the glands [7]. Fat pad develops from subcutaneous mesenchymal cells. Parathyroid hormone-related protein secreted from the mammary epithelium seems to be involved in the bud formation, transition from budding to branching, as well as nipple generation [7]. The precise mechanism for the formation of the ductal lumen is not clear, while nipple arises by modification of the skin and suppression of hair follicles during the fifth month of gestation [4, 7]. Mammary glands in males and females possess equal growth potential and have comparable structure with no clear-cut histologic or functional difference until the onset of puberty [2, 4]. At birth only a few small ducts are present and they have an open lumen. Estrogen and androgen receptors are present in both male and female breasts [2]. The difference in the growth and proliferation of breast tissue in each sex is largely affected by the endocrine environment [6]. Estrogens (estrone and mainly estradiol) strongly stimulate and androgens weakly inhibit mammary gland growth [2, 8].

It is the estrogen surge in prepuberty in girls that initiates the process of mammary development, the thelarche [9]. There are two forms of the estrogen receptor, α and β, each encoded by a separate gen, ESR1 on chromosome 6q24-27 and ESR2 on chromosome 14q22-24, respectively [10]. Estrogen receptor α seems to be more important for the ductal formations [7], but a study revealed a correlation between gynecomastia in adolescents and the estrogen receptor β gene polymorphisms [11]. Female pubertal breast represents mammary tree with substantial number of blind-ended ductules, called acini [7]. Estrogens not only stimulate growth, division, and elongation of the tubular duct system, but they contribute also to the development and maintenance of alveoli at the ends of the ducts [4].

Progesterone is required for the normal process of alveologenesis [4]. In combination with prolactin, progesterone stimulates the differentiation of the alveoli, which synthesize and secrete milk during lactation [7].

Growth hormone (GH) through its receptor in stromal fibroblasts induces insulin-like growth factor 1(IGF1) which in turn signals to the mammary epithelium [12]. Systematically produced IGF1 by the liver also acts in this regard at puberty [7]. The observation that the appearance of pubertal gynecomastia coincides within a year of age of peak height velocity [13] further underlines the significant role of growth hormone for breast enlargement. Even when GH is present, no mammary development is possible in the absence of IGF 1 [9]. On the other hand, the proliferative action of IGF1is inhibited by the insulin-like growth factor-binding protein-5, and this protein is linked to the involution of the mammary gland [7].

Insulin, thyroid hormones, leptin, and cortisol play also a role in mammogenesis. The presence of thyroid hormone receptor has been found in normal human breast [14]. It was speculated that the GH/IGF 1 axis and thyroid hormones interact and influence breast enlargement in puberty [14].

Due to the absence of sufficient quantities of estrogen and progesterone and because of the antimammary action of androgens in normal adult men, no breast tissue can be palpated. There are only histological remnants of the duct system [4].

Prevalence

The prevalence of pubertal gynecomastia varies between 4 and 69 % according to the criteria defined for diagnosis [2, 15]. It may not be as common as previously reported [16].

In the largest cross-sectional study performed to date on adolescent gynecomastia, breast enlargement was not found in boys younger than 10 years [16]. A gradual increase was observed from 8 % at age 11.5 years to 43.8 % at age 13.5 years and peak incidence of 61.1 % occurring in 14-year-old boys [17]. After this age the incidence gradually decreased. The gynecomastia was more frequent in children with pubic hair Tanner stage 3 and 4 and testicular volume between 5 and 10 mL [16]. Pubertal gynecomastia coincides with peak height velocity usually at Tanner stage 3 for pubic hair [13]. These findings suggest that gynecomastia is a mid-puberty event.

Etiology and Pathogenesis of Gynecomastia

The etiology still remains unclear. As estrogens stimulate the breast tissue proliferation and androgens suppress it, gynecomastia is regarded as a sign and consequence of disturbed balance between these two hormonal groups. As early as in 1941, it was suggested that gynecomastia is due to increased estrogen secretion or to decreased androgen production [4].

In normal men only about 15 % of the estradiol and 5 % of the estrone in blood circulation are secreted directly by the testes daily [3]. The rest is produced in extragonadal tissues (fat, muscle, skin, bone, liver, kidneys) by the aromatase, the key enzyme for estrogen biosynthesis, from the precursors testosterone and androstenedione [18, 19]. There is also an interconversion between estradiol and estrone in the extragonadal tissues [3]. Testosterone and estradiol bind to sex hormone-binding globulin (SHBG) and, to a lesser extent, to albumin, and a small quantity is unbound in circulation. Only this free fraction is capable to enter the target cells and exert its biologic action. SHBG has greater binding affinity to testosterone than to estradiol and estrone, and hence when serum levels of this globulin increase, relatively more estrogen is available than testosterone to the tissues which can stimulate male breast growth.

The imbalance in men between estrogens and androgens may result from:

- Increase in estrogens through
  - Direct secretion from the testes or adrenals
  - Extraglandular aromatization of testosterone and androstenedione
  - Displacement of more estrogens than androgens from SHBG by certain factors
  - Decreased or altered metabolism of estrogens
  - Exposure to exogenous estrogens or estrogen-like substances
- Decrease of androgens, especially their free fractions in the circulation through
  - Decreased secretion from the testes
  - Altered metabolism of androgens
  - Increased binding of androgens to SHBG
- Androgen receptor defects due to
  - Mutations in the receptor
  - Displacement of androgens from androgen receptor
- Enhanced sensitivity of breast tissues [18]

Pubertal gynecomastia can be explained with the different dynamics of the estradiol and testosterone in the course of puberty. During mid-puberty, relatively more estrogens may be produced by the testes and peripheral tissues before testosterone secretion reaches adult concentrations [20], and this temporary imbalance may result in gynecomastia. The reason for the differences in androgen and estrogen secretion is not clear. In most cases the alteration that lead to pubertal gynecomastia no longer exists when boys present for evaluation [4]. Pubertal gynecomastia usually resolves spontaneously within 1–3 years [21] when adult estrogen/androgen ratios are achieved [22].

In a longitudinal study Biro et al. found that free testosterone levels and body weight were significantly lower and SHBG higher in boys with gynecomastia [23]. Evaluation of 24-h profiles of steroid adrenal and gonadal hormones in eight boys with delayed puberty and 11 with pubertal gynecomastia showed that estradiol and estrone levels were higher relative to testosterone concentrations in the afternoon and evening (when testosterone levels normally are lowest) and that estradiol–testosterone ratio was significantly elevated in subjects with gynecomastia [24].

No relationship was found between gynecomastia and urban/rural areas of living and residences at different sea level, respectively [16], giving ground for assumption that these environmental factors may not play a role in breast development. No significant difference in incidence was observed when groups of fair-skinned and brunette (white) boys were compared [25].

Sher et al. demonstrated that boys with idiopathic gynecomastia tended to be taller and heavier than average [26], whereas other authors found young men with breast enlargement to be heavier only [27]. Obesity may be associated with increased peripheral conversion of androgens to estrogens and thus with higher prevalence of gynecomastia [28]. It was shown that serum leptin levels were higher in boys with

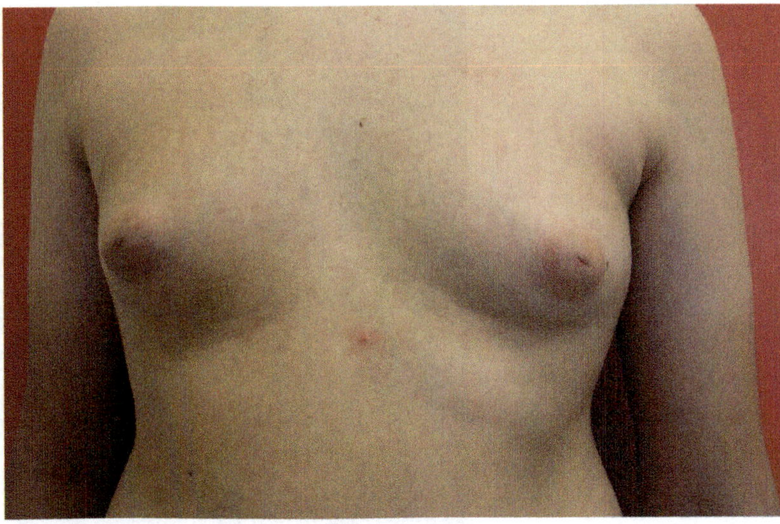

Fig. 13.1 A 14-year-old boy with gynecomastia. His father and grandfather have had bilateral gynecomastia too which had resolved within less than 1 year

pubertal gynecomastia [29] and in other studies was found that leptin increased not only aromatase activity but also activated estrogen receptor α [rev. in 11]. In certain cases leptin receptor gene polymorphism may increase the susceptibility to gynecomastia [11]. Obesity is associated with a significant reduction in SHBG but nevertheless with high incidence of gynecomastia [6]. In contrast, one longitudinal study revealed that boys with pubertal gynecomastia are shorter and leaner [23]. In accordance with the latter, the largest cross-sectional study found that adolescent boys with low BMI are more likely to develop gynecomastia [16]. These both observations suggest that the idea according to which adipose tissue as the site of peripheral conversion of androgens to estrogens is positively correlated with the development of breast tissue in adolescents may not be true. The fact that it is easier to detect gynecomastia in lean boys may also be the cause of the above-described finding.

Approximately half of adolescents with breast enlargement have a positive family history [30] (Fig. 13.1).

Available images of Tutankhamun and his close relatives pharaohs Akhenaten and his father Amenhotep III represent them with enlarged breasts, which gives ground to assume familial gynecomastia in two or three generations [31], but this suggestion has not been proven yet [32]. Tutankhamun died at around the age of 19 years [32]; therefore, his breast enlargement could be regarded as persistent pubertal gynecomastia (Fig. 13.2).

Pubertal gynecomastia is not always a harmless deviation of the norm. In many cases it is a manifestation of underlying medical problems or results from drug side effects and is denoted as pathologic gynecomastia [4, 21, 26].

Approximately half of nonmosaic and a third of mosaic patients with *Klinefelter syndrome* develop gynecomastia during puberty [4]. It is associated with decreased

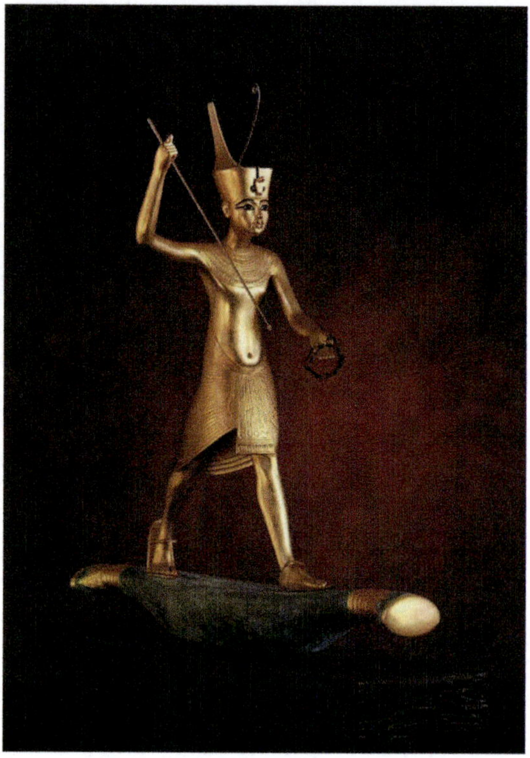

Fig. 13.2 Statue of pharaoh Tutankhamun on a papyrus boat. Pronounced bilateral gynecomastia in the young ruler? (© exhibition TUTANKHAMUN HIS TOMB AND HIS TREASURES)

testosterone production rates and enhanced peripheral aromatization [3]. Gynecomastia may be found also in *XX males*. It can be a sign of the *defects in testosterone biosynthesis* due to deficiencies of enzymes involved in the conversion of cholesterol to testosterone [3]. It was observed that breast enlargement correlates positively with varicocele at the ages at which gynecomastia is most prevalent (12–14 years); therefore, the suggestion arises that adolescent boys with left-sided varicocele are more likely to have gynecomastia [16] (Fig. 13.3). Varicocele can impair Leydig cell production of testosterone and by the resulting estrogen/androgen imbalance cause gynecomastia [33]. In *hypergonadotropic hypogonadism* independently of the form, because of the absent or limited feedback by decreased testosterone, there is increased luteinizing hormone (LH) secretion and the remaining Leydig cells are stimulated to produce estradiol with the effects on the breast tissues [21]. On the contrary, breast enlargement is not usual in *hypogonadotropic hypogonadism* because gonadotropins and sex steroids are low [21].

The highest incidence of *testicular neoplasms* occurs after the end of puberty. Nevertheless they can be the cause of breast development in adolescents [15]. Estradiol production can be stimulated by a human chorionic gonadotropin (hCG)-secreting tumor of gonadal or extra gonadal germ-cell origin (eutopic hCG production) or from lung, gastric, or renal carcinomas (ectopic hCG production) [20]. As a result there is excessive estrogen and deficient androgen action on the breast tissue.

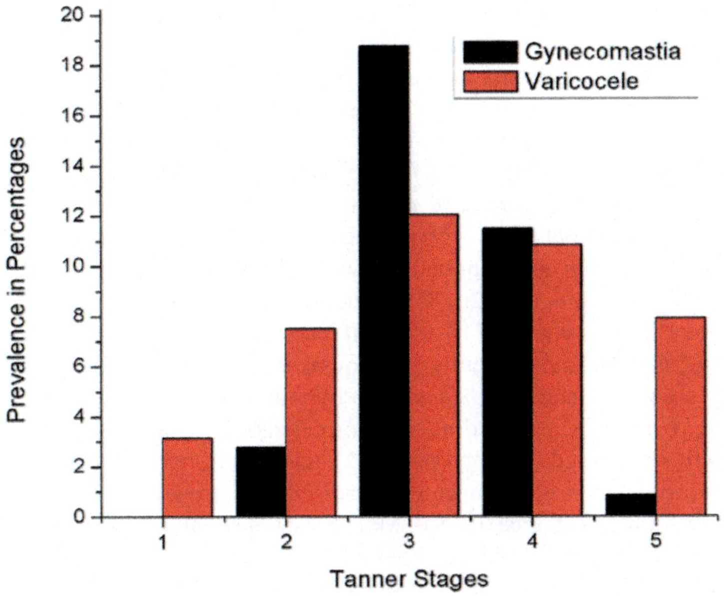

Fig. 13.3 Prevalence of gynecomastia and varicocele according to pubic hair Tanner stages in boys of age 10–19 years. Data are expressed as percentages. (Reprinted from Kumanov Ph, Deepinder F, Robeva R, Tomova A, Li J, Agarwal A. Relationship of adolescent gynecomastia with varicocele and somatometric parameters: a cross-sectional study in 6200 healthy boys. J Adolescent Health. 2007; 41(2): 126–131. With permission from Elsevier)

Sertoli cell tumors may occur in association with multiple intestinal polyps and mucocutaneous pigmentation (Peutz–Jeghers syndrome) [21].

Usually *adrenal tumors* secrete large amounts of androstenedione, dehydroepiandrosterone (DHEA), and dehydroepiandrosterone sulfate (DHEAS) which are then aromatized to estradiol in peripheral tissues. It is also possible that adrenal tumors secrete excessive amounts of estradiol and estrone because of enormous expression of aromatase in the tumor cells [34]. Feminizing adrenocortical tumors are typically malignant [21].

Prolactin receptors are present in male breast tissue [21], but *hyperprolactinemia* usually is not accompanied by gynecomastia. However, in men with gynecomastia, milk is rarely secreted because progesterone is not high enough for breast acinar development to occur [35].

Thyroid hormones alter the estrogen/androgen ratio by two mechanisms: by direct stimulation of peripheral aromatase and consequently estrogen production and also by increasing hepatic SHBG synthesis and hence decrease of free testosterone levels relative to free estrogen concentrations [rev. in 6]. About 30 % of young men with *hyperthyroidism* develop clinically apparent breast enlargement [8]. However, it resolves with treatment that restores euthyroidism [21].

In *liver diseases* hepatic extraction of androstenedione is decreased, and thus there is an increase availability of this substrate for estrogen synthesis [4]. Moreover, in hepatic cirrhosis, serum levels of SHBG are increased [35]. Both alterations have as a consequence male breast enlargement.

The cause of gynecomastia as well as of the testicular dysfunction in patients with *chronic renal failure* is not clear. Breast enlargement in such situation does not respond to treatment [34]. Gynecomastia can develop on several mechanisms in individuals with *acquired immunodeficiency syndrome* (AIDS) [3, 8].

Familial or sporadic *aromatase excess syndrome* manifests itself around the adrenarche and is characterized with prepubertal onset of gynecomastia and incomplete virilization by the end of puberty as well as with accelerated growth in childhood but reduced final height [20, 36]. Mutations in aromatase gene CYP19 which is located on chromosome 15q21.2 [37] can increase aromatase activity resulting in hyperestrogenism and subsequently gynecomastia may arise [38, 39].

During *starvation* and *weight loss*, the hypothalamic-pituitary-gonadal axis is suppressed. With sufficient feeding and normalization of the weight, the gonadal function will be restored ("second puberty"), and like in normal puberty, there is a possibility for transient disturbance in estradiol/testosterone ratio in favor of estradiol with inducing gynecomastia [35]. Male breast may enlarge on the same mechanism during recovery from chronic illness.

Testosterone, an aromatizable androgen, and *androgenic anabolic steroids* are widely used for muscle mass and better sport achievements. They not only diminish testosterone production by suppressing gonadotropin secretion but are substrates for peripheral conversion to estrogens with the resulting altered estrogen/androgen balance and breast enlargement in men [15].

Environmental influence of estrogens or estrogen-like substances may induce gynecomastia. It has been reported that lavender and tea tree oils might be the factor of gynecomastia in prepubertal boys due to their antiandrogenic and weak estrogenic activities [40].

Substantial number of *drugs*, although most of them are rarely used in adolescent years, may cause breast enlargement. Among them besides the estrogens and antiandrogens are also metronidazole, ketoconazole, spironolactone, cimetidine, ranitidine, omeprazole, alkylating agents, vinca alkaloids, cardiovascular drugs, theophylline and some psychoactive agents [28]. Spironolactone and ketoconazole displace steroids from SHBG with estrogens released more easily [3]. Moreover, spironolactone blocks the biosynthesis of testosterone and also inhibits the binding of testosterone and dihydrotestosterone to androgen receptor [3]. Thus, at least on three different mechanisms, spironolactone can cause gynecomastia.

Alcohol increases metabolism and clearance of androgens [6]. Alcohol abuse is associated with elevated levels of SHBG. It has direct toxic effects on the testes [3]. Marijuana and heroin also have been linked to the development of gynecomastia [8, 15].

In some patients there is no alteration in estradiol/testosterone ratio in systemic circulation. It has been proposed that the changes are only *local*, e.g., enhanced aromatization of androgens in subareolar adipose tissue, resulting in elevated estrogen concentration in the breast [20]. Alternatively, enhanced susceptibility of breast tissue to estrogens could also be considered. No identified cause is found in 25 % of patients with gynecomastia [18, 26] and therefore it is signed as *idiopathic*.

This brief survey indicates that all male patients with breast enlargement should undergo complete evaluation.

Histology of Gynecomastia

In gynecomastia of recent onset, the histologic findings include hyperplasia of the ductal epithelium, infiltration of the periductal tissue with inflammatory cells, and increased subareolar fat [20]. When gynecomastia lasts long without or still under hormonal influences, there is progressive fibrosis and hyalinization and regression of epithelial proliferation [4]. Inflammatory reaction wanes [21]. The number of ducts decreases, they disappear but the fibrosis usually remains even when the cause of the gynecomastia is no more active [4]. Hence, pathologic changes correlate with the duration and not with the causes of gynecomastia. The histological appearance of gynecomastia is the same regardless of the cause [21].

Unilateral breast enlargement should be regarded as a stage in the development of the gynecomastia [4].

Outcome

Recently onset gynecomastia is usually accompanied with pain or sensitiveness to clothing. Pubertal gynecomastia has a negative impact on the self-esteem of adolescent boys. In all ages it can lead to psychological distress, decreased participation in social activities, and to depression.

It has not been established that gynecomastia predisposes to breast cancer. Klinefelter syndrome, often associated with breast enlargement, does carry a higher risk for mammary malignancy [21]. However, this malignancy is rare in men [4].

Diagnosis

Diagnosis aims to solve two problems:

- To differentiate true gynecomastia from:
  - Pseudogynecomastia
  - Breast cancer
  - Other processes in breast area: neurofibroma, lymphangioma, hematoma, lipoma, and dermoid cyst [3]
- To determine if the breast enlargement is caused by an underlying disorder or it is idiopathic [5]

A careful medical history should be obtained from the patients and, when necessary, from their parents. The breast should be carefully inspected and palpated. The normal male breast is relatively flat with certain degree of fullness around the nipple-areola complex [2]. The true gynecomastia can be distinguished from breast adiposity simply by palpation. With the patient supine on his back with his hands clasped beneath his head, the examiner grasps the breast between the thumb and forefinger and gradually moves the digits toward the nipple [15, 20]. In case of gynecomastia freely mobile disk of tissue will be palpated concentrically under the nipple and areola [8, 20]. According to some authors, gynecomastia is present when the subareolar disk is about 0.5 cm in diameter [17, 25], and others recommend acceptance of gynecomastia when the diameter is 2 cm [27]. Macrogynecomastia is referred to excessive breast enlargement (>4 cm) [21]. Another method for evaluation of gynecomastia is the use of Tanner stages for breast development in girls during puberty (see Chap. 4, Fig. 4.1). Due to excessive fat and/or connective tissue, the glands can be significantly prominent [5]. In cases of macrogynecomastia, the areola and nipple form a secondary mound over the dome-shaped breast as in Tanner stage 4 female breast development [8]. Obesity may disturb the accurate assessment of the size of gynecomastia. Glandular breast tissue has rubber consistence and is firmer than the surrounding adipose tissue. Gynecomastia of recent onset (less than 6 months' duration) is in most cases tender on palpation [20]. In patients with pseudogynecomastia on the contrary, no such subareolar disk of glandular tissue is palpated [15, 20]. Gynecomastia is usually bilateral and more or less symmetric. Estrogens darken the areolae and therefore some patients with gynecomastia may have change in areolar pigmentation [5].

Physical examination should include height and weight, pubertal development stage, testes size, and palpation of possible testicular masses [2]. Renal and liver function tests should be done along with the assessment of serum levels of LH, testosterone, estradiol, prolactin, DHEAS, and thyreostimulating hormone (TSH) [4, 15]. If both testes are small (testes volumes less than 6 mL), karyotype should be evaluated [22], and in case of asymmetrical gonads, ultrasound of the testes is indicated and the serum levels of tumor markers hCG and α-fetoprotein should be assessed. Elevated levels of hCG and normal findings on testicular ultrasonography are indication for searching for extragonadal hCG secreting tumor [28]. A constellation of accelerated linear growth, high estradiol, low LH, and normal gonadal and adrenal imaging is typical for the increased peripheral aromatase activity (aromatase excess syndrome) [21, 36]. Breast ultrasound is useful for differentiation between adipomastia and gynecomastia [34]. At ultrasound examination, homogenous hypoechoic glandular tissue beneath the nipples may be found or nonhomogenous and hyperechogenic tissue is present with increased amount of adipose and fibrous tissues [39].

One-sided gynecomastia should always be differentiated from breast cancer. The latter is usually very hard on palpation and eccentrically located from the nipple and areola [20]. Pain is less common with breast cancer than with gynecomastia [6]. Skin dimpling and nipple retraction may be present as well as bloody nipple dis-

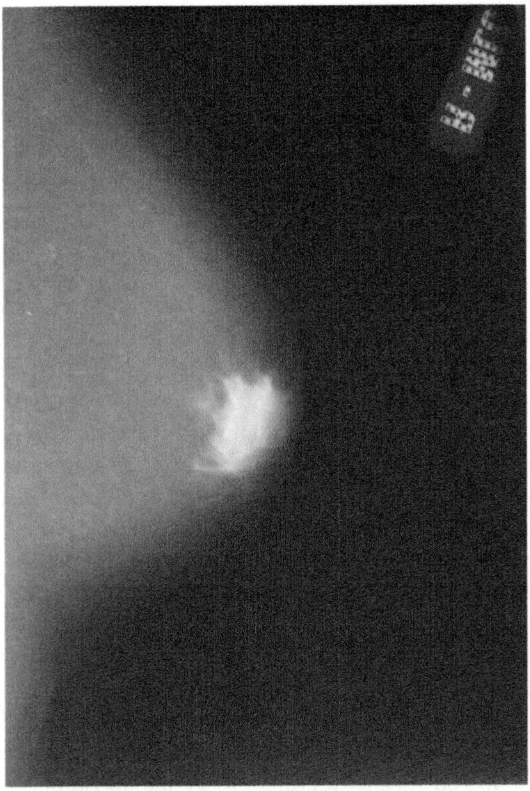

Fig. 13.4 Mammography of a gynecomastia in a 13-year-old boy

charge; these signs can be observed in breast carcinoma but never in gynecomastia [20, 35]. Lymphadenopathy is also suspicious for malignancy [35]. Mammography (Fig. 13.4) is fairly accurate in differentiating between malignant and benign male breast diseases, and this method reduces the need for biopsies [28].

Treatment

No guidelines are still available for the management of gynecomastia [20].

In general, the decision to treat gynecomastia depends on the patient's preferences and on the impact of gynecomastia on his quality of life [1]. Underlying pathological condition should be treated. If the enlargement of the breast is drug induced, discontinuation of the drug is advisable.

Reassurance and watchful waiting are regarded as the mainstay of treatment, given that the breast enlargement is usually a self-limiting condition [22, 30]. If pubertal gynecomastia causes anxiety and embarrassment that are not relieved by explanations and reassurance, it should be treated [8].

Medical therapy is indicated during the initial phase of gynecomastia. It aims to correct the estrogen/androgen imbalance by either blocking the effects of estrogens on the breast with estrogen-receptor modulators or by inhibiting estrogen production with anastrozole or testolactone [2]. Aromatase inhibitors would reduce estrogen effect in all tissues. On the contrary, selective estrogen-receptor modulators tamoxifen and raloxifene have antagonist effect only on breast tissue [30].

The selective estrogen-receptor modulator tamoxifen (10 or 20 mg orally once or twice a day for 3 months) is effective in pain and size reduction of pubertal and adult gynecomastia of recent onset [30, 41, 42]. Adverse events seem to be uncommon [20]. It has been shown that the selective estrogen-receptor modulator raloxifene (60 mg once daily) for 3 months reduces the size of gynecomastia in boys [20, 30]. In a comparative study, they both appeared to be safe and effective in reducing persistent pubertal gynecomastia, with a better response to raloxifene than to tamoxifen [30].

Using the aromatase inhibitor testolactone in a dosage of 150 mg three times daily, Mahoney has found it less effective than tamoxifen in reducing pubertal gynecomastia [8]. In a randomized, double-blind, placebo-controlled study on boys aged 11–18 years, the aromatase inhibitor anastrozole 1 mg daily for 6 months showed no significant difference as compared to placebo in the percentage of patients with breast volume reduction [19]. Since aromatization of androgens is a prerequisite for breast enlargement in many cases, it is not clear why such discouraging results are obtained with aromatase inhibitors [20]. This would suggest that gynecomastia, at least some cases of this heterogeneous abnormality, results not from the altered estradiol/testosterone ratio but from other signaling pathways [19].

Despite some promising observations, no pharmacological agents have been approved for the treatment of gynecomastia [19].

Breast enlargement of longer than 1 year duration is not responsive to medical treatment because of substantial stromal fibrosis. Such cases should undergo surgical removal of the breast tissue and subareolar fat [2, 18, 35]. The available data suggest that the first surgical attempt was undertaken in the seventh century AD by the byzantine physician Paulus Aegineta [2]. After many modifications surgery remains the most effective overall method in treating gynecomastia [3]. The goals should be restoration of adequate male chest shape with limited scar extensions [2]. Complications include skin retraction, scars as well as hematoma and insufficient resection but they all are seldom when the surgeons are experienced [2].

Conclusion

Gynecomastia is not a separate disease. In many cases and in all ages, it may reflect severe underlying conditions. Gynecomastia is often asymptomatic and in adolescents usually resolves spontaneously within 1–3 years. Nevertheless a pathologic process, environmental exposure, or abuse of some substances must be ruled out also in this period of life as well as in preadolescent boys. Due to insufficient studies, there is no consensus recommendation for the treatment of gynecomastia.

References

1. Johnson RE, Kermott CA, Murad MH. Gynecomastia – evaluation and current treatment options. Ther Clin Risk Manag. 2011;7:145–8.
2. Lemaine V, Cayci C, Simmons PS, Petty P. Gynecomastia in adolescent males. Semin Plast Surg. 2013;27:56–61.
3. Mathur R, Braunstein GD. Gynecomastia: pathomechanisms and treatment strategies. Horm Res. 1997;48:95–102.
4. Wilson JD, Aiman J, MacDonald PC. The pathogenesis of gynecomastia. Adv Intern Med. 1980;25:1–32.
5. Kleinberg DL. Gynecomastia and galactorrhea. In: Manni A, editor. Contemporary endocrinology: endocrinology of the breast. Totowa, NJ: Humana press; 1998, p. 359–82
6. Ismail AAA, Barth JH. Endocrinology of gynaecomastia. Ann Clin Biochem. 2001;38:596–607.
7. Macias H, Hinck L. Mammary gland development. Wiley Interdiscip Rev Dev Biol. 2012;1(4):533–57.
8. Mahoney CP. Adolescent gynecomastia differential diagnosis and management. Pediatr Clin North Am. 1990;37(6):1389–404.
9. Ruan W, Kleinberg DL. Insulin-like growth factor I is essential for terminal end bud formation and ductal morphogenesis during mammary development. Endocrinology. 1999;140:5075–81.
10. Enmark E, Gustafsson J-Å. Oestrogen receptors – an overview. J Intern Med. 1999;246:133–8.
11. Eren E, Edgunlu T, Korkmaz HA, Cakir EDP, Demir K, Cetin ES, et al. Genetic variants of estrogen beta and leptin receptors may cause gynecomastia in adolescent. Gene. 2014;541:101–6.
12. Kleinberg DL, Feldman M, Ruan W. IGF-I: an essential factor in terminal end bud formation and ductal morphogenesis. J Mammary Gland Biol Neoplasia. 2000;5(1):7–17.
13. Limony Y, Friger M, Hochberg Z. Pubertal gynecomastia coincides with peak height velocity. J Clin Res Pediatr Endocrinol. 2013;5(3):142–4.
14. Mieritz MG, Sorensen K, Aksglaede L, Mouritsen A, Hagen CP, Hilsted L, et al. Elevated serum levels of free triiodothyronine in adolescent boys with gynecomastia compared with controls. Eur J Endocrinol. 2014;171:193–8.
15. Nordt CA, DiVasta AD. Gynecomastia in adolescents. Curr Opin Pediatr. 2008;20:375–82.
16. Kumanov P, Deepinder F, Robeva R, Tomova A, Li J, Agarwal A. Relationship of adolescent gynecomastia with varicocele and somatometric parameters: a cross-sectional study in 6200 healthy boys. J Adolescent Health. 2007;41:126–31.
17. Güvenc H, Yurdakök M, Kinik E, Büyükgebiz A. The incidence of pubertal gynecomastia in boys living in the Ankara region. Turk J Pediatr. 1989;31:123–6.
18. Braunstein GD. Gynecomastia. N Engl J Med. 1993;328:490–5.
19. Plourde PV, Reiter EO, Jou H C, Desrochers PE, Rubin SD, Bercu BB, et al. Safety and efficacy of anastrozole for the treatment of pubertal gynecomastia: a randomized, double-blind, placebo-controlled trial. J Clin Endocrinol Metab. 2004;89:4428–33.
20. Braunstein GD. Gynecomastia. N Engl J Med. 2007;357:1229–37.
21. Ma NS, Geffner ME. Gynecomastia in prepubertal and pubertal boys. Curr Opin Pediatr. 2008;20:465–70.
22. Lazala C, Saenger P. Pubertal gynecomastia. J Pediatr Endocrinol Metab. 2002;15(5):553–60.
23. Biro FM, Lucky AW, Huster GA, Morrison JA. Hormonal studies and physical maturation in adolescent gynecomastia. J Pediatr. 1990;116:450–5.
24. Large DM, Anderson DC. Twenty-four hour profiles of circulating androgens and oestrogens in male puberty with and without gynecomastia. Clin Endocrinol. 1979;11:505–21.
25. Nydick M, Bustos J, Dale JH, Chester P, Rawson RW. Gynecomastia in adolescent boys. JAMA. 1961;178(5):449–54.

26. Sher ES, Migeon CJ, Berkowitz GD. Evaluation of boys with marked breast development at puberty. Clin Pediatr. 1998;37:367–72.
27. Georgiadis E, Papandreou L, Evangelopoulou C, Aliferis C, Lymberis C, Panitsa C, et al. Incidence of gynaecomastia in 954 young males and its relationship to somatometric parameters. Ann Hum Biol. 1994;21(6):579–87.
28. Johnson RE, Murad MH. Gynecomastia: pathophysiology, evaluation, and management. Mayo Clin Proc. 2009;84(11):1010–5.
29. Dundar B, Dundar N, Erci T, Bober E, Büyükgebiz A. Leptin levels in boys with pubertal gynecomastia. J Pediatr Endocrinol Metab. 2005;18(10):929–34.
30. Lawrence SE, Faught KA, Vethamuthu J, Lawson ML. Beneficial effects of raloxifene and tamoxifen in the treatment of pubertal gynecomastia. J Pediatr. 2004;145:71–6.
31. Paulshock BZ. Tutankhamun and his brothers Familial gynecomastia in the eighteenth dynasty. JAMA. 1980;244(2):160–4.
32. Hawass Z, Gad YZ, Ismail S, Khairat R, Fathalla D, Hasan N, et al. Ancestry and pathology in King Tutankhamun's family. JAMA. 2010;303(7):638–47.
33. Castro-Magana M, Angulo M, Uy J. Elevated serum estradiol associated with increased androstenedione-testosterone ratio in adolescent males with varicocele and gynecomastia. Fertil Steril. 1991;56(3):515–8.
34. Hershkovitz E, Leiberman E. Gynecomastia: a review. Endocrinologist. 2002;12:321–32.
35. Matsumoto AM, Bremner WJ. Testicular disorders. In: Melmed S, Polonsky KS, Larsen PR, Kronenberg HM, editors. Williams textbook of endocrinology. Philadelphia: Elsevier Saunders; 2011. p. 688–816.
36. Stratakis CA, Vottero A, Brodie A, Kirschner LS, DeAtkine D, Lu Q, et al. The aromatase excess syndrome is associated with feminization of both sexes and autosomal dominant transmission of aberrant P450 aromatase gene transcription. J Clin Endocrinol Metab. 1998;83:1348–57.
37. Braunstein GD. Aromatase and gynecomastia. Endocr Relat Cancer. 1999;6:315–24.
38. Shozu M, Sebastian S, Takayama K, Hsu W-T, Schultz RA, Neely K, et al. Estrogen excess associated with novel gain-of-function mutations affecting the aromatase gene. N Engl J Med. 2003;348:1855–65.
39. Czajka-Oraniec I, Zgliczynski W, Kurylowicz A, Mikula M, Ostrowski J. Association between gynecomastia and aromatase (CYP 19) polymorphisms. Eur J Endocrinol. 2008;158:721–7.
40. Henley DV, Lipson N, Korach KS, Bloch CA. Prepubertal gynecomastia linked to lavender and tea tree oils. N Engl J Med. 2007;356:479–85.
41. Derman O, Kanbur NO, Kutluk T. Tamoxifen treatment for pubertal gynecomastia. Int J Adolesc Med Health. 2003;15(4):359–63.
42. Hanavadi S, Banerjee D, Monypenny IJ, Mansel RE. The role of tamoxifen in the management of gynaecomastia. Breast. 2006;15:276–80.

Chapter 14
Pubertal Acne

Devinder Mohan Thappa and Munisamy Malathi

Introduction

Acne, often the first sign of puberty in boys and girls, occurs due to increased sebum production resulting from hormonal surges. Nowadays, the onset of acne in children has been found to occur earlier than has been described in the past as evidenced by the declining age of children seeking treatment for acne over time indicating that puberty is occurring earlier [1, 2]. The appearance of mild acne at the pubertal age group is generally not of concern as it represents what may be called the "adrenal awakening." However, hyperandrogenism and other dermatologic conditions need to be considered in the differential diagnosis when they occur with increased severity warranting detailed evaluation [3]. In addition to the challenging differentiation of the eruptions, treatment also requires special consideration among children of this age group owing to contraindications to the use of certain treatments.

Epidemiology

The epidemiology and demographic profile of acne has changed considerably over the past two decades, to affect children as young as 7 years of age conforming to the documented evidence of earlier onset of puberty [2, 4]. It has been observed that acne was three times higher in pubertal girls and five times higher in pubertal boys when compared with prepubertal children in whom the prevalence of acne was already high [4]. In recent cross-sectional study involving school children from Lithuania, it was observed that 42 % of those aged 7–9 years and 76 % of those aged

D.M. Thappa (✉) • M. Malathi
Department of Dermatology and Sexually Transmitted Diseases, Jawaharlal Institute of Postgraduate Medical Education and Research (JIPMER),
Puducherry, Pondicherry 605006, India
e-mail: dmthappa@gmail.com; mmalthi.dr@live.com

P. Kumanov, A. Agarwal (eds.), *Puberty*, DOI 10.1007/978-3-319-32122-6_14

10–12 years had acne indicating an earlier age at onset [4]. Among premenarchal girls, the prevalence of acne ranges between 61 and 71.3 %, and the prevalence and severity of acne increase with advancing pubertal maturation in boys and girls [5].

Gender and ethnic differences exist in the prevalence of pubertal acne. Acne was found to be more prevalent in girls at younger age with increased prevalence among boys as they reached puberty [6]. Also, a decreasing trend in the age at onset of acne has been observed among white children with no significant changing trend among black children with acne owing to the fact that the onset of puberty is earlier in black individuals and sebum production increases during puberty [7]. Thus the prevalence of pubertal acne is higher among black girls. But as most studies till date have focused on Caucasian and black skin types, there are no such studies in Asian or Hispanic patients for comparison [7].

A family history of acne among first-degree relatives especially mothers has been shown to have the strongest impact on prevalence, age at onset, severity, and treatment success of acne in children. Other risk factors include dietary factors with high glycemic load and dairy products and higher body mass index which may be associated with hyperandrogenism which in turn affects sebum production and follicular keratinization resulting in acne [4].

Etiology and Pathogenesis

Pubertal acne occurs prior to true puberty which is due to maturation of gonads mediated by the hypothalamo-pituitary axis. Prior to puberty, during the period of adrenarche which occurs at the age of 6–7 years in girls and 7–8 years in boys, the adrenal glands secrete increased levels of androgens—dehydroepiandrosterone (DHEA) and dehydroepiandrosterone sulfate (DHEAS)—resulting in reactivation of sebaceous glands. Since DHEAS closely correlates with the initiation of acne, it is known as the "acne hormone" and its levels have been found to correlate with sebum production [5]. However, DHEAS is a weak androgen and is further converted to testosterone, and part of testosterone is converted by 5-alpha reductase to dihydrotestosterone (DHT), which is a more potent androgen, which acts on the skin, penis, prostate, and other tissues. In addition, the skin being an intracrine organ can locally convert DHEA to testosterone and DHT which act on the androgen receptors found in the basal layer of sebaceous glands and follicular keratinocytes, thereby augmenting the androgen-mediated signaling in acne prone skin [8].

During this period, the gonadal androgen secretion is minimal, and ovarian androgen excess should raise the possibility of polycystic ovarian syndrome or rarely ovarian tumors. Low birth weight has been implicated as a risk factor for premature adrenarche, and low birth weight has been associated with higher androgen levels in childhood. Other associations with premature adrenarche include impaired insulin sensitivity, dyslipidemia, and proinflammatory shift of the adipokine profile commonly seen in polycystic ovarian syndrome [5]. The onset of menarche was found to be earlier in girls with severe acne associated with high levels of serum DHEAS. In addition, a high number of comedones, early development of comedones, and high–normal levels of DHEAS, free and total testosterone was found to be predictive for the severity of late inflammatory acne, or persistent acne [5].

The clinical course of acne was found to correspond less closely to plasma androgen levels than it does to growth hormone (GH) and insulin-like growth factor 1 (IGF-1). During puberty, there is an increase in the pulsatile pituitary secretion of GH resulting in a physiological state of transient insulin resistance. GH induces the synthesis and secretion of IGF-1, and all three factors—GH, insulin, and IGF-1—stimulate sebocyte growth and differentiation [8]. IGF-1 enhances the sensitivity of the adrenal gland to ACTH thereby inducing adrenal androgen biosynthesis and production of DHEAS, which results in an increase in sebum production and the development of comedonal acne [8].

Thus acne is considered as an androgen-dependent multifactorial disease originating from the pilosebaceous unit that usually starts at puberty when growth hormone (GH), transient insulin resistance, plasma insulin-like growth factor-1 (IGF-1), and androgen plasma levels are elevated [8].

Whatever may be the initiating factor in pubertal acne, the pathogenesis of acne involves a complex interplay of four main factors [9, 10] (Fig. 14.1).

- *Excess sebum production*: Sebum production which is considered the prerequisite for the formation of microcomedone occurs at the onset of puberty due to activation of the sebaceous glands by androgens.
- *Disturbed keratinization within the follicle*: Hypercornification of the pilosebaceous duct due to the retention of hyperproliferating ductal corneocytes is modulated by androgens. This along with the irritant effect of certain sebaceous lipids and ductal cytokines leads to microcomedone formation. Sebum and keratinocyte debris accumulate in the microcomedone, resulting in macrocomedones, which clinically manifest as closed or open comedones.
- *Colonization of the pilosebaceous duct by the oxygen-tolerant, anaerobic bacterium Propionibacterium acnes (P. acnes)*: Presence of seborrhoea at puberty results in marked increase in ductal colonization of facial skin by *P. acnes* which is likely the prerequisite for acne inflammation.
- *Release of inflammatory mediators into the skin*: *P. acnes* stimulates the release of inflammatory mediators into the surrounding perifollicular dermis which act as chemoattractants to immunocompetent cells resulting in the development of inflammatory acne lesions.

Clinical Features

Acne can be clinically categorized based on the predominant morphology as follows:

(a) Comedonal acne with closed and open comedones ("whiteheads" and "blackheads," respectively)

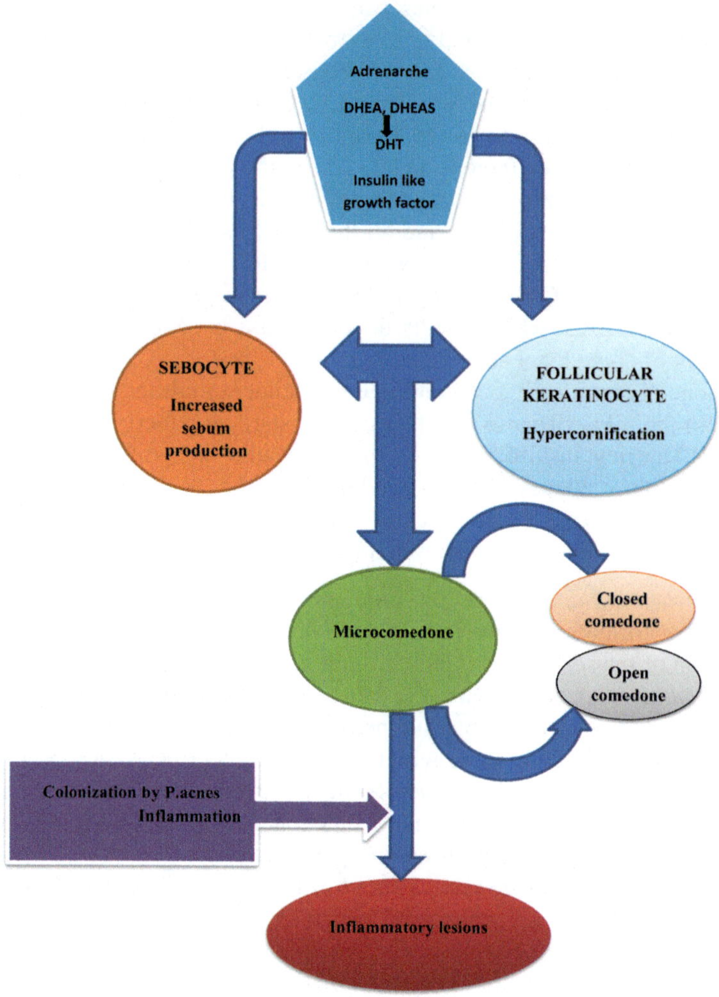

Fig. 14.1 Pathogenesis of acne

(b) Inflammatory acne with erythematous papules, pustules, nodules, or cyst-like nodular lesions
(c) Mixed type with both types of lesions

The microcomedone resulting from hyperactive sebaceous glands and altered follicular growth and differentiation is the clinically unapparent precursor of both comedonal and inflammatory lesions. Comedones occur due to increased cell division and cohesiveness of cells lining the follicular lumen. Abnormal accumulation of these cells mixed with sebum partially obstructs the follicular opening forming the closed comedone or whitehead. In case of larger follicular opening, increased keratin and sebum buildup with oxidization results in open comedone or blackhead. Inflammatory papules and pustules occur as a result of inflammation mediated by follicular colonization with *P. acnes*. Nodular acne, characterized by large inflammatory nodules or pseudocysts, is often accompanied by scarring and sinus tracts [5, 11].

The severity of acne can be graded as mild, moderate, or severe (Table 14.1) based on the number and type of lesions and the depth and extent of skin involved [11]. There are many methods of measuring the severity of acne vulgaris which include simple grading based on clinical examination, lesion counting, and those that require complicated instruments such as photography, fluorescent photography, polarized light photography, video microscopy, and measurement of sebum production. The two commonly used measures are grading and lesion counting. Grading is a subjective method, which involves determining the severity of acne, based on observing the dominant lesions, evaluating the presence or absence of inflammation, and estimating the extent of involvement. Lesion counting involves recording the number of each type of acne lesion and determining the overall severity. However, no universal standard exists for grading acne severity till date [12].

The prevalence and severity of acne increases with pubertal maturation, and hence comedonal acne predominates in preteens with the onset of facial sebum

Table 14.1 Evidence-based recommendations by the American Acne and Rosacea Society for the treatment of pubertal acne

Grade of acne	Clinical presentation	Initial treatment	Inadequate response	Special remarks
Mild	Predominantly comedonal or mixed comedonal and mild inflammatory disease	Over-the-counter products such as benzoyl peroxide (BP) as a single agent, topical retinoids, or combinations of topical retinoids, antibiotics, and BP as individual agents or fixed-dose combinations	Check adherence	Topical antibiotic monotherapy is not recommended
			A topical retinoid or BP may be added to monotherapy with either agent	If topical antibiotic treatment is to be prolonged more than a few weeks, topical BP should be added to optimize efficacy and reduce antibiotic resistance
			Concentration, type, and/or formulation of the topical retinoid may be changed, or the topical combination therapy can be changed to topical dapsone	Comparative studies of dapsone versus other topicals are lacking in pediatric patients

(continued)

Table 14.1 (continued)

Grade of acne	Clinical presentation	Initial treatment	Inadequate response	Special remarks
Moderate	Predominantly inflammatory or mixed comedonal and marked inflammatory lesions	Topical combinations including a retinoid and BP and/or antibiotics, or with combinations that include topical dapsone or with oral antibiotics in addition to a topical retinoid and BP and/or topical antibiotics	Check adherence	Tetracycline derivatives (tetracycline, doxycycline, and minocycline) should not be used in children <8 years of age
			Type, strength, or formulation of the retinoid, BP, or BP-antibiotic component of the topical regimen	Second-generation tetracyclines (doxycycline, minocycline) are preferred to tetracycline in children > 8 years of age because of ease of use, fewer problems with absorption with food, and less-frequent dosing
			Referral to a dermatologist or pediatric dermatologist	Monitor for potential adverse events
				Discontinue (or taper) within 1–2 months once new inflammatory acne lesions stop
				For children <8 years of age and in those with tetracycline allergies, erythromycin, azithromycin, and trimethoprim/sulfamethoxazole should be used

(continued)

production, with increasing inflammatory acne developing during the teen years with the colonization by *P. acnes* [6].

Acne in preadolescent children occurs as a result of normal adrenarche and testicular/ovarian maturation and may precede any other sign of pubertal maturation. In fact the comedonal type of acne can be the first sign of pubertal maturation in

Table 14.1 (continued)

Grade of acne	Clinical presentation	Initial treatment	Inadequate response	Special remarks
Severe	Extensive inflammatory or mixed and nodular lesions	Oral antibiotics and topical retinoids with BP, with or without topical antibiotics, with consideration of hormonal therapy in pubertal females, oral isotretinoin, and dermatologist referral	Check adherence	Prompt initiation of appropriate treatment to prevent scarring
			Change the oral antibiotic agent or the class of antibiotic	Isotretinoin is recommended for severe, scarring, and/or refractory acne in adolescents and may be used in younger patients.
			For female patients, combination oral contraceptive (OC) therapy should be considered. Both males and females unresponsive to topical and oral therapies will benefit from oral isotretinoin	Extensive counseling regarding the avoidance of pregnancy as well as careful monitoring of potential side effects and toxicities
				Withhold OC for acne unassociated with endocrinologic pathology until 1 year after onset of menstruation
				In congenital adrenal hyperplasia, low-dose glucocorticoids are used to suppress the adrenal production of androgens

Based on data from [11]

girls, even preceding pubic hair and areolar development. With the trend toward earlier age of onset of adrenarche and menarche, there appears to be a downward shift in the age at which acne first appears [5].

Pubertal acne usually presents with comedones with or without inflammatory lesions predominantly affecting the central area of the face, involving the mid-forehead, nose, and chin ("T-zone") (Fig. 14.2). Comedones of the ear (concha) can be an early

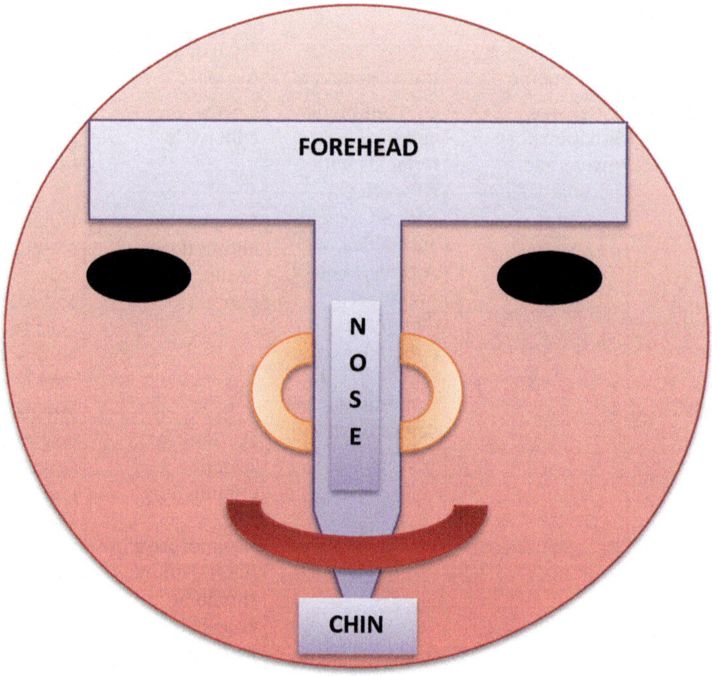

Fig. 14.2 Pubertal acne affects "T"-zone of the face

presentation. Inflammatory acne lesions may involve the face, chest, and back. However, in the case of severe acne with nodules and cysts, the lesions might involve the arms, abdomen, buttocks, and scalp in addition to the face, chest, and back [8].

Since acne may be the first physical sign of pubertal maturation in some girls, the presence of severe acne in prepubertal girls that is unresponsive to treatment and if associated with other signs of excess androgens should raise a suspicion of possible endocrine disorders such as premature adrenarche, polycystic ovarian syndrome, congenital adrenal hyperplasia, or true precocious puberty [6, 11].

In the largest population-based study on pubertal acne involving 6200 Caucasian boys, the interrelations between the presence of acne and several variables associated with somatic growth, pubertal maturation, and environmental conditions (altitude and regions of residence) were studied [13]. They observed that 12–15-year-old boys with acne were taller and heavier than the ones without acne, and they also had increased penile length and circumference as well as larger testicular volumes. However, there were no differences in the somatometric and pubertal characteristics of 17–19-year-old boys with and without acne. Overall, the prevalence of acne among Caucasian boys was 7.74 %. There was no difference in the acne prevalence between the rural and urban inhabitants, but they made an interesting observation that the risk for acne development was significantly higher in adolescent boys living at the altitude under 200 m compared to those living at 500 m or more.

Differential Diagnosis

Pubertal and prepubertal acne needs to be differentiated from childhood granulomatous periorificial dermatitis (characterized by discrete yellow brown papules, lack of pustules, less prominent erythema in the perinasal, periorbital, and perioral areas of the face, and noncaseating granulomatous infiltrate on histologic examination occurs in prepubertal children with history of prior topical corticosteroid application), lupus miliaris disseminatus faciei (presents as firm, yellowish brown or red, 1–3 mm monomorphous smooth-surfaced papules on the face especially eyelids histologically showing caseating epithelioid cell granulomas), childhood granulomatous rosacea (persistent facial erythema of convexities of the face with papular eruption; histologically papules show perifollicular granulomatous response), and acne secondary to hyperandrogenism, Cushing's syndrome, congenital adrenal hyperplasia, gonadal/adrenal tumors, and precocious puberty (adolescent females present with severe, persistent, or recalcitrant form of acne in the setting of other signs of androgen excess like menstrual irregularity and hirsutism or virilizing features like deepening voice, increased muscle mass, and androgenetic alopecia) [5, 11].

Evaluation

Adrenal androgens play an important role in the pathogenesis of acne with the most common identifiable androgenic abnormality associated being a marginal increase in adrenal androgen levels usually within a normal defined range. It has been shown that increasing levels of ovarian androgens and adrenal and testicular androgens at adrenarche may be responsible for early onset of acne at puberty in girls and boys, respectively. Early onset acne before obvious signs of puberty is usually a clinical sign of a normal or accelerated biological adrenarche but may also be the first sign of an underlying hormonal abnormality. Any of the signs of puberty can occur prematurely as an isolated abnormality, and the diagnosis of precocious puberty, precocious pseudopuberty, and premature adrenarche can be controversial because clinical signs may not correlate with measurable standard biochemical markers. However, long-term follow-up of these children with signs of early onset androgen excess, including those with premature adrenarche, appeared to have a risk of metabolic syndrome, thus warranting the need for identification and follow-up of this phenotype of children with stress on lifestyle modifications. Thus most cases of preadolescent acne represent a functional hyperandrogenism that could be the earliest sign of polycystic ovarian syndrome or a metabolic syndrome phenotype and are not associated with virilizing endocrinopathies. But, they are at risk for more severe or prolonged acne in adolescence or adulthood [5, 14].

Concern about preventable sequelae of precocious puberty is often disproportionate to the risk in children with early onset acne in the absence of other signs.

Hence extensive investigations often provoke needless parental anxiety. A left-hand and wrist X-ray for bone age would be a sufficient initial screening test for those with high growth parameters [1].

Hence a focused history and physical examination are sufficient to evaluate the majority of children with acne. Further work-up is generally unnecessary unless there are signs of excess androgen. However, hormonal evaluation is recommended in children with prepubertal acne with associated advanced bone maturation and early pubarche [1, 11, 14].

Treatment

The therapeutic objective in acne is to target the age-appropriate pathogenetic factors which include reduction of sebum production, prevention of microcomedone formation, suppression of *P. acnes*, and reduction of inflammation to prevent scarring. Reduction in existing microcomedones and prevention of the formation of new ones are central to the management of all acne lesions [3, 11]. As regards to pubertal acne, the approach should be to use the least aggressive regimen that is effective while avoiding regimens that encourage the development of bacterial resistance. Though it is unknown whether treatment of pubertal acne can alter *P. acnes* colonization and therefore subsequent inflammatory acne, appropriate treatment in this population is important as early development of comedonal acne is one of the best predictors of later, more severe disease, thereby necessitating early intervention to prevent unwanted sequelae [7, 15].

Educating the child and parents about reasonable expectations and treatment-related side effects can maximize both compliance and efficacy.

Management issues in pubertal acne are of special concern for the following reasons [11]:

(a) Availability of little published evidence regarding the safety and efficacy of many acne medications in pediatric patients as majority of clinical trials for acne are conducted in patients 12 years of age or older.
(b) Few treatment options have been approved for children younger than 12 years of age [16].
(c) Treatment of acne involves several medications targeting the morphological types, severity, and factors involved in pathogenesis resulting in complex drug interactions.
(d) Preadolescent patients tend to produce less sebum, which makes their skin more sensitive to acne treatments than their adolescent counterparts warranting need for supportive therapies to improve tolerability [3].
(e) Systemic side effects and impact of medications on growth and development.
(f) Significant psychosocial impact of acne.
(g) Issues related to treatment adherence.
(h) Knowledge gap in prescribing patterns among pediatricians who commonly encounter pubertal acne compared to dermatologists [15].

To address these issues, the first detailed, evidence-based clinical guidelines for the management of pediatric acne has been recommended by the American Acne and Rosacea Society and endorsed by the American Academy of Pediatrics [11].

As per their recommendations, treatment of uncomplicated preadolescent or pubertal acne (7–12 years of age) is comparable to that of acne in older age groups, and work-up is generally unnecessary unless there are signs of androgen excess, PCOS, or other systemic abnormalities. Nevertheless, it is important to elicit the child's level of concern regarding his or her acne in this age group as it may not always be concordant with parental concern. The consensus recommendations for the various grades of acne are summarized in Table 14.1 [11].

The general measures to be followed include:

(a) Institution of a low glycemic diet.
(b) Twice-daily washing with a gentle soap-free, pH-balanced cleanser.
(c) Use of too harsh cleanser can disrupt skin barrier, thereby increasing the transepidermal water loss, encouraging bacterial colonization, and promoting comedones, and can cause symptoms of burning and stinging.
(d) Avoid overuse of facial toners as they can be irritating, thereby adversely affecting the tolerability of acne medications.
(e) Use of concealing oil-free, noncomedogenic makeup to improve quality of life in females.
(f) Use of noncomedogenic moisturizer that includes a sunscreen to improve tolerability of retinoids.
(g) Use of pea-size amount of retinoids to cover the entire face and not spot treatment as done for other acne medications.

Quality of Life

The pubertal years are a time of significant physical, psychological, and social change. Self-esteem plays a major role in this transition, both psychologically and socially. Acne is perceived to have important negative influence on the self-esteem resulting in long-term personal and social consequences. The documented negative psychosocial effects of acne on self-esteem are significant more so in this age group as they are concerned with their physical appearance and place great importance on the opinions of their peers in this regard. Also, the level of distress may not correlate directly with acne severity; hence effective and early treatment is essential to prevent sequelae and to limit the long-term physical and psychological impact of acne [17].

Prognosis

Acne in children may be a sign of more severe acne with early comedonal prepubertal acne being predictive for severe comedonal acne or a long-term disease later in life. However, in most cases, acne decreases in a few years after the adolescence, while in up to 20 % it can persist beyond the age of 25, with higher prevalence among females [4].

Conclusion

Acne which commonly accompanies normal adrenarche and gonadal maturation is becoming a more common diagnosis in younger, preadolescent children relating to a trend toward children reaching puberty at an earlier age. A focused history and physical examination are sufficient to evaluate majority of these children with the exception of few who have severe acne associated with signs of hyperandrogenism requiring an endocrinological work-up. Treatment of uncomplicated pubertal acne is comparable to that of acne in older age groups except that most of the available treatments are considered off label for this age group thereby necessitating the need for future studies to optimize treatment outcomes in this population.

References

1. Bree AF, Siegfried EC. Acne vulgaris in preadolescent children: recommendations for evaluation. Pediatr Dermatol. 2014;31:27–32.
2. Goldberg JL, Dabade TS, Davis SA, Feldman SR, Krowchuk DP, Fleischer AB. Changing age of acne vulgaris visits: another sign of earlier puberty? Pediatr Dermatol. 2011;28:645–8.
3. Hensley D, Meckfessel MH. Tolerability of a skin care regimen formulated for acne-prone skin in children. Pediatr Dermatol. 2015;32:501–5.
4. Karciauskiene J, Valiukeviciene S, Gollnick H, Stang A. The prevalence and risk factors of adolescent acne among schoolchildren in Lithuania: a cross-sectional study. J Eur Acad Dermatol Venereol. 2014;28:733–40.
5. Antoniou C, Dessinioti C, Stratigos AJ, Katsambas AD. Clinical and therapeutic approach to childhood acne: an update. Pediatr Dermatol. 2009;26:373–80.
6. Tan JK, Bhate K. A global perspective on the epidemiology of acne. Br J Dermatol. 2015;172 Suppl 1:3–12.
7. Bhate K, Williams HC. Epidemiology of acne vulgaris. Br J Dermatol. 2013;168:474–85.
8. Melnik BC. Acne. In: Irvine AD, Hoeger PH, Yan AC, editors. Harper's textbook of pediatric dermatology. 3rd ed. UK: Wiley-Blackwell; 2011. p. 79.1–79.22.
9. Gollnick HP. From new findings in acne pathogenesis to new approaches in treatment. J Eur Acad Dermatol Venereol. 2015;29 Suppl 5:1–7.
10. Kubba R, Bajaj AK, Thappa DM, Sharma R, Vedamurthy M, Dhar S, et al. Acne in India: guidelines for management—IAA consensus document. Indian J Dermatol Venereol Leprol. 2009;75 Suppl 1:1–62.
11. Eichenfield LF, Krakowski AC, Piggott C, Del Rosso J, Baldwin H, Friedlander SF, et al. Evidence-based recommendations for the diagnosis and treatment of pediatric acne. Pediatrics. 2013;131 Suppl 3:S163–86.
12. Tan JK, Jones E, Allen E, Pripotnev S, Raza A, Wolfe B. Evaluation of essential clinical components and features of current acne global grading scales. J Am Acad Dermatol. 2013;69:754–61.
13. Robeva R, Assyov Y, Tomova A, Kumanov P. Acne vulgaris is associated with intensive pubertal development and altitude of residence—a cross-sectional population-based study on 6,200 boys. Eur J Pediatr. 2013;172:465–71.
14. De Raeve L, De Schepper J, Smitz J. Prepubertal acne: a cutaneous marker of androgen excess? J Am Acad Dermatol. 1995;32(2 Pt 1):181–4.

15. Davis SA, Sandoval LF, Gustafson CJ, Feldman SR, Cordoro KM. Treatment of preadolescent acne in the United States: an analysis of nationally representative data. Pediatr Dermatol. 2013;30:689–94.
16. Parikh SA, Davis SA, Krowchuk DP, Feldman SR. Common use of prescription off-label acne therapy in children younger than 12 years old. Pediatr Dermatol. 2014;31:551–5.
17. Krowchuk DP, Stancin T, Keskinen R, Walker R, Bass J, Anglin TM. The psychosocial effects of acne on adolescents. Pediatr Dermatol. 1991;8:332–8.

Chapter 15
Adolescent Varicocele

Ahmad Majzoub and Edmund Sabanegh Jr.

Introduction

A varicocele is the abnormal dilatation of pampiniform plexus of veins in the scrotum [1]. Adolescent varicocele has gained a lot of interest principally because the condition starts around childhood or adolescence, progresses with age, and may affect testicular growth, rendering it the most common cause of adult male infertility.

History of Varicocele

For almost 2000 years, the term varicocele has been linked to testicular ailments. In his treatise "De Medicina," Celsus (25 BC) was the first to associate varicocele to testicular atrophy [2]. With the beginning of the seventeenth century, many believed in the presence of a solid connection between varicocele and infertility [3]. However, caution from the liberal performance of surgery started after a tragic incidence in 1832, when J. Delpech, a well-known professor of surgery, was murdered by a man who suffered from testicular atrophy as a consequence of bilateral varicocele surgery [4]. Since then, awareness to such risk factors triggered a search for more conservative approach to varicocele management through the use of suspensory garments, cold showers, and lifestyle modifications such as moderation in sexual habits [4].

In spite of major surgical advancements in the early 1900s, caution remained a prevailing view to varicocele surgery. Conservative measures were often practiced

A. Majzoub • E. Sabanegh Jr. (✉)
Department of Urology, Glickman Urological and Kidney Institute, Cleveland Clinic Foundation, 9500 Euclid Ave, Cleveland, OH 44195, USA
e-mail: majzoua@ccf.org; sabanee@ccf.org

P. Kumanov, A. Agarwal (eds.), *Puberty*, DOI 10.1007/978-3-319-32122-6_15

by many physicians who believed in their success or were simply not convinced with surgery [4]. Interest in surgery re-immerged only after the introduction of inguinal and retroperitoneal ligature procedures and several reports followed demonstrating effect of varicocele surgery on fertility. In 1952, Tulloch was the first to report appearance of sperm after performing bilateral varicocelectomy to a patient with azoospermia [5]. Many other uncontrolled trials also revealed an improvement in semen parameters after surgery [6] and generated additional interest in surgical technique modification. The introduction of optical magnification and ultrasound probes in 1983 [7] had positive impact on surgical outcome. Different approaches were also explored, such as the subinguinal approach in 1985 [8] and laparoscopic approach in 1992 [9]. Today varicocelectomy is by far the most commonly performed operation for the treatment of male infertility. However, proper patient selection is still the most important factor to maximize patient benefit.

Epidemiology

The prevalence of varicocele varies greatly and is estimated to be in the range of 10–20 % of the general male population [2, 10]. This discrepancy is due to differences in origin and nature of the studied population and more importantly because the condition is often subjectively diagnosed. The condition appears at puberty but can also be present in prepubertal boys [11], as young as 10 years of age [12]. In a study of 6200 boys, Kumanov and colleagues detected varicocele in about 8 % of boys between 10 and 19 years of age [13]. The prevalence was also found to increase with age [14], at a rate of 10 % each decade, afflicting 75 % of men by their eighth decade of life [15]. Varicoceles are much more common in the subfertile population affecting 35 and 80 % of men with primary and secondary infertility, respectively [16]. These reasons mark varicocele as a progressive disease with deleterious effects on testicular function [14, 17].

Few studies revealed an inverse relationship between varicocele and body mass index, denoting a higher prevalence of disease among lean men although this may relate to more ease of diagnosis in the lean population [18, 19]. First-degree relatives are also more commonly affected, suggesting a genetic pattern of inheritance [17].

Etiology

An understanding of the anatomy of the vascular supply of the testes is essential before explaining varicocele etiology. The anatomical position of the testis and its unique vascular supply are crucial for its optimal physiology and contribution to men's reproductive health. A triple arterial supply to the testes exists. The first is the testicular artery (or internal spermatic artery) that originates from the aorta. The second is the cremasteric artery (or external spermatic artery), which originates from the inferior epigastric artery, a branch of the external iliac artery. The third is the deferential (vasal) artery, which originates from the superior vesical artery, a branch of the internal iliac artery.

Venous drainage, on the other hand, is more complicated, with many individual routes. A network of venous communications called the pampiniform plexus exists above the testes and drains through the testicular vein, pudendal veins, and vasal veins [20]. In the inguinal canal, the pampiniform plexus of veins travels in close proximity to the testicular arteries allowing for countercurrent heat exchange, which is thought to be the method by which the arterial blood going to the testis is cooled to temperatures as low as 33 °C [21]. The left testicular vein drains into the left renal vein, while the right testicular vein drains directly into the inferior vena cava. Variations do exist; the left testicular vein can rarely drain to the inferior vena cava or communicates with it before entering the renal vein [22].

Several theories have been proposed in the etiology of varicocele. *Idiopathic* varicocele is a term given when varicocele is thought to result from incompetent or absent unidirectional valves within the gonadal veins. This concept remains debatable. Despite the significant association that some researchers found between varicocele and valvular incompetence in the saphenofemoral junction [23, 24], others have demonstrated the presence of varicocele in patients with competent venous system [25, 26] or even failed to identify the presence of such valves [27, 28].

The predilection of varicocele on the left side triggered an assumption that anatomical differences may be contributing to varicocele etiology. These differences, which are thought to result in higher left venous hydrostatic pressure, include (1) longer left testicular vein by around 8–10 cm than its counterpart [29], (2) perpendicular angle of entry of the left testicular vein into the left renal vein in comparison to a more acute angle of entry of the right vein into the IVC, (3) and presence of a "nutcracker effect" resulting in a higher left renal vein pressure as it is compressed between the superior mesenteric artery and the aorta [30]. Gat and colleagues were able to validate the presence of high left spermatic vein hydrostatic pressure [31].

Animal studies have hypothesized that adolescent varicocele could result from increased arterial blood flow to the testis at puberty. The amount of flow exceeds the venous capacity and results in dilatation and engorgement of the pampiniform plexus of veins [32]. The likelihood of this information should be confirmed with human studies before adopting such a hypothesis.

Varicocele has been associated with several urological and non-urological medical conditions both in adolescents and adults. Examples include premature ejaculation [33], prostatitis [33], ankylosing spondylitis [34], and chronic obstructive pulmonary disease [35]. On a higher level, varicocele was associated with specific somatometric parameters in adolescents. It had a direct relationship with patient's age, height, and penile length and an inverse relationship with testicular volume, BMI, and pubic hair distribution [36]. Furthermore, Kumanov and colleagues detected a possible link between varicocele and iris pigmentation [37].

Secondary varicocele is a term given when the condition occurs as a result of venous compression from retroperitoneal tumors such as sarcomas, lymphomas, or renal tumors. It should be suspected when encountering varicocele on the right side, relatively acute onset, or when the distention does not reside when the patient lies on his back.

Pathophysiology

Several pathophysiologic mechanisms have been proposed to help explain the deleterious effects of varicocele on testicular function. It is likely that not just a single mechanism is responsible, but rather a combination that ultimately results in testicular dysfunction.

Hyperthermia Increased intratesticular temperature secondary to varicocele is the most commonly studied pathophysiology. It has long been observed that minor changes in testicular temperature can affect spermatogenesis [38]. The reason for this is that many of the enzymes responsible for DNA synthesis in the testis are temperature dependent [39], mainly favoring temperatures lower than body temperature. The anatomic position of the testis in the scrotal sac together with the countercurrent cooling mechanism provided by the pampiniform plexus of veins is responsible for testicular temperature regulation [40]. In a varicocele, the resulting blood stasis disrupts the countercurrent cooling effect causing testicular temperature elevation and defective spermatogenesis [41]. Scrotal skin temperature measurement, which reliably reflects testicular temperature [42], was assessed in few studies. In a comparative study, Wright and colleagues confirmed the presence of higher scrotal skin temperature in patients with varicocele with successful reduction to near-normal levels after varicocele ligation [43]. Moreover, scrotal temperature elevation was found to be a more accurate reflection of testicular dysfunction than the grade of varicocele [44].

Adrenal Reflux Reflux of blood down the testicular vein has been demonstrated in patients with varicocele [45]. This triggered the hypothesis that exposure of the testis to adrenal and renal metabolites could be the reason for defective spermatogenesis. Chemicals such as adrenomedullin, catecholamines, cortisol, prostaglandins E and F, and serotonin were suggested. Animal studies on this issue showed conflicting results. Although Camoglio et al. [46] demonstrated worse testicular pathology in varicocele-induced rats with intact adrenal gland than in rats that had adrenalectomy, other studies failed to document the presence of such metabolites at the testicular levels [47].

Endocrine Imbalance Puberty and testicular development are regulated by the hypothalamic-pituitary gonadal axis. Several endocrine disturbances were found to be associated with varicocele, most notable of which are low intratesticular levels of testosterone [48, 49]. Intratesticular testosterone is the most important regulator of spermatogenesis [50]. The exact cause of this finding may be secondary to suboptimal function of Leydig cells often observed with varicocele [48] or from a pattern similar to hypergonadotropic hypogonadism [51]. An abnormal response to gonadotropin-releasing hormone (GnRH) is found with elevated levels of LH resulting in Leydig cell hyperplasia [52]. Sertoli cell dysfunction has also been observed in association with supranormal levels of FSH. These endocrine imbalances were found in all varicocele patients irrespective of their fertility status. Varicocelectomy was associated with normalization of FSH, LH, and intratesticular testosterone levels [49, 53].

Disturbance of Paracrine Regulation In addition to optimal levels of intratesticular testosterone, spermatogenesis is regulated by complex interactions and signals at the cellular level. Germ cell apoptosis is under the control of Sertoli cells through utilization of the Fas system. The Fas is a transmembrane receptor protein expressed on germ cells and is under the control of proapoptotic ligand Fas (FasL) and anti-apoptotic soluble Fas (sFas), both secreted by Sertoli cells [54]. As a result of Sertoli cell dysfunction, patients with varicoceles were found to have higher levels of seminal FasL and lower levels of seminal sFas [55, 56]. Inhibin is another substance produced by Sertoli cells. It has a negative feedback control on pituitary FSH secretion. Additionally it works in a paracrine manner stimulating Leydig cells to produce testosterone. Again adolescents with varicocele were found to have subnormal levels of inhibin B that positively correlated with testicular volume [57].

Free radicals are other forms of paracrine disturbances as they are produced and act locally. They include a wide variety of compounds that are generally divided into reactive oxygen or nitrogen species [58]. Nitrous oxide (NO) is perhaps the most commonly studied substance in varicocele. It was detected in high quantities within the dilated spermatic veins of adolescents with varicocele [59]. Moreover, a direct relation exists between the level of seminal NO and degree of varicocele, i.e., the higher the grade of varicocele, the greater the NO level [60]. NO is synthesized by nitric oxide synthase (NOS) commonly present in neutrophils and macrophages. However under stressful conditions, spermatozoa are also capable of producing NO [61]. Studies on adolescents with varicocele discovered overexpression of NOS in their Leydig cells [62]. Under normal physiologic concentrations, NO produced by Leydig cells diffuses across cellular membranes and stimulates testicular function. However, its overproduction could initiate different pathological consequences. First, it causes vasodilatation of blood vessels resulting in blood stasis [63]; second, it causes prolonged relaxation of peritubular myofibroblasts ultimately affecting the peristaltic activity necessary for sperm transport [63]; third, high levels of NO can inhibit steroidogenesis and reduce testosterone production by Leydig cells [64]; lastly, it could alter Sertoli cell junctions that are fundamental in regulating cellular adhesion, proliferation, migration, and differentiation [65].

Spermatozoa are extremely sensitive to oxidative stress as they lack the necessary enzyme repair systems [66]. As a result, free radicals affect spermatozoa in three main ways: membrane lipid peroxidation, DNA damage, and induction of apoptosis [67]. The spermatozoan membrane is rich in polyunsaturated fatty acids that are susceptible to lipid peroxidation. This process results in loss of intracellular adenosine triphosphate (ATP) causing reduction in sperm viability and motility and alteration of its morphology [68]. Free radicals directly attack the purine and pyrimidine bases destabilizing the DNA molecule and causing anomalies such as point mutations, polymorphisms, deletions, translocations, and even double-stranded breaks [69]. Finally, depending on the degree of the insult, apoptosis will be triggered through the Fas system described above.

Presentation and Diagnosis

Varicocele in the adolescent may present in a variety of ways. Most commonly, it is asymptomatic and often diagnosed during genital examination performed as part of routine sports or school checkups. Sometimes the adolescent notices a scrotal swelling or complains of a dull, bothersome discomfort in the scrotal region, especially after exercise or prolonged standing.

Clinical examination should start while the adolescent is in the standing position preferably in a warm room. The scrotum is inspected for any obvious venous distention around the spermatic cord, which, if seen, denotes the presence of grade 3 varicocele (Fig. 15.1). The scrotum, testes, and cord structures are then gently palpated. A palpable varicocele is described as a feeling of a bag of worms or a squishy tube, which, if felt, indicates the presence of grade 2 varicocele. If nothing is palpable, except for a filling sensation felt between the fingers of the examiner as the patient performs the Valsalva maneuver, a grade 1 varicocele is present.

After examining the patient in the standing position, the patient should be examined supine. Idiopathic varicocele should disappear in the supine position. Persistence of the swelling in supine position, especially on the right side, should raise suspicion for the possibility of secondary causes of varicocele. Retroperitoneal tumors, kidney tumors, and lymphadenopathy are possible causes for secondary varicocele. Additionally, cord thickening due to varicocele should resolve in supine position, whereas a cord lipoma can be suspected if thickening of the cord persists.

Testicular size measurement is crucial to determine whether the varicocele is adversely affecting testicular growth. On palpation one can most effectively gauge whether the right and left sides are grossly symmetric. A prepubertal testis should have a volume of 1–3 mL. A size of >3 mL indicates the initiation of puberty, and this enlargement generally begins before any sign of pubic hair. Because of extensive individual variation in normal growth and development, testicular size is correlated with Tanner stage, growth velocity, and bone age rather than chronological age.

Testicular volume and consistency are an important component of varicocele assessment in the adolescent. Dimensions of the testis can be assessed with caliper measurements in the three dimensions. More commonly, testicular volume can be clinically assessed using a variety of devices including the Prader orchidometer [70], a string of ovoid-shaped beads of increasing sizes, and the Rochester (Takihara) orchidometer [71], a ring of cards with open spaces to accommodate the shape of a

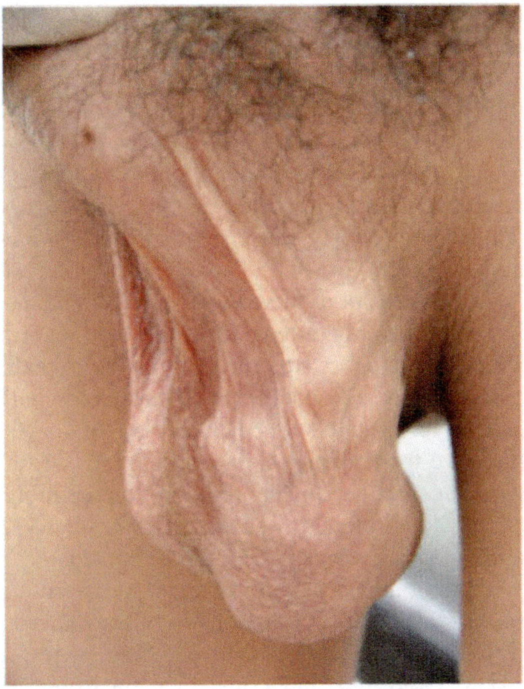

Fig. 15.1 Grade III varicocele in an adolescent (Reprinted from Esteves SC, Miyaoka R, Agarwal A. An update on the clinical assessment of the infertile male. Clinics. 2011; 66 (4): 691–700. With permission from CLINICS)

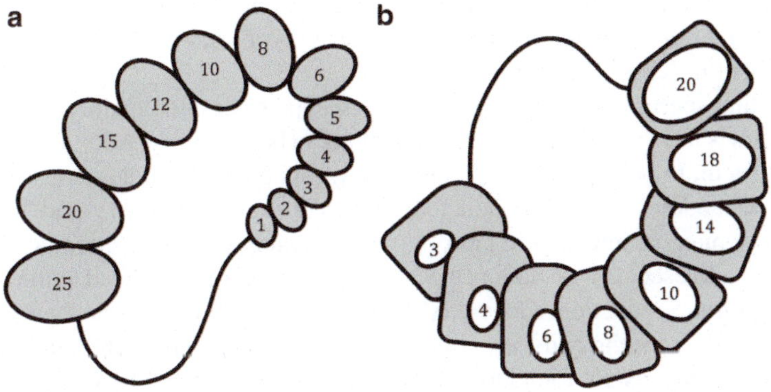

Fig. 15.2 Diagram representing the appearance of (**a**) Prader and (**b**) Rochester orchidometers

testis (Fig. 15.2). The most reliable method, however, for volume calculation is scrotal ultrasound [72]. It has the best correlation with actual testis size [73]. When dealing with adolescent testes, it is important to realize that testicular growth is not necessary identical in both sides. Kolon and colleagues performed yearly ultrasounds on boys who had 15 % testicular size discrepancy attributed to a varicocele. With time, the majority showed resolution of their size discrepancy [74]. This finding suggested that surgery might not be recommended based on one static measurement and inspired the authors to recommend at least two sequential ultrasounds, 6–12 months apart, before surgical decision is made [74]. In addition to testicular volume measurement, duplex ultrasonography is important to accurately evaluate venous flow reversal as well as vein diameter. A diameter of 3 mm is generally accepted as a cutoff value for diagnosing varicocele [75]. Chiou and colleagues developed an ultrasound scoring system aiming to increase the sensitivity and specificity of varicocele detection. Their system incorporated the following criteria: maximal venous dilatation (score 0–3), the presence of a venous plexus, the sum of the diameters of veins in the plexus (score 0–3), and the change of flow on Valsalva maneuver (score 0–3). A total score of 4 or more was used to define the presence of a varicocele [76].

Some have suggested performing serum hormone evaluation on adolescents with varicocele to assess the integrity of the hypothalamic-pituitary gonadal axis. One must take into account, however, the adolescent's developmental stage before interpreting test results. In 2013, as part of the CALIPER study (Canadian Library Initiative for Pediatric Reference Ranges), Konforte and colleagues examined sex hormones in a healthy cohort of children aiming to stratify normal reference ranges of fertility hormones by age and Tanner stage [77]. Their results showed that normal ranges in children can generally be considered low in the adult population.

Finding higher than normal levels of serum LH and FSH may suggest the presence of testicular dysfunction [78]. Testosterone may be also reduced in adolescents with varicocele, although this finding is not specifically investigated in this age group. Goldstein and colleagues measured serum testosterone pre- and post-varicocelectomy in 110 infertile men. Despite finding variable preoperative levels, patients with lower serum testosterone had significant improvement in their testosterone level after varicocele surgery that was proportional with the degree of improvement in semen analysis [50].

Evaluating sperm parameters among adolescents is complex mainly because spermatogenesis is in its initial stages and test results can be transitory. Additionally, the test itself is difficult to be executed by younger boys. As a result, studies assessing semen parameters in adolescents are conducted in boys of Tanner stages IV and V [79–81]. Abnormal semen parameters such as oligospermia and asthenozoospermia were more prevalent in adolescents with varicocele and seem to be directly related to the degree of testicular volume reduction. Generally, volume reduction of greater than 20 % was associated with twice the odds of finding abnormal semen analysis [80], unlike varicocele grade, which was not found to have any significant influential effect [79].

Management

Varicocele in the adolescent population represents a dilemma to the treating urologist. Historically, adolescent varicocele was left untreated, as there was lack of evidence associating it with infertility. The earliest report suggesting benefit from varicocelectomy in the form of reversal of testicular growth arrest came from Kass and Belman in 1987 [82]. Improvements in testicular growth and semen analyses were also detected in several studies done on adolescents [83–85]. More importantly, however, when dealing with adolescent varicocele, concern remains regarding the progressive nature of the condition, which, if left untreated, may continue to affect testicular growth and spermatogenesis [10, 86]. All these reasons signify a potential advantage to low morbidity surgery, but the question remains as to who will benefit most from surgery. It is obviously impractical and not cost effective to perform surgery for all adolescents with varicocele. On the other hand, it is also unacceptable to allow the deleterious effects of this condition to occur if they may be prevented.

In an effort to identify patients who could benefit from treatment, several variables were evaluated to select those who should have a favorable outcome. Currently, areas used to establish criteria for varicocele repair are as follows.

Varicocele Grade Varicocele grade has long been subject to extensive research aiming to identify potential connection with testicular dysfunction. Studies by Diamond and Alukal did not find any significant association between grade of varicocele and degree of testicular hypotrophy or defective semen parameters [79, 87]. Paduch and Zampieri, on the other hand, demonstrated a direct association with testicular growth arrest [88, 89]. The amount of venous reflux, irrespective of the grade of varicocele, was also found to be an important predictor for the development of infertility [90]. The grade of varicocele was not associated with significant testicular regrowth after surgery, as shown by the work of Decastro and colleagues [91]. They verified that the prevalence of testicular catch-up growth after varicocelectomy is high, even for patients in their early 20s [91]. These results imply that the grade of varicocele by itself should not be the sole indication for treatment.

Testicular Volume Testicular growth arrest is an established consequence to varicocele in adolescents [87, 92, 93]. Likewise, its catch-up growth after varicocelectomy is also confirmed [91, 94]. A decrease in testicular volume has long been the best indication for surgical correction of varicocele. However, not every boy with varicocele and testicular growth arrest will be infertile, and testicular growth is not necessarily symmetrical as the previously presented study by Kolon and colleagues indicated [74]. As a result, the search for a test that would better distinguish between adolescents with a varicocele who will develop infertility and those who will remain fertile is warranted. Currently, the most accepted indication for surgery in adolescents is the presence of testicular volume difference of 2 mL [94].

GnRH Stimulation Test The normal physiologic response to GnRH stimulation is an increase in FSH and LH secretion from the anterior pituitary. The rationale behind this test is that the damage to the germinal epithelium results in compensatory stimulation of the pituitary gland and subsequent increase in FSH and LH production. As a result a higher than normal baseline FSH and LH is present with subsequent exaggerated response to GnRH stimulation. In theory, the GnRH stimulation test could distinguish between adolescents with varicocele who have abnormal testicular function and those who have normal spermatogenesis. However, in clinical practice, the GnRH stimulation test is expensive, requires multiple serum samples, and lacks an association between abnormal results, growth arrest, and infertility. While studying prepubertal boys, Fideleff and colleagues noticed that changes in the hormonal profile and responses to GnRH stimulation did not have a consistent pattern especially when correlated with the clinical grades of varicocele [95]. Additionally, it is difficult to relate test results only to testicular dysfunction secondary to varicocele in the adolescent population. Hormonal responses can be exaggerated due to testicular growth during this stage of development [96].

Inhibin B Level Serum inhibin is a protein complex secreted by Sertoli cells. It downregulates FSH synthesis and inhibits FSH secretion. Serum inhibin B measurement in varicocele patients gained interest as it can reflect the integrity of the seminiferous tubules and function of the Sertoli cells. Following GnRH stimulation test, serum inhibin levels failed to aid in stratification of adolescents with varicocele [97]. More recent studies, however, were able to detect significantly lower levels of serum inhibin B in adolescents with varicocele than controls [57, 98, 99], suggesting it as a useful marker of Sertoli cell damage and a potential indication for surgery.

Semen Analysis Varicocele is associated with documented abnormalities in semen analysis. In a meta-analysis evaluating the effect of varicocele on semen samples obtained from adolescents, Nork and colleagues confirmed the presence of abnormalities in sperm density, motility, and morphology [100]. Varicocele was associated with alterations in early spermatid head differentiation during spermiogenesis, prompting some to select patients with high incidence of sperm acrosome and nucleus malformations as appropriate candidates for varicocele correction [101].

Lastly, it should be restressed that the practice of performing prophylactic surgery for every adolescent with varicocele is impractical. Currently accepted indications for varicocelectomy in the adolescent population [102] include:

1. Testicular growth arrest (more than 2 mL of difference or 2 SD from normal testicular growth curves)
2. High-grade varicocele in addition to abnormal semen analysis
3. Symptomatic patients
4. Bilateral varicoceles

Surgical Approaches

Surgical options available for adolescent varicocele are similar to those performed on adults. Several surgical classifications exist and are based on the technique (conventional, microsurgical, laparoscopic, and radiologic embolization) or the level of testicular vein ligation (high or low) or whether the gonadal artery is spared or ligated. Generally, advancements in optical magnification and microscopy in recent years eventually influenced varicocele surgery and were favored by an increasing number of urologists. In 1994, Donovan and colleagues surveyed 720 urologists and found that microsurgery was performed only by 6% of them [103]. In contrast, another survey in 2008 noticed an increasing number of urologists utilizing loop magnification and microsurgery, 48 % and 18 %, respectively [104]. Scrotal varicocelectomy that was once utilized is currently abandoned due to the high incidence of injury to the testicular artery during dissection.

Controversy once existed on whether to spare the testicular artery during the course of varicocele repair. Advocates of total ligation, or nonartery-sparing, techniques claim that sparing the artery can be associated with higher incidence of varicocele recurrence. The main reason for this association is the presence of tiny veins (venae comitantes) along the course of the testicular artery that are usually missed in attempts to spare the artery [105]. However, substantial evidence exists in support of sparing the artery. Damage to the seminiferous tubules with subsequent testicular atrophy is always a possibility with artery ligation [106]. Additionally with the advent use of proper magnification, artery-sparing techniques can be performed without compromising the surgical outcome.

Conventional Varicocelectomy

Retroperitoneal Approach In 1949, Palomo described the retroperitoneal approach for ligation of internal spermatic vessels [107]. A muscle splitting incision is performed at the level of the internal inguinal ring; the vessels are then identified and ligated at a point that has the fewest arterial and venous branching. A modified artery-sparing Palomo technique is later implemented. Unfortunately, it was associated with a high incidence of postoperative recurrence especially in the adolescent population [108]. Moreover artery sparing without optical magnification was found to be difficult in this age group due to the small caliber of the artery.

Inguinal Approach The inguinal approach was described by Ivanissevich [109] in 1960. An incision is made over the inguinal canal followed by opening of the external oblique fascia and delivery of the spermatic cord. The exposed cord is then explored, and once the vas deferens is isolated, the veins are identified and divided. Artery-sparing and nonartery-sparing modifications to this procedure were also described. While an effective technique, it has the disadvantage of requiring the patient to have delayed return to full activity due to the extensive muscular dissection in the inguinal canal.

Subinguinal Approach The subinguinal approach described by Marmar in 1985 [8] is ideally used in adult varicocele, but has gained some acceptance among some pediatric urologists as well. The incision is performed at or near the pubic tubercle avoiding the need to open the external oblique aponeurosis. Advantages of this technique include less pain, smoother recovery, and easier access to the spermatic cord especially among obese patients or those with previous inguinal surgery. However, a greater number of veins are present at such a low level, making the procedure technically challenging.

Microsurgical Varicocelectomy

With the introduction of microsurgery into the field of urology in the mid-1970s [110], it was rapidly utilized to aid in varicocele surgery. The motive for its use was the high incidence of varicocele recurrence and hydrocele formation after conventional surgery. Performing the procedure under magnification allowed for meticulous vein ligation and sparing of lymphatics resulting in lower rates of varicocele recurrence and hydrocele formation, respectively. Microsurgery was used in inguinal and subinguinal approaches with results confirming a superior outcome for varicocelectomy. Reports by Minevich and Goldstein demonstrated a significantly lower recurrence rate and postoperative hydrocele in adolescent patients [111, 112]. These superior surgical outcomes lead many authors to consider microsurgical varicocelectomy as the gold standard technique for varicocele surgery [113].

Laparoscopic Varicocelectomy

The first report on laparoscopic varicocelectomy came from Hagood and colleagues in 1992 [9]. Since that time, this approach has been utilized with acceptable surgical outcomes. Artery-sparing and nonartery-sparing modifications were performed and the vessels can be divided with hemostatic clips or coagulated with bipolar electrode [114].

Although laparoscopic varicocelectomy is a suitable alternative, it has some significant drawbacks such as the need for pneumoperitoneum, prolonged operative time, and higher cost [103]. Additionally complications such as bowel perforation, major vascular injury, pneumothorax, and incisional hernia, while rare, can be catastrophic complications. Varicocele recurrence and postoperative hydrocele rates with laparoscopy are significantly higher than the subinguinal microsurgical approach. In attempts to reduce the incidence of postoperative hydrocele, lymphatic-sparing techniques were introduced. Rizkala and colleagues compared lymphatic sparing to standard laparoscopic varicocelectomy in 97 patients; the postoperative hydrocele rate was 4.5 % in the lymphatic-sparing group in comparison to 43 % in the standard surgery group [115]. Advancements in the field of laparoscopy were also utilized in adolescent varicocele surgery. Natural orifice transluminal endoscopic surgical (NOTES) procedures [116] and laparoendoscopic single-site (LESS) surgery [117] were utilized in varicocelectomy with promising results. Although such procedures can be very attractive surgical options, they need to be validated in large randomized, clinical trials where patient safety, surgical outcomes, and procedure cost are taken as end points.

Angiographic Embolization

Interventional radiologists have also contributed to the management of varicocele through angiographic antegrade or retrograde embolization or sclerotherapy. Although the minimally invasive nature of such a procedure may have some advantages in adults, it certainly had predictable concerns when duplicated in children and adolescents. Technical difficulties were faced resulting in a failure rate of up to 20 % of cases because of aberrant venous anatomy, difficulty in cannulating the testicular vein, and extravasation of contrast during the procedure [118, 119]. Other important concerns in this age group are the need for general anesthesia and radiation exposure while performing the procedure. Although these reasons make percutaneous angioembolization a less favorable procedure for treating adolescent varicocele, recent studies reflecting advancements to this field of medicine indicate that it still can be considered as another potential alternative [120].

Several comparative studies were made to evaluate different surgical approaches in adult varicocele surgery. Al-Said and colleagues compared open, laparoscopic, and microsurgical approaches in 446 varicocelectomies. The incidence of postoperative hydrocele was 2.8 %, 5.4 %, and 0 %, respectively. Varicocele recurrence was seen in 11 % of the conventional group, 17 % of the laparoscopic group, and 2.6 % of the microsurgical group. Compared to preoperative values in the three groups, postoperative semen parameters specifically sperm count and motility were significantly higher in the microsurgical group [121]. In a recent meta-analysis of 35 randomized controlled trials and observational studies, Wang and colleagues examined improvements in semen analysis and reported complication rates in various varicocele treatments [122]. Again, microsurgery had the best improvement in sperm density and sperm motility and the least reported complication rate. In adolescents, however, microsurgery was introduced at a later stage [111], but, despite that, results of recent reviews indicate comparable results to those seen in the adult population [123].

Conclusion

The management of adolescent varicocele can be challenging to the practicing urologist. Over the past decade, tremendous research has helped unveil some of its uncertainties. Longer-term studies are needed to understand the exact influence of varicoceles on future fertility and help identify the best approach for its management.

References

1. Jarow JP. Evaluation of the azoospermic patient. J Urol. 1989;142(1):62–5.
2. Saypol DC. Varicocele. J Androl. 1981;2:61.
3. Redmon JB, Carey P, Pryor JL. Varicocele–the most common cause of male factor infertility? Hum Reprod Update. 2002;8(1):53–8.

4. NoÈske H-D, Weidner W. Varicocele ± a historical perspective. World J Urol. 1999;17:151–7.
5. Tulloch WS. A consideration of sterility factors in light of subsequent pregnancies. Edinb Med J. 1952;59:29–34.
6. Schlesinger MH, Wilets IF, Nagler HM. Treatment outcome after varicocelectomy. Urol Clin North Am. 1994;57(6):1289–93.
7. Wosnitzer M, Roth JA. Optical magnification and Doppler ultrasound probe for varicocelectomy. Urology. 1983;22(1):24–6.
8. Marmar JL, DeBenedictis TJ, Praiss D. The management of varicoceles by microdissection of the spermatic cord at the external ring. Fertil Steril. 1985;43(4):583–8.
9. Hagood PG, Mehan DJ, Worischeck JH, Andrus CH, Parra RO. Laparoscopic varicocelectomy: preliminary report of a new technique. J Urol. 1992;147(1):73–6.
10. Gorelick JI, Goldstein M. Loss of fertility in men with varicocele. Fertil Steril. 1993;59(3):613–6.
11. Buch JP, Cromie WJ. Evaluation and treatment of the preadolescent varicocele. Urol Clin North Am. 1985;12(1):3–12.
12. Oster J. Varicocele in children and adolescents. Acta Paediatr Scand Suppl. 1970;206 Suppl 206:81.
13. Kumanov P, Robeva RN, Tomova A. Adolescent varicocele: who is at risk? Pediatrics. 2008;121(1):e53–7.
14. Canales BK, Zapzalka DM, Ercole CJ, Carey P, Haus E, Aeppli D, et al. Prevalence and effect of varicoceles in an elderly population. Urology. 2005;66(3):627–31.
15. Levinger U, Gornish M, Gat Y, Bachar GN. Is varicocele prevalence increasing with age? Andrologia. 2007;39(3):77–80.
16. Russell JK. Varicocele in groups of fertile and subfertile males. Br Med J. 1954;1(4873):1231–3.
17. Raman JD, Walmsley K, Goldstein M. Inheritance of varicoceles. Urology. 2005;65(6):1186–9.
18. Nielsen ME, Zderic S, Freedland SJ, Jarow JP. Insight on pathogenesis of varicoceles: relationship of varicocele and body mass index. Urology. 2006;68(2):392–6.
19. Chen SS, Huang WJ. Differences in biochemical markers and body mass index between patients with and without varicocele. J Chin Med Assoc. 2010;73(4):194–8.
20. Lechter A, Lopez G, Martinez C, Camacho J. Anatomy of the gonadal veins: a reappraisal. Surgery. 1991;148:1190–4.
21. Turner TT, Lopez TJ. Testicular blood flow in prepubertal and older rates with unilateral experimental varicocele and investigation into the mechanism of the bilateral response to the unilateral lesion. J Urol. 1982;144:1018.
22. Chatel A, Bigot JM, Dectot H, Helenon C. Radiological anatomy of the spermatic veins. Report of 152 retrograde spermatic phlebographies. J Chir. 1978;115:443–50.
23. Ciaccio V, Ficola F, Ceccarelli F, Capodicasa E. Assessment of sapheno-femoral junction continence in 42 patients with primary varicocele. Minerva Chir. 1995;50(5):469–73.
24. Bilgili MY, Basar H, Simsir I, Unal B, Batislam E. Assessment of sapheno-femoral junction continence in patients with primary adolescent varicocele. Pediatr Radiol. 2003;33:603–6.
25. Wishahi MM. Anatomy of the spermatic venous plexus (pampiniform plexus) in men with and without varicocele: intraoperative venographic study. J Urol. 1992;147(5):1285–9.
26. Braedel HU, Steffens J, Ziegler M, Polsky MS, Platt ML. A possible ontogenic etiology for idiopathic left varicocele. J Urol. 1994;151(1):62–6.
27. Dennison AR, Tibbs DJ. Varicocele and varicose veins compared. A basis for logical surgery. Urology. 1986;28(3):211–7.
28. Kass EJ, Reitelman C. Adolescent varicocele. Urol Clin North Am. 1995;22(1):151–9.
29. Shafik A, Bedeir GA. Venous tension patterns in cord veins. I. In normal and varicocele individuals. J Urol. 1980;123(3):383–5.
30. Buschi AJ, Harrison RB, Norman A, Brenbridge AG, Williamson BR, Gentry RR, et al. Distended left renal vein: CT/sonographic normal variant. AJR Am J Roentgenol. 1980;135(2):339–42.
31. Gat Y, Zukerman Z, Chakraborty J, Gornish M. Varicocele, hypoxia and male infertility. Fluid mechanics analysis of the impaired testicular venous drainage system. Hum Reprod. 2005;20(9):2614–9.

32. Li H, Dubocq F, Jiang Y, Tiguert R, Gheiler EL, Dhabuwala CB. Effect of surgically induced varicocele on testicular blood flow and Sertoli cell function. Urology. 1999;53(6):1258–62.
33. Lotti F, Corona G, Mancini M, Biagini C, Colpi GM, Innocenti SD, et al. The association between varicocele, premature ejaculation and prostatitis symptoms: possible mechanisms. J Sex Med. 2009;6(10):2878–87.
34. Hamidi C, Batmaz I, Gumus H, Penbegul N, Cetincakmak MG, Tahtasiz M, et al. The association between varicocele and ankylosing spondylitis via color duplex sonography. Mod Rheumatol. 2014;24(1):162–5.
35. Erdogmus B, Yazici B, Balbay O, Annakkaya AN, Ozdere BA, Bulut I. Association between varicocele and chronic obstructive pulmonary disease. J Clin Ultrasound. 2006;34(2):55–9.
36. Prabakaran S, Kumanov P, Tomova A, Hubaveshki S, Agarwal A. Adolescent varicocele: association with somatometric parameters. Urol Int. 2006;77(2):114–7.
37. Kumanov P, Robeva R, Tomova A. Does an association between the idiopathic left-sided varicocele and eye colour exist? Adv Urol. 2014;2014:524570.
38. Henning H, Masal C, Herr A, Wolf K, Urhausen C, Beineke A, et al. Effect of short-term scrotal hyperthermia on spermatological parameters, testicular blood flow and gonadal tissue in dogs. Reprod Domest Anim. 2014;49(1):145–57.
39. Fujisawa M, Yoshida S, Matsumoto O, Kojima K, Kamidono S. Decrease of topoisomerase I activity in the testes of infertile men with varicocele. Arch Androl. 1988;21(1):45–50.
40. Zorgniotti AW. Testis temperature, infertility, and the varicocele paradox. Urology. 1980;16(1):7–10.
41. Hienz HA, Voggenthaler J, Weissbach L. Histological findings in testes with varicocele during childhood and their therapeutic consequences. Eur J Pediatr. 1980;133(2):139–46.
42. Kurz KR, Goldstein M. Scrotal temperature reflects intratesticular temperature and is lowered by shaving. J Urol. 1986;135(2):290–2.
43. Wright EJ, Young GP, Goldstein M. Reduction in testicular temperature after varicocelectomy in infertile men. Urology. 1997;50(2):257–9.
44. Shiraishi K, Takihara H, Matsuyama H. Elevated scrotal temperature, but not varicocele grade, reflects testicular oxidative stress-mediated apoptosis. World J Urol. 2010;28(3):359–64.
45. Vanlangenhove P, Dhondt E, Everaert K, Defreyne L. Pathophysiology, diagnosis and treatment of varicoceles: a review. Minerva Urol Nefrol. 2014;66(4):257–82.
46. Camoglio FS, Zampieri N, Corroppolo M, Chironi C, Dipaola G, Giacomello L, et al. Varicocele and retrograde adrenal metabolites flow. An experimental study on rats. Urol Int. 2004;73(4):337–42.
47. Turner TT, Lopez TJ. Effects of experimental varicocele require neither adrenal contribution nor venous reflux. J Urol. 1989;142(5):1372–5.
48. Rajfer J, Turner TT, Rivera F, Howards SS, Sikka SC. Inhibition of testicular testosterone biosynthesis following experimental varicocele in rats. Biol Reprod. 1987;36(4):933–7.
49. Ando S, Giacchetto C, Beraldi E, Panno ML, Carpino A, Sposato G, et al. Testosterone and dihydrotestosterone seminal plasma levels in varicocele patients. Acta Eur Fertil. 1982;13(3):113–7.
50. Su LM, Goldstein M, Schlegel PN. The effect of varicocelectomy on serum testosterone levels in infertile men with varicoceles. J Urol. 1995;154(5):1752–5.
51. Kass EJ, Freitas JE, Bour JB. Adolescent varicocele: objective indications for treatment. J Urol. 1989;142(2 Pt 2):579–82. discussion 603-5.
52. Sirvent JJ, Bernat R, Navarro MA, Rodriguez Tolra J, Guspi R, Bosch R. Leydig cell in idiopathic varicocele. Eur Urol. 1990;17(3):257–61.
53. Cayan S, Kadioglu A, Orhan I, Kandirali E, Tefekli A, Tellaloglu S. The effect of microsurgical varicocelectomy on serum follicle stimulating hormone, testosterone and free testosterone levels in infertile men with varicocele. BJU Int. 1999;84(9):1046–9.
54. Riccioli A, Starace D, D'Alessio A, Starace G, Padula F, De Cesaris P, et al. TNF-α and IFN-γ regulate expression and function of the Fas system in the seminiferous epithelium. J Immunol. 2000;165(2):743–9.

55. Fujisawa M, Ishikawa T. Soluble forms of Fas and Fas ligand concentrations in the seminal plasma of infertile men with varicocele. J Urol. 2003;170(6 Pt 1):2363–5.
56. Zedan H, El-Mekhlafi AW, El-Noweihi AM, Abd El-Azim NE, Mostafa T. Soluble Fas and gonadal hormones in infertile men with varicocele. Fertil Steril. 2009;91(2):420–4.
57. Romeo C, Arrigo T, Impellizzeri P, Manganaro A, Antonuccio P, Di Pasquale G, et al. Altered serum inhibin b levels in adolescents with varicocele. J Pediatr Surg. 2007;42(2):390–4.
58. Devine PJ, Perreault SD, Luderer U. Roles of reactive oxygen species and antioxidants in ovarian toxicity. Biol Reprod. 2012;86(2):27.
59. Romeo C, Ientile R, Santoro G, Impellizzeri P, Turiaco N, Impala P, et al. Nitric oxide production is increased in the spermatic veins of adolescents with left idiopathic varicocele. J Pediatr Surg. 2001;36(2):389–93.
60. Shiraishi K, Matsuyama H, Takihara H. Pathophysiology of varicocele in male infertility in the era of assisted reproductive technology. Int J Urol. 2012;19(6):538–50.
61. Aitken RJ, Clarkson JS. Cellular basis of defective sperm function and its association with the genesis of reactive oxygen species by human spermatozoa. J Reprod Fertil. 1987;81(2):459–69.
62. Santoro G, Romeo C, Impellizzeri P, Ientile R, Cutroneo G, Trimarchi F, et al. Nitric oxide synthase patterns in normal and varicocele testis in adolescents. BJU Int. 2001;88(9):967–73.
63. Middendorff R, Muller D, Wichers S, Holstein AF, Davidoff MS. Evidence for production and functional activity of nitric oxide in seminiferous tubules and blood vessels of the human testis. J Clin Endocrinol Metab. 1997;82(12):4154–61.
64. Del Punta K, Charreau EH, Pignataro OP. Nitric oxide inhibits Leydig cell steroidogenesis. Endocrinology. 1996;137(12):5337–43.
65. Santoro G, Romeo C, Impellizzeri P, Cutroneo G, Micali A, Trimarchi F, et al. Immunofluorescence distribution of actin-associated proteins in human seminiferous tubules of adolescent testes, normal and pathologic. J Endocrinol Invest. 2000;23(6):369–75.
66. Saleh RA, Agarwal A. Oxidative stress and male infertility: from research bench to clinical practice. J Androl. 2002;23(6):737–52.
67. Agarwal A, Saleh RA, Bedaiwy MA. Role of reactive oxygen species in the pathophysiology of human reproduction. Fertil Steril. 2003;79(4):829–43.
68. Agarwal A, Virk G, Ong C, du Plessis SS. Effect of oxidative stress on male reproduction. World J Mens Health. 2014;32(1):1–17.
69. Agarwal A, Hamada A, Esteves SC. Insight into oxidative stress in varicocele-associated male infertility: part 1. Nat Rev Urol. 2012;9(12):678–90.
70. Prader A. Testicular size: assessment and clinical importance. Triangle. 1966;7:240–3.
71. Takihara H, Sakatoku J, Fujii M, Nasu T, Cosentino MJ, Cockett AT. Significance of testicular size measurement in andrology. I. A new orchiometer and its clinical application. Fertil Steril. 1983;39(6):836–40.
72. Diamond DA, Paltiel HJ, DiCanzio J, Zurakowski D, Bauer SB, Atala A, et al. Comparative assessment of pediatric testicular volume: orchidometer versus ultrasound. J Urol. 2000;164(3 Pt 2):1111–4.
73. Paltiel HJ, Diamond DA, Di Canzio J, Zurakowski D, Borer JG, Atala A. Testicular volume: comparison of orchidometer and US measurements in dogs. Radiology. 2002;222(1):114–9.
74. Kolon TF, Clement MR, Cartwright L, Bellah R, Carr MC, Canning DA, et al. Transient asynchronous testicular growth in adolescent males with a varicocele. J Urol. 2008;180(3):1111–4. discussion 4-5.
75. Eskew LA, Watson NE, Wolfman N, Bechtold R, Scharling E, Jarow JP. Ultrasonographic diagnosis of varicoceles. Fertil Steril. 1993;60(4):693–7.
76. Chiou RK, Anderson JC, Wobig RK, Rosinsky DE, Matamoros Jr A, Chen WS, et al. Color Doppler ultrasound criteria to diagnose varicoceles: correlation of a new scoring system with physical examination. Urology. 1997;50(6):953–6.
77. Konforte D, Shea JL, Kyriakopoulou L, Colantonio D, Cohen AH, Shaw J, et al. Complex biological pattern of fertility hormones in children and adolescents: a study of healthy children from the CALIPER cohort and establishment of pediatric reference intervals. Clin Chem. 2013;59(8):1215–27.

78. Guarino N, Tadini B, Bianchi M. The adolescent varicocele: the crucial role of hormonal tests in selecting patients with testicular dysfunction. J Pediatr Surg. 2003;38(1):120–3. discussion 120-3.
79. Diamond DA, Zurakowski D, Bauer SB, Borer JG, Peters CA, Cilento Jr BG, et al. Relationship of varicocele grade and testicular hypotrophy to semen parameters in adolescents. J Urol. 2007;178(4 Pt 2):1584–8.
80. Kurtz MP, Zurakowski D, Rosoklija I, Bauer SB, Borer JG, Johnson KL, et al. Semen parameters in adolescents with varicocele: association with testis volume differential and total testis volume. J Urol. 2015.
81. Christman MS, Zderic SA, Kolon TF. Comparison of testicular volume differential calculations in adolescents with varicoceles. J Pediatr Urol. 2014;10(2):396–8.
82. Kass EJ, Belman AB. Reversal of testicular growth failure by varicocele ligation. J Urol. 1987;137(3):475–6.
83. Laven JS, Haans LC, Mali WP, te Velde ER, Wensing CJ, Eimers JM. Effects of varicocele treatment in adolescents: a randomized study. Fertil Steril. 1992;58(4):756–62.
84. Okuyama A, Nakamura M, Namiki M, Takeyama M, Utsunomiya M, Fujioka H, et al. Surgical repair of varicocele at puberty: preventive treatment for fertility improvement. J Urol. 1988;139(3):562–4.
85. Haans LC, Laven JS, Mali WP, te Velde ER, Wensing CJ. Testis volumes, semen quality, and hormonal patterns in adolescents with and without a varicocele. Fertil Steril. 1991;56(4):731–6.
86. Sayfan J, Siplovich L, Koltun L, Benyamin N. Varicocele treatment in pubertal boys prevents testicular growth arrest. J Urol. 1997;157(4):1456–7.
87. Alukal JP, Zurakowski D, Atala A, Bauer SB, Borer JG, Cilento Jr BG, et al. Testicular hypotrophy does not correlate with grade of adolescent varicocele. J Urol. 2005;174(6):2367–70. discussion 70.
88. Paduch DA, Niedzielski J. Semen analysis in young men with varicocele: preliminary study. J Urol. 1996;156(2 Pt 2):788–90.
89. Zampieri N, Zuin V, Corroppolo M, Ottolenghi A, Camoglio FS. Relationship between varicocele grade, vein reflux and testicular growth arrest. Pediatr Surg Int. 2008;24(6):727–30.
90. Zampieri N, Cervellione RM. Varicocele in adolescents: a 6-year longitudinal and followup observational study. J Urol. 2008;180(4 Suppl):1653–6. discussion 6.
91. Decastro GJ, Shabsigh A, Poon SA, Laor L, Glassberg KI. Adolescent varicocelectomy--is the potential for catch-up growth related to age and/or Tanner stage? J Urol. 2009;181(1):322–7. discussion 7.
92. Thomas JC, Elder JS. Testicular growth arrest and adolescent varicocele: does varicocele size make a difference? J Urol. 2002;168(4 Pt 2):1689–91. discussion 91.
93. Diamond DA. Adolescent varicocele. Curr Opin Urol. 2007;17(4):263–7.
94. Paduch DA, Niedzielski J. Repair versus observation in adolescent varicocele: a prospective study. J Urol. 1997;158(3 Pt 2):1128–32.
95. Fideleff HL, Boquete HR, Suarez MG, Ruibal GF, Sobrado PG, Azaretsky M, et al. Controversies in the evolution of paediatric-adolescent varicocele: clinical, biochemical and histological studies. Eur J Endocrinol. 2000;143(6):775–81.
96. Lee PA. Physiology of puberty. In: Becker KL, editor. Principles and practice of endocrinology and metabolism. 3rd ed. Philadelphia: JB Lippincott Co.; 2001. p. 886.
97. Carrillo A, Gershbein A, Glassberg KI, Danon M. Serum inhibin B levels and the response to gonadotropin stimulation test in pubertal boys with varicocele. J Urol. 1999;162(3 Pt 1):875–7.
98. Trigo RV, Bergada I, Rey R, Ballerini MG, Bedecarras P, Bergada C, et al. Altered serum profile of inhibin B, Pro-alphaC and anti-Mullerian hormone in prepubertal and pubertal boys with varicocele. Clin Endocrinol (Oxf). 2004;60(6):758–64.
99. Blevrakis E, Chatzidarellis E, Anyfantakis D, Sakellaris G, Raissaki M, Zoras O, et al. Impact of varicocele on biological markers of gonadal function. Hernia. 2015;19:1–5.
100. Nork JJ, Berger JH, Crain DS, Christman MS. Youth varicocele and varicocele treatment: a meta-analysis of semen outcomes. Fertil Steril. 2014;102(2):381–7.e6.

101. Reichart M, Eltes F, Soffer Y, Zigenreich E, Yogev L, Bartoov B. Sperm ultramorphology as a pathophysiological indicator of spermatogenesis in males suffering from varicocele. Andrologia. 2000;32(3):139–45.
102. Paduch DA, Skoog SJ. Current management of adolescent varicocele. Rev Urol. 2001;3(3):120–33.
103. Donovan Jr JF. Laparoscopic varix ligation. Urology. 1994;44(4):467–9.
104. Sehgal SS, Chu DI, Otto BJ, Acosta DN, Goldstein M. Survey of varicocelectomy: techniques employed by AUA urologists. J Urol. 2008;179(4):657.
105. Hirokawa M, Matsushita K, Iwamoto T, Iwasaki A, Asakura S, Masuda M. Assessment of Palomo's operative method for infertile varicocele. Andrologia. 1993;25(1):47–51.
106. Riccabona M, Oswald J, Koen M, Lusuardi L, Radmayr C, Bartsch G. Optimizing the operative treatment of boys with varicocele: sequential comparison of 4 techniques. J Urol. 2003;169(2):666–8.
107. Palomo A. Radical cure of varicocele by a new technique; preliminary report. J Urol. 1949;61(3):604–7.
108. Levitt S, Gill B, Katlowitz N, Kogan SJ, Reda E. Routine intraoperative post-ligation venography in the treatment of the pediatric varicocele. J Urol. 1987;137(4):716–8.
109. Ivanissevich O. Left varicocele due to reflux; experience with 4,470 operative cases in forty-two years. J Int Coll Surg. 1960;34:742–55.
110. Schultheiss D, Denil J. History of the microscope and development of microsurgery: a revolution for reproductive tract surgery. Andrologia. 2002;34(4):234–41.
111. Minevich E, Wacksman J, Lewis AG, Sheldon CA. Inguinal microsurgical varicocelectomy in the adolescent: technique and preliminary results. J Urol. 1998;159(3):1022–4.
112. Lemack GE, Uzzo RG, Schlegel PN, Goldstein M. Microsurgical repair of the adolescent varicocele. J Urol. 1998;160(1):179–81.
113. Mehta A, Goldstein M. Varicocele repair for nonobstructive azoospermia. Curr Opin Urol. 2012;22(6):507–12.
114. Amendolara M, Antoniello L, Battocchio F. Laparoscopic treatment of varicocele. Chir Ital. 1999;51(3):247–52.
115. Rizkala E, Fishman A, Gitlin J, Zelkovic P, Franco I. Long term outcomes of lymphatic sparing laparoscopic varicocelectomy. J Pediatr Urol. 2013;9(4):458–63.
116. Osorio L, Silva D, Autorino R, Damiano R, Correia-Pinto J, Lima E. Pure NOTES transvesical venous ligation: translational animal model of varicocelectomy. Urology. 2011;78(5):1082–6.
117. Lee SW, Lee JY, Kim KH, Ha US. Laparoendoscopic single-site surgery versus conventional laparoscopic varicocele ligation in men with palpable varicocele: a randomized, clinical study. Surg Endosc. 2012;26(4):1056–62.
118. Thon WF, Gall H, Danz B, Bahren W, Sigmund G. Percutaneous sclerotherapy of idiopathic varicocele in childhood: a preliminary report. J Urol. 1989;141(4):913–5.
119. Clarke SA, Agrawal M, Reidy J. Percutaneous transfemoral testicular vein embolisation in the treatment of childhood varicocele. Pediatr Radiol. 2001;31(7):515–7.
120. Fayad F, Sellier N, Chabaud M, Kazandjian V, Larroquet M, Raquillet C, et al. Percutaneous retrograde endovascular occlusion for pediatric varicocele. J Pediatr Surg. 2011;46(3):525–9.
121. Al-Said S, Al-Naimi A, Al-Ansari A, Younis N, Shamsodini A, A-sadiq K, et al. Varicocelectomy for male infertility: a comparative study of open, laparoscopic and microsurgical approaches. J Urol. 2008;180(1):266–70.
122. Wang J, Xia SJ, Liu ZH, Tao L, Ge JF, Xu CM, et al. Inguinal and subinguinal micro-varicocelectomy, the optimal surgical management of varicocele: a meta-analysis. Asian J Androl. 2015;17(1):74–80.
123. Waalkes R, Manea IF, Nijman JM. Varicocele in adolescents: a review and guideline for the daily practice. Arch Esp Urol. 2012;65(10):859–71.

Chapter 16
Polycystic Ovary Syndrome in Adolescent Girls

Sajal Gupta, Elizabeth Pandithurai, and Ashok Agarwal

Introduction

PCOS: Definition

Polycystic ovary syndrome (PCOS), also called Stein–Leventhal syndrome, is one of the most common disorders of hormonal imbalance in women of reproductive age. The name by itself is a misnomer, as not all women with the syndrome have polycystic ovaries and not all women with polycystic ovaries suffer from PCOS.

Gynecologists Irving F. Stein, Sr., and Michael L. Leventhal first described the disease in 1935 [1]. They noticed ovarian cysts in women with anovulatory cycles and found an association between the two. The combination of symptoms such as oligomenorrhea, infertility, and hirsutism along with bilaterally enlarged polycystic ovaries formed the diagnosis of Stein–Leventhal syndrome. The name was later replaced as "polycystic ovary syndrome." The presence of ovarian cysts and anovulation remained the main diagnostic criteria for the syndrome for many years, until recently, when the multisystem involvement of the disease was understood by the clinicians.

In 1982, Hughesdon reported that the polycystic appearance of the ovaries was caused by an increase in the number of growing follicles measuring less than 10 mm

S. Gupta (✉)
Andrology Center, Cleveland Clinic,
10681 Carnegie Avenue, Cleveland, OH 44195, USA
e-mail: guptas2@ccf.org

E. Pandithurai
Department of Urology, Cleveland Clinic,
10681 Carnegie Avenue, Cleveland, OH 44195, USA

A. Agarwal
American Center for Reproductive Medicine, Cleveland Clinic,
Cleveland, OH, USA

P. Kumanov, A. Agarwal (eds.), *Puberty*, DOI 10.1007/978-3-319-32122-6_16

in diameter. These follicles are arrested at various stages of development. Because an arrested ovarian follicle looks like a cyst, it should be considered normal. It is only the increase in the number of follicles that is considered pathologic, with polycystic ovarian syndrome being the major underlying cause. Multifollicular ovaries have been reported as a normal feature of puberty, and these changes recede with onset of regular menstruation [2, 3].

Epidemiology

The disease is frequently misdiagnosed in adolescent girls because signs and symptoms commonly overlap with those of normal puberty, and they are often missed completely. The hormonal and metabolic changes that occur during puberty increase the incidence of PCOS in adolescent girls and may also contribute to the pathogenesis of PCOS in this patient population [4]. After the onset of the first menstrual cycle, adolescent girls enter a transient state of anovulation, which is considered physiological. However, in certain adolescents, regular menstrual cycles fail to occur within 2–3 years of menarche and they remain anovulatory. In those cases, the possibility of PCOS must be explored [5].

The prevalence of PCOS is determined by the diagnostic criteria being used. According to diagnostic criteria outlined by the NIH/NICHD, PCOS affects 4–8 % women of reproductive age [6]. Using NIH adult criteria, the prevalence of PCOS in adolescent girls aged 15–19 years is approximately 1 %, although this may be an underestimation as PCOS is an underdiagnosed condition, especially in non-overweight girls [7]. According to Michelmore et al. [5] the prevalence of PCOS in women aged 18–25 years is 8 % [5]. Overall, PCOS is the most common endocrine disorder in females, affecting roughly 5–10 % of all women of reproductive age [8].

Clinical Features of PCOS

The onset of symptoms predominantly occurs during puberty [9]. PCOS may manifest as early as the first decade of life as premature pubarche or menarche.

Oligomenorrhea in the early postpubertal years, although very common, may be an early symptom of PCOS, particularly in overweight girls with hirsutism or acne [10]. Signs and symptoms that occur during adolescence include hyperandrogenism such as acne, hirsutism, alopecia, weight gain [11, 12], and menstrual disturbances as well as insulin resistance that is evident by skin pigmentation (acanthosis nigricans). Most of these symptoms contribute to psychosocial aspects of the disease, which include lowered self-esteem, social anxiety, psychological stress, impaired well-being, and quality of life. Recent studies have also shown that adolescent girls with PCOS have sleep disorders including excessive daytime sleepiness and sleep-disordered breathing [4].

There are numerous underlying mechanisms linking obesity and PCOS. Hence, women with PCOS are mostly obese, and obesity exacerbates the clinical features of PCOS [13]. Trent et al. reported that adolescent girls with PCOS had a higher BMI than their healthy peers. The significantly elevated BMI in such girls decreased their quality of life [14].

Diagnostic Criteria

Although PCOS is the most common endocrine disorder in reproductive age women, the diagnosis is challenging. Three societies have published criteria for the diagnosis of PCOS—the NIH/NICHD (1990), ESHRE/ASRM (Rotterdam), and the Androgen Excess Society (AES) (2006) (Table 16.1). Although the Rotterdam criteria are widely used for the diagnosis of PCOS in women, their use in adolescent girls is under debate. Hence, the NIH and AES criteria are considered more useful for the diagnosis of PCOS in adolescents [15].

The ESHRE/ASRM (European Society of Human Reproduction and Embryology/American Society for Reproductive Medicine) criteria (Table 16.1) state that the diagnosis of PCOS must include two of the following symptoms—clinical and/or biochemical hyperandrogenism, polycystic ovaries, and oligo-/anovulation—and exclude any other condition with androgen excess or related disorders [6]. Ultrasound criteria include an ovarian volume (OV) of threshold 10 cm^3 and 12 or more follicles measuring 2–9 mm in diameter, and these were considered diagnostic for PCOS by the ESHRE/ASRM group [16].

According to NIH/NICHD (National Institute of Child Health and Human Disease/National Institute of Child Health and Human Development) (Table 16.1), the criteria for the diagnosis of PCOS include clinical and/or biochemical hyperandrogenism with menstrual dysfunction and exclude other conditions with androgen excess or related disorders [6]. The AES 2006 criteria (Table 16.1) for the diagnosis of PCOS include

Table 16.1 Diagnostic criteria for PCOS in women

Diagnostic criteria for PCOS in Women (NIH/NICHD)1990 [8]	Diagnostic Criteria for PCOS in Women ESHRE/ASRM(Rotterdam Criteria) 2003 (includes two of the following) [8]	Diagnostic criteria for PCOS in Women (Androgen Excess Society) 2006 [8]
1. Clinical and/or biochemical hyperandrogenism (excluding other androgen excess or related disorders) 2. Menstrual dysfunction	1. Clinical and/or biochemical hyperandrogenism (excluding other androgen excess or related disorders) 2. Oligo-ovulation (or) anovulation 3. Polycystic ovaries	1. Clinical and/or biochemical hyperandrogenism (excluding other androgen excess or related disorders) 2. Ovarian dysfunction and/or polycystic ovaries

Table 16.2 Diagnostic criteria for PCOS in adolescents

Diagnostic criteria of PCOS in adolescents (Sultan and Paris) {at least 4 out of the 5 following criteria} [18]	Diagnostic Criteria of PCOS in adolescents (Bruni et al.,) [27]	Diagnostic Criteria of PCOS in adolescents (Legro RS et al.,) [3]
1. Oligomenorrhea or amenorrhea 2 years after menarche 2. Signs of clinical hyperandrogenism such as persistent acne or severe hirsutism 3. Increased plasma testosterone>50 ng/dl, increased LH/FSH ratio 4. Insulin resistance/hyperinsulinemia evident as acanthosis nigricans, abdominal obesity, glucose intolerance 5. Polycystic ovaries on ultrasound scan showing enlarged ovaries, peripheral microcysts, increased stroma.	1. Clinical hyperandrogenism (Hirsutism) +/– 2. Biochemical hyperandrogenism and 3. Oligomenorrhea	1. Clinical and/or biochemical hyperandrogenism (excluding other pathologies) and 2. Persistent oligomenorrhea

clinical or biochemical hyperandrogenism with ovarian dysfunction and/or polycystic ovaries, and the criteria exclude other androgen excess or related disorders [6].

Diagnostic Criteria in Adolescents

There is no current consensus on the diagnosis of PCOS in adolescent girls. Studies done in the United States and Europe have shown that adolescent girls with PCOS had clinical, metabolic, and endocrine features similar to that of adult women with PCOS [17]. Sultan and Paris have suggested that adolescent PCOS could be defined by at least four of the five following criteria: (1) oligomenorrhea or amenorrhea 2 years after menarche; (2) signs of clinical hyperandrogenism such as persistent acne and severe hirsutism; (3) increased plasma testosterone >50 ng/dl (1.735 nmol/l) and increased LH/FSH ratio; (4) insulin resistance/hyperinsulinemia evident as acanthosis nigricans, abdominal obesity, and glucose intolerance; and (5) polycystic ovaries upon ultrasound showing enlarged ovaries, peripheral microcysts, and increased stroma [18] (Table 16.2). According to a study done by Bruni et al., PCOS in adolescents was best characterized by clinical hyperandrogenism (hirsutism) and/or biochemical hyperandrogenism and oligomenorrhea [15] (Table 16.2). Legro et al. suggest that PCOS in adolescents can be diagnosed by (1) the presence of clinical and/or biochemical hyperandrogenism (excluding other pathologies) and (2) persistent oligomenorrhea. They clearly stated that the anovulatory symptoms and ovarian morphology cannot be taken into account for the diagnosis of PCOS in adolescents as it can be a normal finding during reproductive maturation [3] (Table 16.2). Third PCOS consensus report concluded that the criteria for diagnosis of PCOS in adolescent girls differ from those used for older women of reproductive age group [19]. Chinese adolescent girls with PCOS were noted to have a mean ovarian volume of 6.74 cm^3 and a maximum ovarian volume of 7.82 cm^3, which is lesser than 10 cm^3, as per the Rotterdam criteria [20].

Pathogenesis of PCOS

Endocrine Disorder

Women with PCOS have several endocrine disturbances including hyperinsulinemia, hyperglycemia, glucose intolerance, dyslipidemia, and obesity, which are considered as characteristic components of metabolic syndrome. There is a strong association between insulin resistance, obesity, and metabolic syndrome in PCOS. Hyperandrogenemia is also very commonly seen in peripubertal PCOS associated with obesity.

Insulin Resistance

The role of decreased insulin sensitivity in the pathogenesis of the disease has gained attention in recent years. There is significant insulin resistance seen in individuals with PCOS [21]—about 50–70 % of individuals with PCOS have insulin resistance contributing to its symptoms and long-term complications. Abdominal adipose tissue seen in adolescents with PCOS impairs the action of insulin. In addition, increased levels of androgen also impair glucose uptake, which again contributes to insulin resistance and increased deposition of visceral fat [15].

Elevated levels of pro-inflammatory cytokines such as TNF-alpha seen in women and adolescent girls with PCOS induce insulin resistance by decreasing glucose transporter type 4 (GLUT-4) expression leading to decreased transport of glucose and the development of hyperinsulinemia [22]. Insulin resistance and obesity enhance follicular excess noticed in patients with PCOS through the dysregulation of anti-Müllerian hormone pathway or via hyperandrogenemia pathway [23]. Elevated IL-6 levels induce the production of acute phase reactant C-reactive protein, which has been noted to be associated with increased incidence of cardiovascular events, insulin resistance, type 2 diabetes, and metabolic syndrome [24].

It should also be kept in mind that it is completely physiological to have increased insulin resistance during the peripubertal period. During adolescence, production of growth hormone increases, which is compensated by increased secretion of insulin, leading to reduced insulin sensitivity. Insulin resistance during adolescence can also be partly caused by increased oxidation of fat and reduced oxidation of glucose [25].

Alterations in GnRH, LH/FSH Ratio

Gonadotropin-releasing hormone (GnRH) stimulates the release of LH and FSH from the pituitary gland. FSH controls the growth of the ovarian follicles, especially the granulosa cells. FSH acts on the granulosa cells of the ovary and converts androgens from the theca cells of the ovary to estradiol with the help of the enzyme aromatase. LH controls the theca cells of the ovary, which are responsible for producing androgens. High GnRH pulse frequency favors production of LH and low GnRH pulse frequency favors FSH production [26].

During a normal menstrual cycle, the GnRH pulse frequency gradually increases during the first half of the cycle—the follicular phase—which is controlled by FSH. The GnRH pulse frequency peaks in the second half of the cycle, increasing LH production and decreasing FSH production. Further, the estradiol production during the first half of the cycle reaches a threshold and causes the midcycle LH surge, which induces ovulation. After ovulation, the corpus luteum develops, which generates the production of progesterone. The hormone progesterone sends feedback to the hypothalamus and subsequently slows GnRH pulse frequency, favoring FSH production and initiating the next cycle.

In PCOS, there is persistently high pulse frequency of GnRH resulting in elevated levels of LH and decreased levels of FSH, thereby elevating the LH/FH ratio. This in turn stimulates ovarian androgen synthesis leading to hyperandrogenemia in individuals with PCOS [27]. The relatively low levels of FSH impair follicular development [26].

Hyperandrogenemia

Hyperandrogenemia plays a vital role in the pathophysiology of PCOS. According to a cross-sectional case-control study done by Coviello et al., adolescent girls with PCOS had a higher prevalence of metabolic syndrome than their healthy peers. The study noted that hyperandrogenemia was an independent risk factor for metabolic syndrome irrespective of obesity and insulin resistance [28].

PCOS in adolescence is thought to be a precursor to PCOS later in life. Girls with increased androgen levels also have reduced hypothalamic sensitivity to progesterone feedback [26], and hence, there is no slowing of GnRH pulse frequency. LH levels remain high, leading to increased androgen levels.

GnRH pulse generators are a group of neurons in the hypothalamus that generate release of GnRH in a pulsatile fashion. Blank et al. hypothesized that excess androgen levels during the peripubertal period may decrease the sensitivity of the GnRH pulse generator to sex steroid inhibition in liable individuals, leading to increased GnRH pulse frequency and thereby alterations in gonadotropin secretion, ovarian androgen synthesis, and ovulatory function. These abnormalities may advance over time to clinical hyperandrogenism and chronic oligo-ovulation typically seen in adult patients with PCOS [26].

Hyperandrogenemia seen in patients with PCOS was thought to cause low-grade inflammation by increasing sensitivity to glucose-induced oxidative stress and promoting the transcription of pro-inflammatory cytokines TNF-alpha and IL-6. These pro-inflammatory cytokines stimulate steroidogenic enzymes in the ovaries, increase the extent of androgen production, and promote central obesity through the activation of hypothalamic–pituitary–adrenal axis; this leads to insulin resistance that may in turn cause hyperandrogenism [29, 30].

Hyperinsulinemia

Insulin resistance and its compensatory hyperinsulinemia are clearly linked to anovulation and hyperandrogenism in adolescents with PCOS. These girls have an ovarian androgenic hyperresponsiveness to circulating insulin [31]. It is to be noted that a reciprocal relationship exists between hyperinsulinemia and hyperandrogenism. Evidence suggests administration of androgens can induce insulin resistance in both men and women. On the other hand, insulin stimulates androgen production in ovarian theca cells which is evident in patients with PCOS [32]. It is also a universal finding that adolescent girls with PCOS have elevated levels of free testosterone and lower levels of sex hormone-binding globulin [10]. It can be attributed that hyperinsulinemia in individuals with PCOS lowers sex hormone-binding globulin and thereby enhances the free testosterone fraction. Study done by Ormazabal P. et al. suggests that testosterone may play a negative role on the metabolic effects of insulin on endometrial stromal cell cultures in women with PCOS and may favor insulin resistance in the endometria of such patients [32].

Obesity: Cause or Effect of PCOS?

Strong evidence suggests that growth patterns in early life are associated with the risk of metabolic syndrome in adulthood [33]. Obesity during adolescence may cause changes in the hypothalamic–pituitary axis and insulin secretion as well as insulin sensitivity *which* can predispose individuals to the endocrine and metabolic changes seen in individuals with PCOS. These changes include impaired glucose tolerance, insulin resistance, dyslipidemia, decreased leptin secretion, menstrual irregularities, and infertility [4]. Levels of several pro-inflammatory cytokines including TNF-alpha and IL-6 are elevated with obesity and PCOS possibly due to hyperandrogenemia and/or excess adipose tissue, but this still needs further research [15]. Obese young girls with PCOS tend to have severe symptoms.

According to a study, young girls with a higher than normal BMI during childhood had an increased risk of menstrual disturbances such as oligomenorrhea and a diagnosis of PCOS during young adulthood (age 24) [34]. A large cohort study conducted in 244 randomly selected postmenarchal girls reported polycystic ovarian morphology in 61.1 % of obese girls and in 32.1 % of normal weight girls, suggesting that obesity is a contributing factor of PCOS [34]. In another study, adolescent girls (age 14) were diagnosed with PCOS using the Rotterdam criteria and 33 % showed class III obesity by age 24 compared to 8 % of girls without the diagnosis of PCOS. This suggests that PCOS is a predicting factor of class III obesity [34]. Other predictors of class III obesity are low sex hormone-binding globulin (SHBG), metabolic syndrome, oligomenorrhea, high childhood insulin levels, and increased calculated free testosterone (cFT) which again are identified as PCOS phenotypes. According to the abovementioned studies, it is important that young girls who are obese or who have PCOS have to be monitored closely considering the long-term complications such as metabolic syndrome [15].

Ovarian Dysfunction

PCOS is a syndrome of ovarian dysfunction that includes hyperandrogenism and polycystic ovarian morphology. Studies have noted that ovarian enlargement is a key feature of PCOS. A typical ovary with PCOS is two to five times larger than a normal ovary [20]. Evidence suggests that PCOS is a functional disorder in which anovulation is a consequence of overproduction of ovarian androgen [35]. Adolescent girls and adults with PCOS have similar clinical and biochemical profiles. Ninety-five percent cases of functionally typical PCOS have classic PCOS, which is evident by hyperandrogenic anovulation with polycystic ovarian morphology [36].

Valproic Acid and PCOS

Valproic acid causes ovarian dysfunction by increasing ovarian androgen synthesis, thereby contributing to the hyperandrogenemia seen in girls with PCOS.

Adolescent girls frequently suffer from mental health issues such as bipolar disorder and may be prescribed chronic psychotropic drugs. Valproic acid is an anticonvulsant and also a mood-stabilizing drug that is widely used to treat adolescent girls with epilepsy and bipolar disorder and for migraine prophylaxis. The association between valproic acid use and PCOS was initially suggested in 1993 in a study where women with epilepsy who were treated with valproic acid showed more irregularities in their menstrual cycle than women using other anticonvulsants. The study also noted that the menstrual irregularities were more pronounced in the women who were started on valproic acid during adolescence; 80 % of the women started on valproic acid before the age of 20 were noted to have polycystic ovaries [37].

In a study conducted in women who were treated with valproic acid for epilepsy, 7 % of them developed features of PCOS [38]. Another study noted that 10 % of women treated with valproic acid for bipolar disorder developed PCOS [39]. In both of these studies, the association between PCOS and valproic acid use was strongest in females between the ages of 13 and 25. Hence, it is to be noted that adolescent girls are more prone to develop PCOS with valproic acid use. It can be suggested that the immature HPO axis in adolescents may leave them more prone to the iatrogenic effects of valproic acid. However, the cause remains unclear. The most well-studied proposed mechanism of action involves a direct increase in ovarian androgen biosynthesis by theca cells [40].

When similar doses of valproic acid used to treat bipolar disorder and epilepsy treatment were introduced into cultures of human ovarian theca cells, there was increased transcription of ovarian androgens. Various studies suggest that valproic acid may inhibit the metabolism of testosterone and thereby contribute to features of PCOS [41]. It may also have a central effect on GnRH or an indirect effect of obesity and insulin resistance that may induce the development of PCOS [42].

In summary, valproic acid therapy in adolescent girls is linked to PCOS. The risk for developing PCOS should be discussed before starting therapy with valproic acid. Menstrual patterns and signs of hyperandrogenism prior to initiation of treatment should be documented. Patients who are maintained chronically on valproic acid must be monitored closely for menstrual irregularities and signs of PCOS.

Hereditary Predisposition

Several studies have suggested that there is an increased risk of PCOS in adolescent girls with a family history of PCOS [18]. Girls with low birth weight and those with a family history of diabetes mellitus or premature cardiovascular disease are noted to have increased risk for developing PCOS [10]. Metabolic perturbations start early in adolescence and also exist in adolescent relatives of women with PCOS, even before clinical signs of PCOS become evident. A study by Li et al. reported risk factors associated with PCOS in adolescent Chinese girls—early menarche (<12 years), family histories of menstrual disorders, diabetes, and hypertension [17]. Twin studies suggest that the etiology of PCOS is strongly heritable [43]. In a genetic case-control study conducted in South India by Thathapudi et al., LH–chorionic gonadotropin hormone receptor (LHCGR) (rs2293275) polymorphism was found to be associated with PCOS; this study suggested that it could be used as a relevant molecular marker to identify girls at risk of developing PCOS and may provide an understanding about the etiology of the disease [44].

A Chinese study by Sun et al. suggested that genetic factors may affect the metabolic aspects of PCOS. The THADA gene is associated with lipid metabolism, whereas the DENND1A gene may be involved in insulin metabolism in patients with PCOS [45]. A study by Zhao et al. confirmed that SNP rs13429458 in the THADA gene is significantly associated with the risk of developing PCOS [46]. Identifying these genes in adolescent girls with a family history of PCOS may help physicians to evaluate their disease risk.

Long-Term Complications

Adolescents with PCOS are at a higher risk for comorbidities such as impaired glucose tolerance, metabolic syndrome, hypertension, dyslipidemia, diabetes, and endometrial hyperplasia [6,47]. Endometrial hyperplasia, if not treated, can lead to endometrial cancer. Adolescent girls with PCOS are also likely to be at increased risk for cardiovascular disease later in life [48]. The presence of obesity in adolescents with PCOS further adds to this complication [9] as it is associated with thickening of the intima media of the carotid artery. Adolescent girls with PCOS tend to have a higher body mass index and systolic blood pressure than healthy girls, which increases their risk for carotid artery disease to that of adult women with the disease [49]. Psychiatric issues such as depression, anxiety, bipolar disorder, and binge eating disorder are also noted to be among the long-term complications seen in individuals with PCOS [6]. Early diagnosis, prevention, and treatment are therefore important.

Diagnosis of PCOS

The diagnosis of PCOS during adolescence is important in order to monitor and screen for the development of type 2 diabetes and metabolic and reproductive complications [31]. Hyperandrogenism in adolescents can be determined biochemically by measuring levels of calculated free testosterone (cFT) and dehydroepiandrosterone.

Physiologically, morphological features such as ovarian volume and antral follicle count can be evaluated by the use of transabdominal ultrasonography, although they are operator dependent and of limited value for use in overweight adolescents. The use of transvaginal or transrectal ultrasound could be considered, but their use would be unethical in adolescents who are not yet sexually active [15]. With the use of ultrasound, ovarian volume and morphology such as the location, number of follicles, and stromal area can be assessed [50]. Patients with PCOS are noted to have multiple (>10) peripheral follicles, and the stromal volume positively correlates with hyperandrogenemia seen in those patients [50], although the ultrasonographic findings as mentioned in the Rotterdam criteria may not be sensitive for diagnosis of PCOS in adolescents.

Physiologically, it is normal for adolescents to have acne, anovulation, menstrual irregularities, and increased ovarian volume during the peripubertal period. Thus, specific diagnostic criteria to adolescent PCOS must be established. It is also normal for adolescents to have reduced insulin sensitivity. So, a specific cutoff value for screening tests such as fasting glucose and oral glucose tolerance also should be established [27].

Anti-Müllerian hormone (AMH) level is a good measure to assess both the quantity and quality of ovarian follicle pool. There is an initial increase in their levels until early adulthood with slow decrease with advancing age until it becomes undetectable roughly 5 years prior to menopause [51]. In a study conducted by Tomova A et al., AMH levels were noticed to be greatly elevated in women (mean age 26.59 ± 1.10 years) with PCOS. Furthermore, their levels decreased by 16.27 % after metformin therapy [23]. However, we need further studies on adolescent girls to evaluate the use of AMH levels as a biomarker for diagnosis of PCOS in adolescents and also to evaluate the efficacy of metformin use in such patients. More studies need to be conducted to explore the use of other biomarkers which will lead to non-invasive diagnosis for screening girls who are at greater risk for developing PCOS.

Management of PCOS

There is lack of standardized care in the management of adolescent PCOS. The long-term effects of pharmacological treatment in adolescents have not yet been evaluated, and hence, drugs should be used with caution. Overdiagnosis and treatment of the disease are possible. Overdiagnosis may lead to unnecessary use of medication and cause unnecessary psychological stress for the patient. On the other hand, pubertal changes are similar to those seen with PCOS and the disease can be under- or misdiagnosed. Underdiagnosis can put the patient at risk for long-term metabolic and reproductive complications [52]. The management of PCOS in adolescence is primarily targeted to treat menstrual irregularities, cutaneous hyperandrogenism, insulin resistance, and obesity.

Lifestyle Modification

Insulin resistance contributes to 50–70 % of the symptoms of PCOS. Most adolescent girls with PCOS are obese, which contributes to insulin resistance. Hence, weight loss is an important treatment strategy. Weight loss has been noted to improve symptoms of PCOS such as menstrual irregularities, hyperandrogenemia, and infertility. It can be achieved by lifestyle modifications such as exercise and diet control. In two randomized placebo-controlled clinical trials conducted by Hoeger et al., lifestyle modification alone leads to a reduction in the free androgen index, with an increase in sex hormone-binding globulin (SHBG), leading to decreased biochemical hyperandrogenism in obese adolescents with PCOS [53].

Metformin

Recent studies have reported that metformin, when combined with lifestyle modifications, resulted in modest weight loss and restored the menstrual cycle. Increase in insulin sensitivity and improvements in lipid profiles were observed [48, 49].

Metformin also plays a role in ovulation induction. A randomized, double-blind placebo-controlled trial conducted in 22 adolescent girls with PCOS, by Bridger et al., compared 12 weeks of treatment with metformin versus placebo in combination with lifestyle counseling. Metformin significantly decreased total testosterone concentrations and established regular cyclical menses [23]. It was also noted that metformin increased HDL cholesterol levels, but there were no significant changes in body weight or insulin sensitivity [54].

Ibanez and de Zegher conducted a series of clinical trials and reported that treatment with metformin improves insulin sensitivity, corrects dyslipidemia and hirsutism, and establishes cyclical menses in Catalan girls presenting with precocious pubarche [48]. A study done by De Leo et al. confirmed the positive effects of metformin on menstrual periods and suggested that the drug can be administered in young obese women with PCOS to improve hyperandrogenic symptoms such as hirsutism and acne and to restore ovulation [5]. A study by Genazzani et al. showed that metformin modulates ovarian function and affects the secretion of LH by reducing the hyperandrogenic state. The highest rate of endocrine changes was noted in hyperinsulinemic, hyperandrogenic, nonobese PCOS patients [55]. Hence, the study postulates that it is suitable to use metformin even in nonobese patients. The beneficial effect of metformin on hyperandrogenic states in adolescents due to PCOS could be due to the restoration of ovulation and the normalization of estrogen levels [5]. Lactic acidosis is one of the feared adverse effects of metformin, which is rarely reported in adolescents.

Oral Contraceptives

Combined oral contraceptive pills are considered the first-line treatment to regulate menstrual cycles in women with PCOS who are not seeking pregnancy. They also protect the endometrium from cancer. Combination oral contraceptives such as ethinyl estradiol (EE) with drospirenone (EE/D) have been noted to improve symptoms of hyperandrogenism. Progestin-only pills or cyclical progestins can be considered for use in those with contraindications to combined oral contraceptives [56].

Oral contraceptives aid in the treatment of hirsutism along with treating menstrual irregularities. However, more severe cases of hirsutism require antiandrogen pills along with oral contraceptive pills [56]. Cyproterone is a progestogen with antiandrogenic activity, and it should be administered in combination with an oral contraceptive pill to treat hirsutism [10].

In spite of these positive effects, there are concerns about oral contraceptives increasing insulin resistance, which would be an undesirable side effect, particularly in girls with PCOS. It was also noted that the clinical symptoms recur once therapy is stopped [5]. A review conducted by Ibanez and de Zegher stated that while oral contraceptives treat symptoms such as hirsutism and menstrual irregularities in patients with PCOS, hyperinsulinemia may remain unchanged or may even worsen. In adolescents, therefore, the PCOS spectrum can be normalized by combining oral contraceptives with flutamide–metformin.

Flutamide

The combination of flutamide–metformin helps treat hyperinsulinemia or hyperandrogenism, thereby preventing or reversing hirsutism, acne, and irregular menses. In contrast, oral contraceptives mask hirsutism, acne, or irregular menses, and hyperinsulinemia may remain unaltered or may worsen. The combination of flutamide and metformin can help in such cases. However, flutamide cannot be used in sexually active adolescents owing to the risk of embryotoxicity, and under those circumstances, oral contraceptives in the form of estro-progestagen or a non-endocrine method of contraception can be added to the flutamide–metformin combination [57].

In another study by the same group, use of thiazolidinediones such as pioglitazone in addition to flutamide, metformin, and oral contraceptives improved markers of cardiovascular health in young women [58]. Studies have suggested that flutamide, an androgen receptor blocker, restores progesterone sensitivity and hence improves hyperandrogenic symptoms of PCOS [26].

Spironolactone

Medications such as spironolactone and finasteride also improve hyperandrogenemia in adolescent girls with PCOS [6]. Spironolactone is an aldosterone antagonist primarily used to treat hypertension. However, it also has an antiandrogenic effect and hence improves hirsutism [10]. The use of spironolactone in adolescents still needs further clinical study. Breast tenderness and menstrual irregularities have been reported when it is used long term. Pregnancy should be avoided during its use, and it is suggested that spironolactone be used in combination with oral contraceptives in order to improve clinical effectiveness [10].

Progestogens

Progestogens such as medroxyprogesterone acetate, norethisterone, dydrogesterone, and progesterone are useful in managing adolescents whose main complaints are irregularities in menstrual cycles with no evidence of hyperandrogenemia. Progestogens are given on a cyclical basis for 14 days every month in order to ensure withdrawal bleeding. Therapeutic treatment with progestogens protects against endometrial cancer caused by prolonged estrogenic action [10].

Cosmetic Measures

Young girls with diagnosis of PCOS and clinically evident hirsutism can seek cosmetic therapy such as laser photoepilation to eliminate unwanted hair [59].

Psychosocial Interview

A psychosocial interview should take into consideration the psychological aspects of the adolescent by way of using psychosocial screening tools such as interviewing the adolescent regarding several of such factors: education, employment, eating, exercise, peers, and mental health. The assessment of these factors needs to be the basis for the management plan [60]. The quality of life in young women with PCOS is affected by several factors such as weight gain, acne, hirsutism, stress due to menstrual irregularities, and worries about future ability to have children. This can lower their self-esteem and confidence and leave them feeling self-conscious. Motivational interviewing techniques should be used. The clinician should address the concerns of the adolescent first, ask about their plan of lifestyle changes, and then review the steps and address any barriers [60]. This approach along with pharmacological management can help improve clinical outcomes in adolescent girls with PCOS.

Conclusion

PCOS is a heterogeneous disease characterized by endocrine, reproductive, metabolic, and psychosocial abnormalities. The disease has hereditary risk factors and a complex pathogenesis. The hormonal and metabolic changes that normally occur during peripubertal period should be differentiated from the clinical features of PCOS before diagnosing the disease in adolescents. It is important to manage the disease to avoid complications such as impaired glucose tolerance, mental health issues, and long-term complications such as metabolic syndrome, diabetes, hypertension, increased cardiovascular risk, infertility, and endometrial hyperplasia leading to endometrial cancer. Specific diagnostic criteria and optimal diagnostic methods to specifically screen adolescents should be established. A more holistic approach involving the psychosocial support to the adolescent along with lifestyle modifications and pharmacological management will result in improved clinical outcomes in the management of adolescent girls with PCOS.

References

1. Stein Sr IF. The Stein–Leventhal syndrome: a curable form of sterility. N Engl J Med. 1958;259(9):420–3.
2. Dewailly D, et al. Definition and significance of polycystic ovarian morphology: a task force report from the Androgen Excess and Polycystic Ovary Syndrome Society. Hum Reprod Update. 2014;20(3):334–52.
3. Legro RS, et al. Diagnosis and treatment of polycystic ovary syndrome: an Endocrine Society clinical practice guideline. J Clin Endocrinol Metab. 2013;98(12):4565–92.
4. El-Sharkawy AA, et al. Effect of metformin on sleep disorders in adolescent girls with polycystic ovarian syndrome. J Pediatr Adolesc Gynecol. 2014;27(6):347–52.

5. De Leo V, et al. Metformin treatment is effective in obese teenage girls with PCOS. Hum Reprod. 2006;21(9):2252–6.
6. Sirmans SM, Pate KA. Epidemiology, diagnosis, and management of polycystic ovary syndrome. Clin Epidemiol. 2013;6:1–13.
7. Christensen SB, et al. Prevalence of polycystic ovary syndrome in adolescents. Fertil Steril. 2013;100(2):470–7.
8. Azziz R, et al. The Androgen Excess and PCOS Society criteria for the polycystic ovary syndrome: the complete task force report. Fertil Steril. 2009;91(2):456–88.
9. Anderson AD, Solorzano CM, McCartney CR. Childhood obesity and its impact on the development of adolescent PCOS. Semin Reprod Med. 2014;32(3):202–13.
10. Mastorakos G, Lambrinoudaki I, Creatsas G. Polycystic ovary syndrome in adolescents: current and future treatment options. Paediatr Drugs. 2006;8(5):311–8.
11. Beltadze K, Barbakadze L. Diagnostic features of polycystic ovary syndrome in adolescents (review). Georgian Med News. 2015;238:32–4.
12. Azziz R. Controversy in clinical endocrinology: diagnosis of polycystic ovarian syndrome: the Rotterdam criteria are premature. J Clin Endocrinol Metab. 2006;91(3):781–5.
13. Naderpoor N, et al. Obesity and polycystic ovary syndrome. Minerva Endocrinol. 2015;40(1):37–51.
14. Trent M, et al. Overweight status of adolescent girls with polycystic ovary syndrome: body mass index as mediator of quality of life. Ambul Pediatr. 2005;5(2):107–11.
15. Vilmann LS, et al. Development of obesity and polycystic ovary syndrome in adolescents. Horm Res Paediatr. 2012;78(5–6):269–78.
16. Jonard S, Robert Y, Dewailly D. Revisiting the ovarian volume as a diagnostic criterion for polycystic ovaries. Hum Reprod. 2005;20(10):2893–8.
17. Li L, et al. Clinical and metabolic features of polycystic ovary syndrome among Chinese adolescents. J Pediatr Adolesc Gynecol. 2012;25(6):390–5.
18. Sultan C, Paris F. Clinical expression of polycystic ovary syndrome in adolescent girls. Fertil Steril. 2006;86 Suppl 1:S6.
19. Fauser BC, et al. Consensus on women's health aspects of polycystic ovary syndrome (PCOS): the Amsterdam ESHRE/ASRM-Sponsored 3rd PCOS Consensus Workshop Group. Fertil Steril. 2012;97(1):28–38. e25.
20. Chen Y, et al. The role of ovarian volume as a diagnostic criterion for Chinese adolescents with polycystic ovary syndrome. J Pediatr Adolesc Gynecol. 2008;21(6):347–50.
21. Yavuz Taslipinar M, et al. Endothelial dysfunction and insulin resistance in young women with polycystic ovarian syndrome. Turk J Med Sci. 2014;44(5):787–91.
22. Gonzalez F. Inflammation in polycystic ovary syndrome: underpinning of insulin resistance and ovarian dysfunction. Steroids. 2012;77(4):300–5.
23. Tomova A, et al. Anti-Mullerian hormone in women with polycystic ovary syndrome before and after therapy with metformin. Horm Metab Res. 2011;43(10):723–7.
24. Ridker PM, et al. C-reactive protein, the metabolic syndrome, and risk of incident cardiovascular events: an 8-year follow-up of 14 719 initially healthy American women. Circulation. 2003;107(3):391 7.
25. Hannon TS, Janosky J, Arslanian SA. Longitudinal study of physiologic insulin resistance and metabolic changes of puberty. Pediatr Res. 2006;60(6):759–63.
26. Blank SK, et al. Neuroendocrine effects of androgens in adult polycystic ovary syndrome and female puberty. Semin Reprod Med. 2007;25(5):352–9.
27. Bruni V, et al. Polycystic ovary syndrome in adolescence. Ann N Y Acad Sci. 2010;1205:175–84.
28. Coviello AD, Legro RS, Dunaif A. Adolescent girls with polycystic ovary syndrome have an increased risk of the metabolic syndrome associated with increasing androgen levels independent of obesity and insulin resistance. J Clin Endocrinol Metab. 2006;91(2):492–7.
29. Samy N, et al. Clinical significance of inflammatory markers in polycystic ovary syndrome: their relationship to insulin resistance and body mass index. Dis Markers. 2009;26(4):163–70.
30. Alemzadeh R, Kichler J, Calhoun M. Spectrum of metabolic dysfunction in relationship with hyperandrogenemia in obese adolescent girls with polycystic ovary syndrome. Eur J Endocrinol. 2010;162(6):1093–9.

31. Carreau AM, Baillargeon JP. PCOS in adolescence and type 2 diabetes. Curr Diab Rep. 2015;15(1):564.
32. Ormazabal P, et al. Testosterone modulates the expression of molecules linked to insulin action and glucose uptake in endometrial cells. Horm Metab Res. 2013;45(9):640–5.
33. Wells JC, Chomtho S, Fewtrell MS. Programming of body composition by early growth and nutrition. Proc Nutr Soc. 2007;66(3):423–34.
34. Glueck CJ, et al. Sex hormone-binding globulin, oligomenorrhea, polycystic ovary syndrome, and childhood insulin at age 14 years predict metabolic syndrome and class III obesity at age 24 years. J Pediatr. 2011;159(2):308–13. e2.
35. Rosenfield RL, et al. Antimullerian hormone levels are independently related to ovarian hyperandrogenism and polycystic ovaries. Fertil Steril. 2012;98(1):242–9.
36. Rosenfield RL. The polycystic ovary morphology-polycystic ovary syndrome spectrum. J Pediatr Adolesc Gynecol. 2015;28(6):412–9.
37. Isojarvi JI, et al. Polycystic ovaries and hyperandrogenism in women taking valproate for epilepsy. N Engl J Med. 1993;329(19):1383–8.
38. Morrell MJ, et al. Hyperandrogenism, ovulatory dysfunction, and polycystic ovary syndrome with valproate versus lamotrigine. Ann Neurol. 2008;64(2):200–11.
39. Joffe H, et al. Valproate is associated with new-onset oligoamenorrhea with hyperandrogenism in women with bipolar disorder. Biol Psychiatry. 2006;59(11):1078–86.
40. Nelson-DeGrave VL, et al. Valproate potentiates androgen biosynthesis in human ovarian theca cells. Endocrinology. 2004;145(2):799–808.
41. Herzog AG. Temporolimbic epilepsy and polycystic ovary syndrome. Fertil Steril. 1996;65(1):210–11.
42. Joffe H, Hayes FJ. Menstrual cycle dysfunction associated with neurologic and psychiatric disorders: their treatment in adolescents. Ann N Y Acad Sci. 2008;1135:219–29.
43. Welt CK, Duran JM. Genetics of polycystic ovary syndrome. Semin Reprod Med. 2014;32(3):177–82.
44. Thathapudi S, et al. Association of luteinizing hormone chorionic gonadotropin receptor gene polymorphism (rs2293275) with polycystic ovarian syndrome. Genet Test Mol Biomarkers. 2015;19(3):128–32.
45. Sun M, et al. Correlation analysis between polycystic ovary syndrome susceptibility genes and metabolic phenotypes. Zhonghua Fu Chan Ke Za Zhi. 2014;49(6):441–5.
46. Zhao H, et al. Family-based analysis of susceptibility loci for polycystic ovary syndrome on chromosome 2p16.3, 2p21 and 9q33.3. Hum Reprod. 2012;27(1):294–8.
47. Stankiewicz M, Norman R. Diagnosis and management of polycystic ovary syndrome: a practical guide. Drugs. 2006;66(7):903–12.
48. Williams RM, Ong KK, Dunger DB. Polycystic ovarian syndrome during puberty and adolescence. Mol Cell Endocrinol. 2013;373(1–2):61–7.
49. Glueck CJ, et al. Obesity, free testosterone, and cardiovascular risk factors in adolescents with polycystic ovary syndrome and regularly cycling adolescents. Metabolism. 2006;55(4):508–14.
50. Senaldi L, et al. Is ultrasound useful in the diagnosis of adolescents with polycystic ovary syndrome? J Pediatr Endocrinol Metab. 2015;28(5–6):605–12.
51. Broer SL, et al. Anti-Mullerian hormone: ovarian reserve testing and its potential clinical implications. Hum Reprod Update. 2014;20(5):688–701.
52. Powers SE, et al. Trends in standard workup performed by pediatric subspecialists for the diagnosis of adolescent polycystic ovary syndrome. J Pediatr Adolesc Gynecol. 2015;28(1):43–6.
53. Hoeger K, et al. The impact of metformin, oral contraceptives, and lifestyle modification on polycystic ovary syndrome in obese adolescent women in two randomized, placebo-controlled clinical trials. J Clin Endocrinol Metab. 2008;93(11):4299–306.
54. Bridger T, et al. Randomized placebo-controlled trial of metformin for adolescents with polycystic ovary syndrome. Arch Pediatr Adolesc Med. 2006;160(3):241–6.
55. Genazzani AD, et al. Metformin administration is more effective when non-obese patients with polycystic ovary syndrome show both hyperandrogenism and hyperinsulinemia. Gynecol Endocrinol. 2007;23(3):146–52.

56. Spritzer PM, et al. Novel strategies in the management of polycystic ovary syndrome. Minerva Endocrinol. 2015;40(3):195–212.
57. Ibanez L, de Zegher F. Low-dose flutamide-metformin therapy for hyperinsulinemic hyperandrogenism in non-obese adolescents and women. Hum Reprod Update. 2006;12(3):243–52.
58. Ibanez L, et al. Combined low-dose pioglitazone, flutamide, and metformin for women with androgen excess. J Clin Endocrinol Metab. 2007;92(5):1710–4.
59. Gacaferri Lumezi B, et al. Mixed form of hirsutism in an adolescent female and laser therapy. Iran Red Crescent Med J. 2014;16(6), e9410.
60. Mani H, Potdar N, Gleeson H. How to manage an adolescent girl presenting with features of polycystic ovary syndrome (PCOS); an exemplar for adolescent health care in endocrinology. Clin Endocrinol (Oxf). 2014;81(5):652–6.

Chapter 17
Growth Hormone and Steroid Assays' Problems in Childhood and Puberty

Dobrin A. Svinarov

Growth Hormone Disorders: Analytical and Interpretative Challenges

Growth hormone (GH) and insulin-like growth factor-I (IGF-I) are the most important laboratory parameters used in the diagnosis of GH secretion disorders, assessment of children with short stature, and monitoring of replacement therapy with GH and IGF-I. Therefore, clinicians should be permanently updated by their laboratories on the analytical weaknesses and problems of GH and IGF-I assays and how they affect the accuracy of patient assessment, as well as of the ongoing progress for standardization and harmonization of these assays. GH, also known as somatotropin, is secreted by anterior pituitary somatotropic cells under the regulation of two hypothalamic factors: GH-releasing hormone (GHRH) and somatotropin release-inhibiting hormone, with stimulation being predominant over suppression. GH has direct metabolic actions on protein metabolism: increased uptake of amino acids in tissues (anabolic effect), and on lipid metabolism: activation of lipolysis and elevation of free fatty acids (catabolic effect). GH effects on growth are indirect—it induces the secretion of IGF-I (known previously as somatomedin C) from GH responsive tissues—predominantly liver cells. Growth-promoting effects of IGF-I are mostly a result of autocrine and paracrine actions. Elevated IGF-I acts centrally to reduce hypothalamic release of GHRH, thus reducing GH secretion in a negative feedback mechanism. Apart from GH stimulation, IGF-I levels are influenced by thyroid hormones, sex steroids, chronic disease, and nutritional status. Therefore, growth can be impaired even with GH sufficiency in cases of hypothyroidism, sex steroid deficiency, chronic illness, and malnutrition. GH stimulates the production of two other proteins: IGF-binding protein-3 (IGFBP-3) and acid-labile subunit, which may form

D.A. Svinarov (✉)
Department of Therapeutic Drug Management and Clinical Pharmacology, Alexander Hospital, Medical University of Sofia, St. G. Sofiiski 1 Blvd, 1431 Sofia, Bulgaria
e-mail: dsvinarov@yahoo.com

P. Kumanov, A. Agarwal (eds.), *Puberty*, DOI 10.1007/978-3-319-32122-6_17

circulating complexes with IGF. There are six IGFBPs of which IGFBP-3 is the major serum carrier of IGF-I. In addition to GH and IGF-I, IGFBP-3 measurement is also considered for the diagnosis of GH disturbances in childhood and puberty [1, 2].

Problems with GH Immunoassays (IAs)

Controversies in the diagnosis and management of GH-related disorders in childhood and puberty are multifactorial, and this chapter will address only those that are related to GH analysis in the clinical laboratory: heterogeneous nature of GH, its biological variability, problems with IAs, the lack of standardization and of definitive analytical technology, and the role of liquid chromatography coupled to mass spectrometry (LC–MS).

GH is a heterogenic molecular species. It is synthesized as a single-chain polypeptide composed of 191 amino acids with a molecular mass of 22 KDa but exists in the cells and in the circulation in a variety of forms: (1) GH1 (GH-N) and GH2 (GH-V) are full-size 22-KDa molecules encoded by two genes, the first produced primarily in pituitary and the second in placenta. GH1 represents 85–90 % of circulating GH and is its' active form. (2) A 20-KDa GH isoform is derived by GH1 as a result of deletion of amino acids 32–46, has less biological activity, and shows a propensity to dimerize. It accounts for 5–10 % of GH in blood [2]. (3) "Big GH" is a dimeric moiety of the 20-KDa isoform. (4) "Big–big GH": approximately 50 % of GH is bound to its protein transporter—GH-binding protein (GHBP) that is the cleaved N-terminal extracellular domain of the GH receptor (GHR). The circulating complex (GH-GHBP) is sometimes called "Big–big GH" [1]. A small amount (5–8 %) of GH is carried by a low-affinity protein, and the rest is in free (unbound) state. (5) There are also oligomeric forms of GH, which could potentially interfere in some analytical platforms.

Labeled immunochemical analysis is by far the predominant analytical technology for measuring GH. As for most other hormones, IAs progressed from radioimmunoassay to non-isotopic methods utilizing enzyme or luminescent labels (fluorescent, chemiluminescent, and electrochemiluminescent) and from the use of polyclonal to monoclonal antibodies. Nowadays, a variety of both earlier and recently introduced assay kits are commercially available, employing isotopic and non-isotopic labels, and all of them suffer from the same pitfalls. The presence of GH variants and the use of different antibodies, different calibration materials, different labels, and different assay reagents lead to significant discrepancies among the results given by the different IAs [3–5]. Some of the antibodies are quite specific for the 22-KDa GH, and others cross-react with the 20-KDa isoform and its dimers, while the interference of some GH oligomers is not clearly established. Measurement of the 20-KDa isoform has no clinical significance, but it has been shown to be useful for the assessment of GH doping in sports. Overall, affinity of most antibodies is high enough to compete with GHBP, provided the incubation time is sufficient to allow for the dissociation of GH-GHBP complexes. Therefore, those assays give a good approximation of the total GH concentration. The clinical value of free (unbound) GH is not established, although there are IAs developed to measure free GH [2]. Inter-assay variability of IAs was substantially improved over the last years, but still differences in results remain significant enough to lead to misdiagnosis and inappropriate patient management [4, 6] and inability to create generally accepted harmonized clinical guidelines for diagnosis and treatment of GH-related disorders in childhood and puberty. Several international research and professional societies have organized an expert workshop to define criteria, strategies, and ways to implement harmonization of GH and IGF-I assays and created recommendations and requirements for improving assay comparability, which were published in year 2011 [7], and can be summarized as follows: (1) Preanalytical conditions should be strictly adhered to—serum is the preferred specimen for analysis; separation of serum from blood cells is recommended within 2 h of collection, stability at room temperature is proven for 8 h, and if specimens are not tested within that time, they should be stored at 2–8 °C during the same day or frozen at −20 °C for longer periods. Stability at −20 °C is proven for several weeks (no more than 30 days for IGF-I). (2) The most important requirement is by far the need for common calibration. All manufacturers should use a single universally accepted international reference recombinant human GH Standard, IS 98/574, and IS 02/254 WHO recombinant IGF-I reference standard, both of them available from National Institute of Biological Standards and Control (NIBSC), and demonstrate traceability to those standards. Results should be reported in mass units, i.e., μg/L. (3) Commutability of calibrators and control materials should be achieved and validated—the matrix used should be identical to or as close as possible to nonpathologic human serum. (4) Antibodies used in GH assays should be of high affinity and specificity for the 22-KDa form of GH. These assays should have sufficient reproducibility and accuracy, especially at the lower end of the measured interval, with a lower limit of GH quantification (LLOQ) of 0.05 μg/L (CV of <20 %). (5) Interferences should be validated explicitly, including cross-reactivity with 20-KDa GH, GH 2, therapeutic GH analogs, and especially interference of GHBP. (6) Laboratories should use internal quality control (QC) materials from different manufacturer (independent from assay producer) and should participate in an accredited proficiency testing system/external quality assessment program at an international level. Further, development of a reference measurement procedure based on LC–MS is strongly needed and should be utilized for the establishment of acceptance criteria for all IAs intended for clinical use [6]. Manufacturers must inform laboratories for all of the above components and for every change in assay platforms that may influence clinical diagnostic and therapeutic decisions. Laboratories must communicate that information to clinicians and explain the way assay performance could affect patient care [7].

Problems with IGF-I and IGFBP-3 Immunoassays

Unlike GH, serum concentrations of IGF-I and IGFBP-3 are stable throughout the day, and therefore, they can be measured at any time. Total IGF-I is measured via IAs based on the same principles, showing the same historical development as described above for GH assays, but all techniques include a step for dissociation of IGF-I from its binding proteins prior to analysis [1, 2]. Manufacturers should validate the efficiency of that process separately and demonstrate the influence of diseases affecting serum concentrations of IGFBP, such as diabetes, GH disorders, and hepatic or renal impairment, on the total IGF-I concentration measured [4, 7]. Serum concentrations of IGF-I vary with age, sex, and degree of sexual maturation of the child. Unfortunately, there is an overlap of the normal range of serum IGF-I concentrations in young children with the levels found in children with GH deficiency (GHD). In addition, children with malnutrition, hypothyroidism, chronic illness, renal failure, steroid deficiency, and diabetes also have low IGF-I concentrations. On the other hand, IGF-I levels rise dramatically during puberty. Therefore, reference intervals in childhood and puberty should be assessed for data normality, presented in percentiles (2.5–97.5 percentiles) after transformation, and reported as SD scores—the number of SDs a given result is deviated from the age-adjusted mean. Narrow age ranges (e.g., every 3 years) and Tanner stages should be considered, with sufficient number of individuals included and sex-specific reference values for ages between 6 and 18 years [7, 8]. IGFBP-3 does not need a dissociation step from a binding protein, and its concentration is much higher compared to that of IFG-I or GH. Therefore, IAs are generally simpler than those for GH and IGF-I. In addition, IGFBP levels vary to a lesser extent with age, sex, and degree of sexual maturation [1] and are less affected by nutritional status of the child. Based on the above considerations, it was thought until recently that simultaneous measurement of IGF-I and IGFBP-3 could be potentially superior to the assessment of IGF-I alone. However, multiple studies reported a very poor diagnostic sensitivity of IGFBP (approximating 50 %), with no difference of its concentrations between GHD and non-GHD subjects and no advantage over measurement of IGF-I alone [4].

The Role of LC–MS in the Analysis of GH, IGF-I, and IGFBP-3

This technique allows recognition and quantification by mass rather than by epitope and provides the most sensitive and selective analytical results in biology and medicine. It has the potential to circumvent many of the problems associated with IAs for GH, IGF-I, and IGFBP-3 [8, 9]. Several methods for ID-MS (isotope dilution mass spectrometry: MS using stable isotope labeled internal standards, which renders highest possible reliability) determination of these peptides have been described [10–14], with excellent accuracy and precision and lack of interference by GHBP or other constituents of human serum. Application of LC–MS would allow the establishment of reproducible, method-independent, comparable, and unified reference intervals and cut off limits and would ultimately give a chance for the development of clinically unambiguous and generally recognized guidelines for the management of GH-related disorders in childhood and puberty. It was already noted that ID-MS is also the ultimate technique for the development of reference measurement procedures for GH and IGF-I—a key factor for the standardization and harmonization of newer generation IAs.

Clinical Significance

The following brief discussion will focus only on those interpretative challenges in the management of GH-related disorders of childhood and puberty, which are related to the analytical problems of GH, IGF-I, and IGFBP-3 assays. Clinically important states of GH excess or deficiency are rare and difficult to diagnose, with GHD being considerably more challenging and laboratory dependent, compared to GH excess. GH is stored in the pituitary cells after synthesis and is secreted in several (usually seven to eight) pulses per day with some "spikes" after meals or exercise, but most pulses (by number and intensity) occur at night after onset of sleep, with peak values reached during deepest sleep [1, 2] and very low concentrations between pulses. This pattern of secretion and its short half-life makes random measurements of GH non-informative and misleading for assessment of sufficiency or insufficiency. Therefore, diagnosis of GHD requires a combination of provocative screening and stimulation tests and measurement of GH, IGF-I, and in some cases IGFBP-3. Although uncommon itself, GH excess in childhood (gigantism) is much less common than acromegaly, and its' diagnosis is made predominantly by physical appearance (striking acceleration of linear growth) and magnetic resonance imaging [1, 2]. In contrast to GH, IGF-I half-life is much longer, and its concentrations are much less variable during the day. Therefore, a random single measurement of IGF-I is considered to accurately reflect its production. As mentioned previously, IGF-I concentrations are influenced by age, sexual maturation, nutritional status, and several disease states.

There are two general approaches in diagnosing and management of GHD [1]. The first one is preferred by physicians, who believe that physiological variety of GH and reported discrepancies of the non-standardized GH measurements hamper the clinical value of its analysis. This approach relies solely on the measurement of IGF-I level, and diagnosis is considered proven if IGF-I is low and is combined with low growth velocity. The second, more traditional approach comprises a two-step testing of GH concentrations after pharmacologic stimulation with any of the following: clonidine, glucagon, L-dopa, insulin, arginine, pyridostigmine, and GHRH, applied alone or in combination. Physical stimuli of GH secretion, including sleep and exercise, are usually avoided, due to lack of reproducibility. The first step (screening) involves measurement of GH after a single pharmacologic challenge. If the GH rises above the cutoff value for GHD (usually around 7 μg/L, see billow), GH sufficiency is accepted with no need for further measurements. The second step is considered definitive for the diagnosis of GHD and requires a combination of two stimulatory tests, because after a single challenge only 80 % of normal children will respond sufficiently, while after a two-test provocation, this percentage rises over 95 %. The major pitfall in the traditional approach is the analytical uncertainty of GH IAs and method-dependent cutoff values, which differ significantly even with different batches of the same assay. Irrespective of the well-defined requirements for methodological improvement outlined above, there is no GH assay on the market that meets the criteria for standardization and harmonization. Therefore, the recent publication of Wagner et al. [15] plays a key role in the effort to establish comparative harmonized cutoff values for some of the most often used IAs. In this work, the cutoff concentrations for the diagnosis of GHD for six commercial IAs and for an ID-MS-based assay were reexamined, based on the retesting of serum samples of children with GHD and children with no GHD, all of which have undergone stimulation tests. The optimal cutoff value for one of the IAs was identified and converted via regression analysis to comparable cutoff values for the other five assays. An ID-MS-based cutoff concentration was independently derived by analysis of a subset of patients and regression comparison to the same IA. The calculated cutoff limits ranged from 4.32 to 7.77 μg/L. These huge differences demonstrate the unacceptable variability of results obtained by IAs for one sample and the ultimate need for assay-specific cutoffs for the diagnosis of GHD. In addition, comparison of the IAs to ID-MS provides long-term validity of the established cutoff values and helps to detect gaps in the traceability chain, which is a critical unmet requirement of assays' manufacturers.

Interpretation of IGF-I results is greatly facilitated by the recent publication of Bidlingmaier et al. [16], presenting the results of a remarkable international project for the development and validation of a new IA conforming to international recommendations and its application to establish reference intervals for IGF-I from birth to senescence. The major results of this important work could be summarized in regard to assay characteristics and the reported IGF-I reference values. The new assay is calibrated against the recommended standard (02/254). It is very sensitive (limit of detection 4.4 μg/L) and has a broad dynamic range (10–1200 μg/L), with excellent accuracy (92–104 %) and precision (total analytical CV <9 %), and explicitly demonstrated lack of interference from the six IGFBPs and other matrix constituents. Sample material requirements, preanalytical, post-analytical, short-term, and long-term stability, and comparison with other assays complete the validation profile of this new, reliable IA technique. Generation of reference intervals is performed under strict adherence to the most rigorous international guidelines. Reference ranges in childhood and puberty are derived from the conducted multicenter study, with 4252 samples (1884 males, 2368 females) of newborns, children, and adolescents, obtained from seven pediatric cohorts from Canada, the United States, and Europe, with the significant contribution of the Canadian Laboratory Initiative on Pediatric Reference Interval Database (CALIPER and CALIPER new), providing a total of 1948 (1148 males) samples. The pediatric population was ethnically diverse and deemed to be metabolically stable. Pediatric reference values are calculated for each year of life from birth to the age of 20, separately for males and females. Additionally, assessment according to Tanner stages is presented, based on one of the largest cohorts (Danish Cohort, $n = 854$). This publication is a free-access paper, and all clinicians dealing with interpretation of IGF-I concentrations should use it.

Briefly, IGF-I concentrations in cord blood correlated to birth weight but were not different between sexes. After that, concentrations declined and remained lower than at birth during the first year of life (from 57 to 77 μg/L, 2.5th percentile, to 126–157 μg/L, 97.5th percentile). Thereafter, IGF-I increased and reached a pubertal peak both in girls and boys at 15 years (from 127 to 152 μg/L, 2.5th percentile, to 554 μg/L, 97.5th percentile) and relatively fast decline until the age of 21–25 (from 93 to 115 μg/L, 2.5th percentile, to 342–355 μg/L, 97.5th percentile). IGF-I peak was similar in adolescents when data were stratified to chronological age but occurs slightly earlier in girls, when considering stratification according to Tanner stages. During puberty, reference interval was broader in girls, indicating a higher variability of IGF-I concentrations. In both sexes, the lower limit of reference interval (the 2.5th percentile) was lower when calculated on chronological age, compared to the calculation based on Tanner stage, which indicates that reference values adjusted for pubertal development can be useful, especially if IGF-I is low. Body mass index (BMI) extremities and comorbidities had no significant influence on the reference intervals.

Problems of Steroid Assays: Immunochemical Methods or LC–MS/MS

Steroid hormones are synthesized from cholesterol in the adrenal cortex, the gonads, and the placenta, and many of them are of great clinical importance [17]. Abnormal concentration of steroids in children and adolescents may be indicative of ambiguous genitalia in infants, hypogonadism, precocious puberty, oligomenorrhea, hirsutism in females, feminization in males, metabolic and electrolyte disturbances, and rarely, steroid hormone-producing neoplasms [18]. The adrenal gland is composed of the adrenal medulla (inner layer) and cortex (outer layer). The cortex is further composed of three layers: zona glomerulosa, which produces mineralocorticoids such as 11-desoxycorticosterone, corticosterone, and aldosterone, and zonae fasciculata and reticularis, which together are the source of glucocorticoids (11-desoxycortisol, cortisol) and of adrenal androgens dehydroepiandrosterone (DHEA), DHEA-sulfate (DHEAS), and androstenedione. Testosterone is produced by the Leydig cells of the testes, and female sex hormones, estradiol and progesterone, are synthesized in the ovaries. Estradiol could be derived from testosterone by aromatization of ring A (CYP19A1). The same aromatase catalyzes the transformation of androstenedione to estrone, which is also a precursor of estradiol. Estriol is derived from placenta, and its measurement is important in the assessment of fetal status [17, 19, 20]. Biochemical pathways of steroid hormones are far more complex, and as a result, over 300 precursors and metabolites circulate in the body fluids together with the active hormones, in a variety of concentrations and biological activity but with very similar structure. Therefore, analytical methods for steroids need to pose sufficient selectivity and sensitivity to allow for measurement of the steroid of interest, without cross-reactivity and interference, a requirement that is very difficult to achieve.

Free Versus Total Steroid Measurement

Steroid hormones circulate in blood bound to carrier proteins, which regulate their activity. Total concentration of hormones that are highly protein bound depends on the concentration of the protein carrier and therefore may vary significantly, while their unbound (free) concentrations remain within physiologic limits. Measurement of free steroids is a much better indicator of their functional activity—it is the free hormone that binds to the steroid receptor and elicits the biochemical action, but methods that are able to separate free from bound fraction and to reliably measure the unbound hormone are very difficult to develop and validate. There is a need of a preanalytical phase to separate bound and free fraction, which utilizes two techniques—equilibrium dialysis (reference technique) or ultrafiltration. The first procedure is very slow and expensive, and both techniques should strictly be adhered to; otherwise, a disruption of the physiologic ratio between free and bound hormone could occur [19, 20]. After the introduction of very sensitive LC–MS instruments, the required high sensitivity for free steroid analysis is not an issue [17], but until recently, alternative indirect approaches for estimation of unbound concentrations were predominantly employed in the clinical laboratories. These included measurement of specific protein carriers [cortisol-binding globulin (CBG), sex hormone-binding globulin (SHBG), and albumin] and usage of mathematical algorithms for calculation of free concentrations: "selective" precipitation of the tightly bound form or direct (analog tracer) radioimmunoassay. In the past, measurement of urinary cortisol (also providing an estimate of free hormone concentration) has been used for as a screening test for Cushing disease [19]. All indirect methods for assessment of free steroid concentrations give approximation for the unbound fractions and not true values [21, 22]. Therefore, when alternative and new techniques are available, they should be preferred for routine work.

Measurement of saliva steroid concentrations is a practical and convenient way to assess the free steroid fraction. Saliva can be viewed as a natural plasma ultrafiltrate, where only unbound steroids can transfer from plasma. It is obtained noninvasively, which is a special advantage in childhood. In general, most steroids of clinical significance can be measured in saliva. For some steroids, such as cortisol, estriol, and progesterone, measurement of salivary concentration is documented to be a good indicator of the free plasma concentration [19, 20]. The best established and accepted application for hormone analysis in saliva is the use of salivary cortisol in the diagnosis of Cushing syndrome. In pediatric medicine, saliva has proven very beneficial for diagnosing and monitoring of congenital adrenal hyperplasia (most commonly caused by 21-hydrohylase deficiency) via the measurement of salivary 17α-hydroxypreogesterone and androstenedione. In addition to estrogens and gestagens, a special focus for assessment of male hypogonadism is testosterone analysis in saliva, which demonstrates a very high correlation with free testosterone in serum [20, 21]. The predominant advantages of saliva steroid analysis in childhood include the noninvasiveness of sampling procedure, ability for multiple collections, and, unlike venipuncture, availability of samples obtained without unwanted adrenal stress. At the same time, special attention is required regarding standardization of collection devices and procedures, patient compliance to collection procedures, pre-analytical stability of steroids in saliva, and usage of standardized and validated assays [23]. Interpretation of salivary steroid concentrations requires the establishment of special reference intervals.

Immunochemical Assays' Problems for Steroid Hormones

The introduction of IAs nearly 50 years ago allowed for the first time the direct measurement of active hormones in human plasma instead of measuring their inactive metabolites by colorimetric methods in urine or application of cumbersome in vivo bioassays. Thus, IA platforms opened a new era in endocrine research, clinical diagnostics, and patient measurement [24]. Earlier, first-generation methods employed nonspecific polyclonal antibodies and sample pretreatment, such as solvent extraction, chromatographic purification, and pre-concentration. These "indirect" techniques were slow and tedious but provided relatively sufficient specificity and sensitivity—the pretreatment step compensated for the nonspecificity of polyclonal antibodies. Later, in favor of speed, automation, and simplification, newer generation, "direct" IAs, utilizing monoclonal antibodies and enzyme or luminescent labels, replaced the older techniques. Unfortunately, together with high capacity, high speed, and wide availability, the newer "direct" methods sacrificed the requirements for sensitivity and specificity of steroid measurements. Employment of monoclonal antibodies was not sufficient to assure the required reliability. Interference with chemically similar steroid precursors, metabolites, exogenous compounds, and protein carriers, in combination with nonstandard calibration, and lack of standardization and traceability introduced unacceptably high intra-assay and inter-assay variability of currently used IAs [17, 19, 20]. The magnitude of this problem is exemplified with results from one of the external quality assessment programs, exhibiting a threefold to ninefold between-laboratory difference for a single challenge [17]. Therefore, general requirements to manufacturers, listed for GH and IGF-I, fully apply for steroid IAs—need for traceable calibrators, relevant validation for interferences, achievement of clinically needed selectivity and sensitivity, traceability of results to reference measurement procedures (ID-MS), etc. The majority of recent publications, textbooks, and guidelines demonstrate nonlinearity and lack of accuracy of the different IAs [1, 2, 17, 24–26] and recommend their replacement by LC–MS where possible, especially for the following steroids: measurement of cortisol secretion in serum, 24-h urine sample, or midnight saliva [24]; total testosterone in women, in children, and in hypogonadal men; estradiol in clinical situations with expected low levels of less than 10 or 5 pmol/L (healthy men, children, postmenopausal women) [1, 17, 19, 20, 24, 27, 28]. In conclusion, there is no doubt that MS will be the routine method principle for quantification of all steroids in the near future, but the technological transfer will not happen in 1 day and in all places. IAs will continue to be part of the analytical arsenal of clinical laboratories, especially when manufacturers of these assays fulfill the previously mentioned requirements for adequate validation and traceability. For instance, current testosterone IAs are still (and will be) acceptable for determination of higher concentrations in men; IAs perform satisfactory for estradiol in the assessment and management of women with infertility problems [20, 24].

Steroid Analysis by Mass Spectrometry

MS has been used for steroid analysis for more than 70 years, and therefore, it is not correct to appreciate it as the "new guy" in that analytical field. In 1960s, gas chromatography–mass spectrometry (GC–MS) was the major tool for the investigation of steroid metabolism and assessment of steroid profiles in health and disease [24]. Despite of the significant complexity, GC–MS still remains the preeminent discovery technique of choice in the clinical research of steroid metabolome, even in the era of LC–MS/MS. Our current knowledge on inborn errors of steroid metabolism and the identification of nearly all steroid metabolite disorders is based on GC–MS [24, 29]. In the last 15 years, the great technological advance of triple quadrupole LC–MS/MS resulted in the introduction of methods with unbeatable sensitivity and selectivity and extended linearity range, which are much simpler to use in the routine clinical laboratories compared to GC–MS and at the same are based on the current reference (definitive) analytical principles [17, 29–32]. LC–MS/MS reference measurement procedure for testosterone, which will serve for standardization of routine methods (MS and immunoassays), has already been proposed, and such procedures for other steroid hormones are expected to appear in the near future [33, 34]. Further significant advantages of LC–MS/MS include relatively high throughput and the ability to perform panel steroid profiling with simultaneous measurement of precursors, active hormones, and metabolites in a single sample, thus amplifying enormously the informative value of laboratory results, with ultimate improvement of patient care [17, 30, 35]. For instance, assessment of androgen status requires quantification of testosterone and dihydrotestosterone [36], but immunoassays, being single-analyte platforms, do not provide that. Simultaneous analysis of multiple steroids reduces significantly the required sample volume, compared to IAs. Small sample size is especially important in pediatric endocrinology—the ability to obtain more than ten quantitative results from 100 to 200 μL of plasma is easily achievable [17, 33]. However, it should be clearly understood that analysis by LC–MS/MS does not automatically mean reliable results and superiority over IAs. MS is in its early phase of clinical application, roughly at the same stage that IAs were many years ago, when labor-intensive manual testing dominated and automatic immunochemistry analyzers were not available [24]. Among the disadvantages of LC–MS/MS, which currently limit its wider use in routine clinical laboratories, are expensive equipment; fairly labor-intensive sample preparation ("indirect" technique) and requirement for a highly competent and robustly trained staff, compared to immunoassay platforms; lack of standardization (most laboratories develop their own "in-house" methods); and occasional interferences and matrix effects, which require rigorous validation [17, 29, 33]. Manufacturers are trying to develop mass spectrometers that are like clinical chemistry analyzers—more user-friendly, technically, and methodologically standardized and thus appropriate to meet the requirements of the high-throughput medical laboratories. Until that happen, LC–MS/MS will be a preferred routine armamentarium in the larger laboratories, where the expertise and the larger sample workload will provide cost-effectiveness in the effort to overcome the problems of current IAs for steroid analysis.

Interpretation of Results and Reference Intervals

It is fair to admit that pediatric reference values for steroid hormones are not well defined—a situation that challenges diagnostic sensitivity and interpretation of results, especially in cases with mild to modest elevations. Current reference intervals are usually derived based on very small groups of children, which limits the establishment of adequate age-specific and sex-specific differences. In addition, the technological transfer from IAs to LC–MS/MS is underway but not completed: all data, based on IAs, are method dependent and hence only valid for the respective assay; reference intervals based on LC–MS/MS are method independent and could be used more universally, but with mentioned limitations—lack of wide availability of the technique and need for standardization. Of particular importance is also the lack of agreement and comparability between LC–MS/MS and IA results, the latter being significantly higher (often several fold). Therefore, pediatric endocrinologists should communicate closely with the laboratories, requiring information on the particular assays used for steroid analysis and how those assays refer to published reference interval data. This chapter will briefly summarize some of the most convincing and most recent studies presenting pediatric reference values for steroid hormones. Konforte et al. [18] published their results for seven fertility hormones in children and adolescents as part of the CALIPER study, utilizing a new IA platform. These authors present data obtained from 1234 recruited participants and correctly state the advantages and limitations of their work: well-defined assay characteristics with improved sensitivity, compared to other IAs; database still valid for the IA used only, with the need for validation for other IAs; assay used not traced to higher metrology class technique, i.e., ID-MS; and limited number of participants for some age subgroups and for Tanner stage-specific partition, which is based on self-reported Tanner stage. Notably, authors declare that the results for testosterone are not much different from those obtained by LC–MS/MS in the same laboratory. In addition, the results for estradiol, but not for progesterone, are comparable to previously published data, based on LC–MS/MS [20]. Their Tanner-specific results for estradiol could be summarized as follows: for males, upper limits are practically the same for Tanner stages I–III (<70 pmol/L) and for Tanner stages IV and V (<130 pmol/L); female reference values are fully stratified, <70 pmol/L for Tanner stage I,

Table 17.1 Age-specific pediatric reference values for some serum steroids (method: LC–MS/MS, study as part of the CALIPER program)

Steroid	Age	Upper limit (nmol/L)
Cortisol	0–2 years	530
	3–6 years	270
	7–14 years	360
	15–18 years	510
Corticosterone	<1 month	20
	<1 year	15
	1–6 years	4
	7–14 years	9.2
	15–18 years	15
11-Desoxycortisol	<1 year	5.3
	1–6 years	1.0
	7–18 years	2.3
17-Hydroxyprogesterone	0–14 days	4.8
	<1 year	3.4
	1–11 years	1.0
	12–13 years	2.0
	14–18 years	4.0
21-Hydroxyprogesterone	<1 year	0.8
	1–2 years	0.25
	2–11 years	0.15
	12–18 years	0.24

Modified from Kyriakopoulou L, Yazdanpanah M, Colantonio DA, et al. A sensitive and rapid mass spectrometric method for the simultaneous measurement of eight steroid hormones and CALIPER pediatric reference intervals. Clin Biochem. 2013;46:642–651. With permission from Elsevier

<90 pmol/L for Tanner stage II, <300 pmol/L for Tanner stage III, 50–520 pmol/L for Tanner stage IV, and 70–760 pmol/L for Tanner stage V. The same group has published another part of their study, based on LC–MS/MS method for simultaneous measurement of eight steroids, again as part of the CALIPER program, with reported pediatric reference intervals of a total of 337 specimens [37]. In this work, progesterone values were found to be significantly lower, compared to the previously mentioned immunoassay, and similar between boys and girls until the age of 12 years, with female levels began increasing thereafter. Table 17.1 compiles and summarizes their results for five of the steroids that did not require partitioning based on sex. Data have shown that in addition to the known diurnal variation, cortisol changed with age, increasing after the age of 7 years old. Slightly different, compared to other reports, were the findings of this group for corticosterone, which exhibited the highest concentrations between birth and 1 year of life, declining gradually thereafter. Elevation of 11-desoxycortisol, 17-hydroxyprogesterone, and 21-hydroxyprogesterone is of importance for the detection of the respective hydroxylase deficiencies.

Kushnir et al. [38] have published pediatric and adult reference intervals for the major androgen steroids, testosterone, androstenedione, and DHEA, based on a reference population of over 2500 participants, utilizing a validated LC–MS/MS method. Their Tanner-specific stratification is derived from the largest number of observations in each subgroup—over 120 samples for each Tanner stage and results could be summarized as follows. At Tanner stage I, there were no clinically significant sex differences for the three steroids, with upper limits of 0.5–0.6 nmol/L for testosterone, 1.1–1.8 nmol/L for androstenedione, and 8.2–9.6 nmol/L for DHEA. In girls, the three androgens reached adult values at Tanner stage III (0.3–2.2 nmol/L for testosterone, 1.3–7.8 nmol/L for androstenedione, 3.7–27.3 nmol/L for DHEA), while in boys adult values (5.6–29.5 nmol/L for testosterone, 0.9–3.7 nmol/L for androstenedione, 4.3–23.4 nmol/L for DHEA) were reached later—at Tanner stages IV–V. The greatest increase was observed during the transition to Tanner stage II for females and to Tanner stage III for males. At Tanner stage II, the upper reference limit for testosterone was already significantly higher in boys, 10.5 nmol/L, compared 1.4 nmol/L for girls. Levels of androstenedione were approximately twice higher in females since Tanner stage II and thereafter, and for DHEA, the major sex differences were observed at Tanner stages II and III.

References

1. Winter WE, Bazydlo LAL, Harris NS. Quick guide to endocrinology. Washington, DC: AACC Press; 2013.
2. Winter WE, Jialal I, Vance ML, et al. Pituitary function and pathophysiology. In: Burtis CA, Ashwood ER, Bruns DE, editors. Tietz textbook of clinical chemistry and molecular diagnostics. St. Louis: Elsevier Saunders; 2012. p. 1803–45.
3. Boulo S, Hanisch K, Bidlingmaier M, et al. Gaps in the traceability chain of human growth hormone measurements. Clin Chem. 2013;59:1074–82.
4. Murray PG, Dattani MT, Clayton PE. Controversies in the diagnosis and management of growth hormone deficiency in childhood and adolescence. Arch Dis Child. 2014. doi:10.1136/archdischild-2014-307228.
5. Van Helden J, Hermsen D, Von Ahsen N, et al. Performance evaluation of a fully automated immunoassay for the detection of human growth hormone on the Elecsys immunoassay system. Clin Lab. 2014;60:1641–51.
6. Wieringa GE, Sturgeon CM, Trainer PJ. The harmonisation of growth hormone measurements: taking the next steps. Clin Chim Acta. 2014;432:68–71.
7. Clemmons DR. Consensus statement on the standardization and evaluation of growth hormone and insulin-like growth factor assays. Clin Chem. 2011;57:555–9.
8. Gomez-Gomez C, Iglesias EM, Barallat J, et al. Lack of transferability between two automated immunoassays for serum IGF-I measurement. Clin Lab. 2014;60:1859–64.
9. Junnila RK, Strasburger CJ, Bidlingmaier M. Pitfalls of insulin-like growth factor-I and growth hormone assays. Endocrinol Metab Clin North Am. 2015;44:21–34.
10. Cox HD, Lopes F, Woldemariam GA, et al. Interlaboratory agreement of insulin-like growth factor 1. Concentrations measured by mass spectrometry. Clin Chem. 2014;60:541–8.
11. Such-Sanmartín G, Bache N, Bosch J, et al. Detection and differentiation of 22kDa and 20kDa growth hormone proteoforms in human plasma by LC-MS/MS. Biochim Biophys Acta. 1854;2015:284–90.

12. Oran PE, Trenchevska O, Nedelkov D, et al. Parallel workflow for high-throughput (>1,000 samples/day) quantitative analysis of human insulin-like growth factor 1 using mass spectrometric immunoassay. PLoS One. 2014;9:e92801.
13. Arsene CG, Henrion A, Diekmann N, et al. Quantification of growth hormone in serum by isotope dilution mass spectrometry. Anal Biochem. 2010;401:228–35.
14. Barton C, Kay RG, Gentzer W, et al. Development of high-throughput chemical extraction techniques and quantitative HPLC-MS/MS (SRM) assays for clinically relevant plasma proteins. J Proteome Res. 2010;9:333–40.
15. Wagner IV, Paetzold C, Gausche R, et al. Clinical evidence-based cutoff limits for GH stimulation tests in children with a backup of results with reference to mass spectrometry. Eur J Endocrinol. 2014;171:389–97.
16. Bidlingmaier M, Friedrich N, Emeny RT, et al. Reference intervals for insulin-like growth factor-1 (IGF-I) from birth to senescence: results from a multicenter study using a new automated chemiluminescence IGF-I immunoassay conforming to recent international recommendations. J Clin Endocrinol Metab. 2014;99:1712–21.
17. Soldin S, Soldin OP. Steroid hormone analysis by tandem mass spectrometry. Clin Chem. 2009;55:1061–6.
18. Konforte D, Shea JL, Kyriakopoulou L, et al. Complex biological pattern of fertility hormones in children and adolescents: a study of healthy children from the CALIPER cohort and establishment of pediatric reference intervals. Clin Chem. 2013;59:1215–27.
19. Bertholf RL, Jialal I, Winter WE. The adrenal cortex. In: Burtis CA, Ashwood ER, Bruns DE, editors. Tietz textbook of clinical chemistry and molecular diagnostics. St. Louis: Elsevier Saunders; 2012. p. 1847–904.
20. Isbell TS, Jungheim E, Gronowski AM. Reproductive endocrinology and related disorders. In: Burtis CA, Ashwood ER, Bruns DE, editors. Tietz textbook of clinical chemistry and molecular diagnostics. St. Louis: Elsevier Saunders; 2012. p. 1945–90.
21. Turpeinen U, Hämäläinen E, Haanpää M, et al. Determination of salivary testosterone and androstenedione by liquid chromatography-tandem mass spectrometry. Clin Chim Acta. 2012;413:594–9.
22. Fritz KS, McKean AJS, Nelson JC, et al. Analog-based free testosterone test results linked to total testosterone concentrations, not free testosterone concentrations. Clin Chem. 2008;54: 512–6.
23. Gröschl M. Current status of salivary hormone analysis. Clin Chem. 2008;54:1759–69.
24. Taylor A, Keevil B, Huhtaniemi IT. Mass spectrometry and immunoassay; how to measure steroid hormones today and tomorrow. Eur J Endocrinol. 2015;173:D1–12. European Society of Endocrinology, Manuscript EJE-15-0338.
25. Benton SC, Nuttal M, Nardo L, et al. Measured dehydroepiandrosterone sulfate positively influences testosterone measurement in unextracted female serum: comparison of 2 immunoassays with testosterone measured by LC-MS. Clin Chem. 2011;57:1174–83.
26. Huang X, Spink DC, Schneider E, et al. Measurement of unconjugated estriol in serum by liquid chromatography–tandem mass spectrometry and assessment of the accuracy of chemiluminescent immunoassays. Clin Chem. 2014;60:260–8.
27. Stanczyk FZ, Lee JS, Santen RJ. Standardization of steroid hormone assays: why, how, and when. Cancer Epidemiol Biomarkers Prev. 2007;16:1713–9.
28. Handelsman DJ, Newman JD, Jimenez M, et al. Performance of direct estradiol immunoassays with human male serum samples. Clin Chem. 2014;60:510–7.
29. Krone N, Hughes BA, Lavery GG. Gas chromatography/mass spectrometry (GC/MS) remains a pre-eminent discovery tool in clinical steroid investigations even in the era of fast liquid chromatography tandem mass spectrometry (LC/MS/MS). J Steroid Biochem Mol Biol. 2010;121:496–504.
30. Handelsman DJ, Wartofsky L. Requirement for mass spectrometry sex steroid assays in the Journal of Clinical Endocrinology and Metabolism. J Clin Endocrinol Metab. 2013;98:3971–3.
31. Kushnir MM, Rockwood AL, Roberts WL, et al. Liquid chromatography tandem mass spectrometry for analysis of steroids in clinical laboratories. Clin Biochem. 2011;44:77–88.

32. Ketha H, Kaur S, Grebe S, Sihgh RJ. Clinical applications of LC-MS sex steroid assays: evolution of methodologies in 21st century. Curr Opin Endocrinol Diabetes Obes. 2014;21:217–26.
33. Botelho JK, Shaklady C, Cooper HC, et al. Isotope-dilution liquid chromatography–tandem mass spectrometry candidate reference method for total testosterone in human serum. Clin Chem. 2013;59:372–80.
34. Rosner W. Another reference measurement procedure for total testosterone—what's the fuss? Clin Chem. 2013;59:338–9.
35. Koal T, Schmiederer D, Pham-Tuan H, et al. Standardized LC-MS/MS based steroid hormone profile-analysis. J Steroid Biochem Mol Biol. 2012;129:129–38.
36. Shiraishi S, Lee PWN, Leund A, et al. Simultaneous measurement of serum testosterone and dihydrotestosterone by liquid chromatography–tandem mass spectrometry. Clin Chem. 2008;54:1855–63.
37. Kyriakopoulou L, Yazdanpanah M, Colantonio DA, et al. A sensitive and rapid mass spectrometric method for the simultaneous measurement of eight steroid hormones and CALIPER pediatric reference intervals. Clin Biochem. 2013;46:642–51.
38. Kushnir MM, Blamires T, Rockwood LA, et al. Liquid chromatography–tandem mass spectrometry assay for androstenedione, dehydroepiandrosterone, and testosterone with pediatric and adult reference intervals. Clin Chem. 2010;56:1138–47.

Chapter 18
Psychosocial Development of Adolescents With and Without Deviations

Yolanda N. Evans

Overview

Adolescence is an intense period of transition. The experience is one that many adults tend to move past without looking back. There is the awkwardness of a maturing body that may feel foreign and betraying as it morphs from looking like a child into that of an adult. At the same time the maturing brain begins to grasp abstract concepts while simultaneously seeking out behaviors that yield high rewards. With all of this change occurring, it can be challenging to distinguish normal from the deviations of adolescent development. Our culture is often avoidant, afraid of, or shows little patience for children going through adolescence. As adults, we interact with adolescents hoping for mature responses, but may find that their actions are often different than those expected of adults. Why do teens act this way? During adolescence, behavior often occurs because there is a consequence that is of benefit to the youth [1]. Though the medical community emphasizes the harm that can come from deviations from normal adolescent development, it may be challenging to engage the youth in behavior change if they are receiving social benefits. The neuropsychological changes that occur during adolescent development have become better understood over the past decade. The limbic system of the brain, which controls rewards and emotions, matures faster than the prefrontal cortex, the logic center of the brain. This reward center maturation may translate into ongoing harmful behaviors if the stimulus to continue a behavior, and thus receive a reward, is great enough. While the neurologic and cognitive changes take longer to mature, the physical maturity can contribute to adult-like behaviors in the form of both peer and sexual relationships.

Y.N. Evans (✉)
Department of Pediatrics, Seattle Children's Hospital/University of Washington, 4540 Sand Point Way NE, Suite 200, Seattle, WA 98105, USA
e-mail: yolanda.evans@seattlechildrens.org

P. Kumanov, A. Agarwal (eds.), *Puberty*, DOI 10.1007/978-3-319-32122-6_18

Normal Development

A key part of the transition from childhood to adulthood is the development of identity. This formation of identity includes the maturation of intellect, morality, ethnicity, spirituality, and sexuality. The three stages of adolescent development are an outline of the journey to discovering identity [2].

Early Adolescence: Ages 10–14 Years

During the early stage of adolescence, youth begin to exhibit separation from the family. This is the time when it is normal for children to be embarrassed being seen with their parents in public, and they may ask to go out with peers unaccompanied. They are preoccupied with their own body as the physical changes of puberty are underway. Youth begin to identify with their ethnic background, and cultural biases regarding gender, size, religion, ability, and race may lead to preferential interactions with like-minded peers. While youth in this stage have concrete thinking, they are gaining the ability to perceive and truly understand the consequences of their actions. However, this understanding of consequence may be ignored if the reward from risky behavior is great enough. It is during this stage that adolescents may begin to experiment with behaviors, such as substance use. Some youth may initiate sexual activity, but the majority of teens are just beginning to find themselves attracted to another individual in a sexual way [3].

Middle Adolescence: Ages 14–17 Years

During middle adolescence, the physical changes of puberty are ending. Romantic relationships intensify as sexual maturity is achieved. This is the peek of conflict with family as the individual struggles to develop a sense of self. Normal conflict with family can appear in a variety of ways. For some adolescents, they challenge the authority of their parents by defying set rules such as curfew or household chore completion. Others take on political stances that are the opposite of the family. The teen wants to be seen as an autonomous being, yet this is the peek of conforming to peers. Risky behavior heightens, such as substance use, sexual activity, violence, and driving. Though teens push away from family, this is often the time when parental guidance is most needed as the rates of suicide, homicide, sexually transmitted infections, and substance use all increase with this age group [3].

Late Adolescence: Ages 17 and Older

Late adolescence is the developmental stage where identity is beginning to solidify. This age group is less reliant on peer acceptance and may resume seeking counsel from family regarding values. This is the time when education and vocational goals are explored, which provides the developing youth the opportunity to practice autonomy as they make decisions that will shape their future employment and earning potential. Adolescents transition from high school to the pursuit of university or college studies. They may opt to join the military or look at a vocational training program. Romantic relationships also change during this stage. Instead of intense feelings of desire and attachment, older adolescents are beginning to understand the need for mutual support, trust, and intimacy in order to allow relationships to thrive.

The normal stages of adolescence and development of self identity occur over a relatively short time period and when coupled with rapid changes in physical maturity equate to a potentially tumultuous portion of an individual's life. Normal adolescents experiment, push limits, and challenge authority; all are required to reach the goal of recognizing the individual's identity. To aid in this development, society as a whole should encourage pursuit of vocational interests, teach and model healthy romantic relationships, and encourage adolescents through mentorship.

Deviations from Normal Development

Deviations from normal psychosocial development include, but are not limited to, the following: mood disorders such as depression and anxiety [4], violence [5], substance abuse [6–8], and risky sexual behavior [9]. The Youth Risk Behavior Surveillance System (YRBSS) conducted by the US Centers for Disease Control (CDC) was developed in 1990 to look at trends in behavior among teens that contribute to significant morbidity and mortality [3]. The behaviors reported by the YRBSS provide an overview of deviations from normal development in adolescents in the United States. In the survey, adolescents in grades 9–12 were asked questions related to behavior. The most recent survey completed in 2013 addresses adolescent suicidal ideation, violence, substance abuse (including alcohol, marijuana, and tobacco), risky sexual activity, and unhealthy eating behaviors. The following is a summary of the findings.

Suicide

Among those who responded, 17 % seriously considered suicide and 8 % attempted suicide in the 12 months prior to the survey.

Violence

Violent behaviors were categorized by carrying a weapon (17.9 %), carrying a weapon on school property (5.2 %), being in a physical fight (24.7 %), being bullied on school property (19.6 %), being bullied electronically (14.8 %), and being physically forced to have sexual intercourse (7.3 %).

Substance Use

Substance abuse was asked in a variety of ways. Sixty-six percent reported having at least one alcoholic drink in their lifetime, and 20.8 % had at least five drinks in a row during the 30 days prior to the survey. Marijuana use has increased with 31.3 % having used in 1991 versus 40.7 % ever used in 2013. Of those surveyed, 23.4 % reported current use of marijuana.

Sexual Activity

Since 2001, there has been no change in the percentage of youth who reported sexual activity. In 2013, 46.8 % reported that they had ever had sex, 15 % having had more than five lifetime partners, 34 % reporting current sexual activity, 59.1 % used a condom during the last sexual encounter, and 22.4 % had drank alcohol or used drugs before their last sexual encounter.

Eating Behaviors

Breakfast was not eaten by 13.7 % in the week prior to the survey and only 38 % ate breakfast all 7 days prior to the survey. In the 30 days prior to the survey, 13 % did not eat for 24 h in order to lose weight and 4.4 % vomited or took laxatives in order to lose weight.

Contributing Factors to Deviations

Environment and community, family and peer interactions, and individual traits are all factors that can contribute to normal adolescent development. Deviations from normal development in one or more of these factors can lead to psychosocial challenges during puberty. For example, the presence of living in a high-risk neighborhood, having low parental monitoring, and engaging with high-risk peers impacts the probability of a youth engaging in risky behaviors [10]. The following information will discuss variations in each of the above factors and the effect on social characteristics among adolescents.

Individual

Adolescence is characterized by the increasing ability to think abstractly and control behavioral impulses while at the same time seek rewards from behavior and novel experiences. The limbic system matures at a faster pace than the prefrontal cortex which is the area in control of abstract thoughts, consideration of consequences, and logic. This maturation of the emotional control without the mature logic center of the brain likely adds to the stereotypical poor impulse control, high-risk behaviors associated with adolescence [11, 12]. The adolescent brain changes are associated with activation of the regions of the brain associated with rewards and attenuation of areas sensitive to aversive stimuli. The pruning and molding that occurs allows the adolescent to ultimately develop into an adult that encounters aversive stimuli and thus avoids the associated risk [13], but this takes time to mature. Why is it that some teens perform behaviors that can have high rewards and high risks, while others are content to exert autonomy but limit risk taking? Is this difference related to the rate of maturation of the brain, temperament, personality type, or a combination of all three? How might extracurricular activities such as music performance, speaking a second language, or sports participation play a role in deviations from normal psychosocial development?

Temperament and personality type are apparent during childhood and vary little over the course of growth and development [14, 15]. Children who have optimistic thinking styles have been associated with resilience from depression and anxiety [16]. It is reasonable to expect that certain temperaments would be more averse to risk-taking behavior. People who regularly work with teens may benefit from encouraging certain styles of behavior and minimizing others. For example, decreasing or minimizing anxious personality traits (i.e., perfectionism) and maximizing optimism may lead to fewer risk-taking behaviors. Of course, personality type is not the sole factor contributing to behavior. A study exploring white matter integrity in the limbic and prefrontal regions of the brain compared adolescent substance users to nonusers. Early-onset substance use is associated with regular use as an adult [6]. While mid-adolescence is the time when brain changes are at their highest, many high-risk behaviors, such as substance use, peak during emerging adulthood. In the study, those with lower white matter integrity at baseline were associated with a greater chance of initiating substance use by mid-adolescence, and lower white matter predicted future risk-taking behaviors [17]. This combination of brain composition and temperament likely translates into some of the differences in risk-taking behavior observed during the teen years. While both may have genetic contributions, environmental factors likely play a large role in development as well.

Environment and Family

There is no question that the environment in which a youth grows can have profound impacts on health, educational attainment, career, and adult life circumstances. Growing up in a violent community may lead to physical harm as well as external violent behaviors or internal mood disorder. One study of 728 children and families found that for boys, growing up in a violent community with a high-conflict family exacerbated the negative effects of community violence, yet growing up in the violent community with a low-conflict family was protective from negative effects of community violence (depression, anxiety, and risk-taking behaviors). For girls, the family did not moderate the effects of the violent community [5, 18].

Unsupportive environments or changes in environment, whether via immigration or community violence, can affect mood and self-esteem. In the United States, the 2012 Census data found that roughly one fifth of all households spoke a language other than English at home [19]. Acculturation, variation in peer or family expectations from that of the new culture, may lead to adolescents making choices that negatively impact their health. The need to learn a new language, adjust to new cultural norms, and learn new cultural idioms may lead to initial social isolation. Efforts to conform to peers may lead to modified mood in the form of low self-esteem or depression [20].

In combination with environment, the opposite of supportive parenting can have negative effects on behavior. One study examining a national longitudinal data set of adolescent twin and sibling pairs asked if maltreatment by parents caused conduct problems or if conduct problems led to parents treating them poorly. The findings were more consistent with the latter. Parents tended to react to unwanted behavior in a negative way [21]. Parenting styles that promote autonomy instead of negatively controlling motives have been positively associated with adolescent personal well-being [22]. Thus, the external environment in which a child develops into adolescence in addition to the family environment can shape development.

Peers

There is a body of literature on the importance of human relationships for adolescent development and well-being [23, 24]. As children enter adolescence, relationships change and teens begin to exhibit identities that conform to cultural expectations. For males in the USA, this may manifest as masculine ideals, decrease in emotional expression, and increase in individualism. For females, this may appear as a shift toward a more demure exterior. Peer influence plays a significant role in what is viewed as normative and changes in friendships impact behavior. A study using a national longitudinal data set examined the risk behavior of alcohol use and peers in an effort to determine if adolescents would exhibit dangerous behavior (increased alcohol consumption) in order to gain popularity. The study found that alcohol consumption leads to an increase in popularity among white males and females [7]. When adolescents perceive benefits from their actions, they will proceed with the behavior even if it is dangerous. Even in the setting on non-risky behavior, peer presence is impactful during adolescence. A novel study used functional magnetic resonance imaging (fMRI), an imaging study that looks at the blood flow to the brain, to examine teens ages 14–19 years on a card-guessing task that incorporated reward and non-reward tasks. In the setting of completing the task in the presence of same-age peers, teens exhibited greater ventral striatal activation, the part of the brain involved in rewards, than adults (ages 25–35) on the same task [25]. This activation of reward circuitry is evidence for biomechanical impact of the presence on peers for behavioral choices.

Summary

Pubertal development encompasses both cognitive and physical changes which can deviate from the norm. Health-risk behaviors generally increase during adolescence and then level off and diminish into adulthood [26]. Adolescent development can be modified by many factors, from peer relationships to environment, and these factors can contribute to either positive (normal) outcomes or negative (deviations) outcomes. Brain development may play a role in deviations from the norm, as some adolescents may indeed be more susceptible to risk-taking behavior, but there are also factors that may be amenable to intervention, such as peer dynamics, parental support, and community. Parental monitoring and parental communication have been associated with promoting less risk taking [27] and teens may be more susceptible to seeking out immediate rewards when in the presence of peers [28] Providers who routinely engage in care with adolescence should be aware of the influences on normative behavior and risk taking in order to address deviations from the norm.

Guidelines for Providing Care to Adolescents

Adolescents are less likely than younger children to be seen by a healthcare provider. In early childhood, it is recommended that infants visit a provider multiple times per year for routine well-child care screening. As children age, they are still evaluated by a healthcare provider yearly. These visits offer the healthcare provider the opportunity to provide anticipatory guidance to parents, address concerns about development, and screen for behaviors that may impact health. As children enter adolescence, healthcare utilization plummets, with only about a third receiving one healthcare visit a year [29].

Confidentiality is a major barrier to youth seeking out healthcare. If the youth does not trust their healthcare provider, they will not come in for visits. In a large study of adolescents using a national data base with over 18,000 respondents, boys with suicide attempt, depression, and suicidal ideation were more likely to report confidentiality concerns as a reason for not seeking healthcare. Girls with depression, history of sexually transmitted infection, nonuse of birth control at their last sexual encounter, and past alcohol use were also more likely to report confidentiality as the rationale for not seeking care [30]. These youth have the risky behaviors that are most likely to threaten normal development.

When healthcare practitioners provide confidential care, the number of topics addressed in the encounter increases [31], and adolescents are more likely to come in for visits. So how do we accomplish this? First, the healthcare provider must understand the confidentiality laws in their state. All 50 states and the District of Columbia have confidentiality laws in place for minors (under age 18 years) for provision of services related to mental health, substance abuse, and reproductive health. In the patient encounter, an approach that allows the parents to have their concerns heard and addressed, while at the same time allows the youth to have time alone with the provider, can be a challenge. One approach that works well is to split the visit. Initially meet with the youth and parents together. Ask the accompanying adults what their concerns are and what they would like covered during the visit. Let them know that you will spend a few minutes alone with their adolescent as part of your standard practice. After you address the parent concerns, have them step out of the room. When in the room with the adolescent alone, ensure confidentiality, but also let them know the limits to confidentiality laws. An example of how to inform the adolescent about confidentiality is the following:

> Provider: "Everything we talk about can remain between you and me, but there are a few exceptions. If I am concerned about your safety, I have to tell someone. This includes if you tell me you have a plan to end your life, if you have a plan to hurt someone else, or if someone has hurt you."

The provider should take the opportunity to screen for risky behaviors when speaking with the youth in confidence. Your encounter may be the only opportunity for the adolescent to discuss normal and abnormal adolescent development during the teen years. Ask about the home environment, their educational pursuits, activities of interest, and eating patterns. Screen for depression, anxiety, suicidal ideation, and substance use. Inquire about their peers and what activities they enjoy. Screen for sexual debut and sexual identity. If the youth provides an answer outside of the provider's scope of practice, refer to an appropriate practitioner to address the concern and schedule a follow-up with the youth to ensure the issue has been addressed.

References

1. Willoughby T, Good M, Adachi P, Hamza C, Tavernier R. Examining the link between adolescent brain development and risk taking from a social-developmental perspective. Brain Cogn. 2013;83:315–23.
2. HealthyChildren.org. American Academy of Pediatrics. 2015. https://www.healthychildren.org/English/ages-stages/teen/Pages/Stages-of-Adolescence.aspx. Accessed 15 Oct 2015.
3. Centers for Disease Control and Prevention. Youth risk behavior survey. 2013. Accessed 14 Sept 2015. http://www.cdc.gov/healthyyouth/data/yrbs/index.htm
4. Arbeit MR, Johnson S, Champine R, Greenman K, Lerner J, Lerner R. Profiles of problematic behaviors across adolescence: covariations with indicators of positive youth development. J Youth Adolesc. 2014;43(6):971–90.
5. McKelvey LM, Whiteside-Mansell L, Bradley R, Casey P, Conners-Burrow N, Barrett K. Growing up in violent communities: do family conflict and gender moderate impacts on adolescents' psychosocial development? J Abnorm Child Psychol. 2011;39(1):95–107.
6. Griffin KW, Bang H, Botvin GJ. Age of alcohol and marijuana use onset predicts weekly substance use and related psychosocial problems during young adulthood. J Subst Use. 2010;15(3):174–83.
7. Ali MM, Amialchuk A, Nikaj S. Alcohol consumption and social networking ties among adolescents: evidence from add health. Addict Behav. 2014;39(5):918–22.
8. Dayan J, Bernard A, Oliac B, Mailhes A, Kermarrec S. Adolescent brain development, risk-taking, and vulnerability to addiction. J Physiol Paris. 2010;104(5):279–86.
9. Samek DR, Iacono W, Keyes M, Epstein M, Bornovalova M, McGue M. The developmental progression of age 14 behavioral disinhibition, early age of sexual initiation, and subsequent sexual risk-taking behavior. J Child Psychol Psychiatry. 2014;55(7):784–92.
10. Wang B, Deveaux L, Li X, Marshall S, Chen X, Stanton B. The impact of youth, family, peer, and neighborhood risk factors on developmental trajectories of risk involvement from early through middle adolescence. Soc Sci Med. 2014;106:43–52.
11. Geier CF. Adolescent cognitive control and reward processing: implications for risk taking and substance use. Horm Behav. 2013;64(2):333–42.
12. Luciana M. Adolescent brain development in normality and psychopathology. Dev Psychopathol. 2013;25(4 Pt 2):1325–45.
13. Spear LP. Adolescent neurodevelopment. J Adolesc Health. 2013;52(2 Suppl 2):S7–13.
14. Neumann C, Wampler M, Taylor J, Blongen D, Iacono W. Stability and invariance of psychopathic traits from late adolescence to young adulthood. J Res Pers. 2011;45(2):145–52.
15. Meeus W, Van de Schoot R, Kilmstra T, Branje S. Personality types in adolescence: change and stability and links with adjustment and relationships: a five-wave longitudinal study. Dev Psychol. 2011;47(4):1181–95.
16. Patton GC, Tollit M, Romaniuk H, Spence S, Sheffield J, Sawyer M. A prospective study of the effects of optimism on adolescent health risks. Pediatrics. 2011;127(2):308–16.
17. Jacobus J, Thayer R, Trim R, Bava S, Frank L, Tapert S. White matter integrity, substance use, and risk taking in adolescence. Psychol Addict Behav. 2013;27(2):431–42.
18. Wickrama KA, Noh S. The long arm of community: the influence of childhood community contexts across the early life course. J Youth Adolesc. 2010;39(8):894–910.
19. USA Quick Facts. United States Census Bureau. 2015. http://quickfacts.census.gov/qfd/states/00000.html. Accessed 14 Sept 2015.
20. Greene ML, Way N, Pahl K. Trajectories of perceived adult and peer discrimination among Black, Latino, and Asian American adolescent: patterns and psychological correlates. Dev Psychol. 2006;42(2):218–36.
21. Schulz-Heik RJ, Rhee S, Silvern L, Haberstick B, Hopfer C, Lessem J. The association between conduct problems and maltreatment: testing genetic and environmental mediation. Behav Genet. 2010;40(3):338–48.

22. Smits I, Soenens B, Vansteenkiste M, Luyckx K, Goosens L. Why do adolescents gather information or stick to parental norms? Examining autonomous and controlled motives behind adolescents' identity style. J Youth Adolesc. 2010;39(11):1343–56.
23. Osterman KF. Students' need for belonging and school community. Rev Educ Res. 2000;70:323–67.
24. Connell JP, Wellborn JG. Competence, autonomy, and relatedness: a motivational analysis of self-system processes. In: Gunnar MR, Sroufe LA, editors. Self processes and development, vol. 23. Hillsdale, NJ: Erlbaum; 1995. p. 43–77.
25. Smith AR, Steinberg L, Strang N, Chein J. Age differences in the impact of peers on adolescents' and adults' neural response to reward. Dev Cogn Neurosci. 2015;11:75–82.
26. Mahalik JR, Levine Coley R, McPherran Lombardi C, Doyle Lynch A, Markowitz A, Jaffee S. Changes in health risk behaviors for males and females from early adolescence through early adulthood. Health Psychol. 2013;32(6):685–94.
27. Dever BV, Schulenberg J, Dworkin J, O'Malley P, Kloska D, Bachman J. Predicting risk-taking with and without substance use: the effects of parental monitoring, school bonding, and sports participation. Prev Sci. 2012;13(6):605–15.
28. Weigard A, Chein J, Albert D, Smith A, Steinberg J. Effects of anonymous peer observation on adolescents' preference for immediate rewards. Dev Sci. 2014;17(1):71–8.
29. Irwin CE, Adams S, Park M, Newacheck P. Preventive Care for Adolescents: few get visits and fewer get services. Pediatrics. 2009;123(4):e565–72.
30. Lehrer JA, Pantell R, Tebb K, Shafer M. Forgone healthcare among U.S. adolescents: association between risk characteristics and confidentiality concern. J Adolesc Health. 2007;40:218–26.
31. Gilber AL, Rickert VI, Aalsma MC. Clinical conversations about health: the impact of confidentiality in preventive adolescent care. J Adolesc Health. 2014;55(5):672–7.

Chapter 19
Substance Use in Adolescence

Candice E. Van Skike, Shannon L. Zandy, and Douglas B. Matthews

Introduction

Drug experimentation during adolescence is relatively common [1] and drug use during this time is increased, as the rate of past month illicit drug use in adolescents and young adults is nearly three times that of adults [2]. The initiation and progression of substance use during adolescence is influenced by the distinctive behavioral and neurobiological alterations occurring during this developmental period. Various environmental and psychosocial factors also contribute to the initiation of drug use in adolescents. For instance, personality and psychological factors such as impulsivity, autonomy, depression, and anxiety are all associated with drug use. Additionally, a family history of substance abuse is a contributor to use and dependence [3], but that effect can be mediated by adolescent novelty seeking [4]. This behavior, involving risk taking and sensation seeking, increases during adolescence, which is seen in humans [5, 6] and rodents [7]. This parallels drug intake behavior, with adolescent humans [8] and rodents [9–11] consuming more of the substances per occasion than adults.

C.E. Van Skike
Department of Pharmaceutical Sciences, University of Kentucky,
789 S. Limestone Street, BioPharm Complex 498, Lexington, KY 40536, USA
e-mail: CEVanSkike@gmail.com

S.L. Zandy
Department of Pharmacy, The University of Texas at Austin,
2409 University Ave, Stop A1915, Austin, TX 78712, USA
e-mail: szandy@utexas.edu

D.B. Matthews (✉)
Department of Psychology, University of Wisconsin - Eau Claire,
HHH 273, Eau Claire, WI 54701, USA
e-mail: matthedb@uwec.edu

P. Kumanov, A. Agarwal (eds.), *Puberty*, DOI 10.1007/978-3-319-32122-6_19

The progression of drug use is driven by drug responses that are unique to this developmental period. For most drugs of abuse, adolescents generally are more sensitive to the rewarding effects of drugs and also experience less aversive consequences than adults [12]. Furthermore, exposure to drugs of abuse during adolescence permanently changes responses to drug use in the future even after a period of abstinence [13–16]. Perhaps because of these unique age-dependent effects, there is a clear association between an early age of onset and future substance use disorders [17, 18]. Therefore, adolescence can be thought of as a period of enhanced vulnerability to substance use and abuse [12].

The adolescent neurobiology is distinct from that of the adult. The adolescent brain is continuing to develop, with brain regions developing at different rates. For instance, activity in the nucleus accumbens, an area important in reward processing, peaks early during adolescence and correlates with increased laboratory risk-taking behavior [19]. The prefrontal cortex, a region that governs cognitive control, develops later than reward-processing regions [20]. It has been speculated that this offset in development of reward and control brain regions underlies the increased risk taking during adolescence, although recent data does not provide support for this theory on an individual basis [20]. Additionally, the molecular targets of drugs of abuse, called receptors, have differential expression patterns and subunit composition that are differentially altered by brain region, age, and drug exposure. The unique neurobiology of the adolescent likely underlies the enhanced vulnerability of the adolescent to substance use and abuse.

With these generalizations in mind, this chapter will review the epidemiology of adolescent drug use, factors contributing to initiation, and the adolescent-specific neurobiological and behavioral consequences of several commonly used drugs during adolescence: nicotine, alcohol, and marijuana. While significant variability exists between all drugs during adolescence, we hope these three serve as hallmark drugs where the reader gains a valuable insight into how drugs impact this developmental window. We consider both human and animal studies to provide a thorough look at the effects of drug use during this time period. Human studies elucidate the epidemiology of drug use and provide data regarding the effects of individual patterns of intake. While reflective of the actual population, the research is limited by the wide variability of intake patterns and polysubstance use. Preclinical research allows for experimental control and manipulation of specific drugs of abuse and patterns of exposure. This permits the study of the behavioral, neurochemical, cellular, and molecular effects of these drugs under specific conditions. We cover both research approaches, as they complement each other when taking a comprehensive look at substance use during adolescence.

Nicotine

Smoking is a leading cause of preventable morbidity and mortality globally and continues to significantly impact public health in the United States. Smoking initiation occurs most often during adolescence and early use of cigarettes is associated with increased risk of dependence later in life [18]. Conventional cigarette smoking is declining overall among American teenagers with 8 % of eighth, tenth and 12th grade students combined reporting smoking in the prior month [1]. However, there has been a substantial rise in popularity of electronic cigarettes (e-cigarettes) among adolescents. Specifically, the prevalence of e-cigarette use in the last 30 days is more than twice that of regular cigarettes in eighth and tenth grade students and fewer of these students associate significant risks with e-cigarettes compared to conventional cigarettes [1]. This is a concern as e-cigarettes may be a more attractive nicotine delivery method for adolescents. Even low rates of nicotine use during adolescence increases the risk of dependence in adulthood, highlighting the need to understand the factors contributing to early use [21].

There are many environmental and psychosocial factors contributing to smoking initiation in adolescents. Environmental factors, such as exposure to smoking from family members and peers, influence initiation and escalation of smoking in adolescence. For example, parents and the number of friends who smoke is associated with a 30 and 44 % increase in likelihood of adolescent smoking, respectively [22]. Autonomy also plays a significant role in contributing to nicotine use in the adolescent population. As parental involvement declines and decision-making autonomy increases, adolescents are more likely to become smokers, which is shown across ethnic, gender, and socioeconomic groups [23]. In addition, psychological factors such as depression and anxiety are commonly associated with adolescent smoking. Depression and anxiety have been shown to predict initiation of smoking, nicotine dependence, and decreased success at smoking cessation. Young adults that reported elevated depression symptoms as adolescents were found to have significantly higher lifetime smoking rates [24].

Clinical reports suggest an enhanced sensitivity to the positive subjective effects of nicotine may contribute to initiation and continued tobacco use in adolescence. In particular, adult smokers that began smoking during adolescence describe more positive effects and fewer unpleasant side effects of their first smoking episode than smokers that initiated smoking in adulthood [25]. In addition to enhanced positive effects, adolescents may be more resistant to negative effects of nicotine withdrawal, which is a significant predictor of relapse in adult smokers. However, in acute abstinence, adolescent smokers exhibited minimal withdrawal symptoms that were not associated with reports of dependence or biological measures of use [26]. This might indicate that nicotine withdrawal symptoms may not influence maintenance of smoking behavior in adolescents as it does in the adult population. This has important implications for clinical identification and treatment of adolescent nicotine users, as the severity of nicotine withdrawal symptoms is prevalent in current diagnostic criteria and the focus of many available treatment options.

Given that 90 % of adult smokers were under 18 when they had their first cigarette [27], this suggests that there is something unique about the adolescent developmental period that confers increased rates of addiction. Consistent with this notion, preclinical studies indicate that nicotine exposure during the adolescent developmental period perpetuates nicotine use [10, 13], as well as other drugs of abuse [28]. Specifically, voluntary nicotine intake is higher in adolescent rodents compared to adults [9, 10]. Although nicotine pharmacokinetics is altered in adolescent rats [29], studies suggest the age-dependent intake patterns are based on altered motivational properties of nicotine [10]. Indeed, adolescent rodents are more sensitive than adults to the rewarding effects of nicotine [30]. This increased reward during adolescence persists into adulthood even after a period of abstinence [13–15] and corresponds to increased nicotine self-administration later in adulthood compared to adults that were nicotine naïve during adolescence [10]. Furthermore, nicotine exposure during adolescence, but not adulthood, sensitizes future behavioral responses to other drugs of abuse like cocaine [13, 28], THC [31], and alcohol [32].

The altered short- and long-term consequences of nicotine use during adolescence have a neurobiological basis: the adolescent brain is undergoing maturation [33], so the neurobiological response to nicotine is differentially modulated due to both development and drug exposure. Chronic nicotine exposure alters nicotinic acetylcholine receptor (nAChR) expression in the brain of humans [34] and rodents [35]. Of particular interest due to their ubiquitous expression in mammalian brain [36] and role in nicotine dependence and reinforcement [37] are the α4β2-containing (α4β2*) nAChRs [38]. The α4β2* receptors are differentially expressed throughout the brain based on age and brain region, with an average of 50 % greater radioligand binding to these receptors in adolescent rats [39]. Additionally, adolescents have more α4β2* receptors on dopamine cell bodies and terminal regions than adults [39], and since nicotine-induced dopamine release is mediated by the α4β2* receptors [40], the overexpression of α4β2* receptors in these regions may contribute to the enhancement of the nicotine-induced reward seen during adolescence. Nicotine use upregulates α4β2* and α7 receptors, which are involved in acquisition and dependence [41]. While the upregulation of these receptors is reduced in adolescents versus adults [39], these changes are more persistent and ubiquitous throughout different brain regions in adolescents [42]. This distinct pattern of nAChR expression and nicotine-induced upregulation during adolescence may contribute to the initiation and persistence of nicotine use during adolescence.

Many factors contribute to smoking initiation; however, both human and preclinical research indicates that adolescents have an enhanced sensitivity to nicotine reward. Furthermore, nicotine exposure during adolescence alters future responses to other drugs of abuse, yielding a predisposition toward the development of a substance use disorder.

Ethanol

Alcohol is the most widely used drug by adolescents. Two-thirds of high school students have consumed alcohol by graduation and more than a quarter of students report drinking by eighth grade [1]. Binge drinking (defined as consuming five or more drinks per drinking session for males and four or more per session for females) is the most common drinking pattern among adolescents, often drinking more on average in one session than adults [8]. This is particularly concerning as binge drinking is associated with detrimental effects on brain development and cognition and increased rates of alcohol dependence. The rate of alcohol use dramatically increases between ages 12 and 20, which directly translates into an increase in alcohol use disorders. In fact, the highest prevalence of alcohol dependence occurs in ages 18–20, often referred to as "emerging adulthood," the period immediately following adolescence [43]. As with other drugs of abuse, age of onset for alcohol use is a significant predictor for future alcohol-related problems. Adolescents that began drinking prior to the age of 14 were shown to have a fourfold greater rate of alcohol dependence than individuals that did not begin drinking until after 20 years old [17].

Aside from rates of alcohol dependence, research has begun to show adolescents with a history of alcohol use differ significantly on cognitive and neural measures compared to those with little or no alcohol use. Studies show alterations in gray and white matter brain structure, poorer neurocognitive performance, and altered brain activation patterns [44]. For example, adolescents with 2 years of heavy drinking history showed abnormalities in brain activation during a spatial working memory task, which was positively correlated to the amount of alcohol use and hangover symptoms reported [45]. There also may be significant gender considerations to be made for consequences of adolescent alcohol use. Females are more vulnerable to alcohol-induced neurotoxicity [46, 47], an effect that begins to emerge during puberty.

In addition to neurocognitive abnormalities that result from alcohol use, it is also important to highlight neurobiological differences and genetic risks that can increase susceptibility to early initiation of alcohol drinking or heavy patterns of use during adolescence. Poorer performance on tests of inhibitory control in early adolescence prior to any alcohol or drug use was significantly related to heavy alcohol use in later adolescence. Additionally, lower baseline activation and structural differences predict future heavy alcohol use in adolescents [48]. Interestingly, twin studies suggest that environmental influences such as access to alcohol have a large influence on the age that adolescents initiate alcohol use. However, a family history of alcohol misuse has a stronger influence than environmental factors on the amount of alcohol consumed in a session and escalation patterns [49]. Together, these findings suggest that alcohol use in adolescence negatively impacts cognition, brain structure and function, and future health outcomes. Current and future research is leading toward unique opportunities to target prevention and treatment strategies specific to various risk factors within the adolescent population.

Preclinical models also indicate that there is a neurobiological predisposition to excessive binge-like alcohol consumption during adolescence. Indeed, much like adolescent humans [8], adolescent rodents will self-administer greater quantities of alcohol per unit weight than adults [11]. This is likely underscored by age-dependent effects of ethanol on behavior and neurophysiology. Specifically, adolescents are less sensitive to ethanol-induced motor impairments [50], which serve as feedback cues to attenuate consumption within a single drinking session [51]. Changes in cerebellar electrophysiology [50] suggest a neurological correlate for this behavioral difference. Furthermore, adolescents are more sensitive to the ethanol-induced reward and less sensitive to the adverse effects, like acute withdrawal or hangovers [51, 52]. These altered neurobiological responses create a predisposition toward excessive binge-like alcohol use in the adolescent.

This susceptibility is particularly concerning because adolescents are especially vulnerable to ethanol-induced neurotoxicity, as well as age-specific long-lasting neuroadaptations. For example, after binge alcohol exposure, the adult brain has increased gene expression involved with mechanisms of repair and protection against oxidative damage, while adolescents have decreased expression of these genes and increased proapoptotic gene expression [53]. Some of the ethanol-induced neuroadaptations extend into adulthood and are associated with persistent behavioral changes. For instance, adolescent chronic alcohol exposure yields persistent reductions of hippocampal volume [54], decreased neurogenesis [55], and increased cell death [55]. This is correlated with an increase in disinhibitory behavior [55], suggestive of altered risk-taking behavior. In fact, chronic ethanol exposure increases risk preference in adolescent, but not adult, rats even after nearly 3 weeks of abstinence [56]. Alcohol reward is also altered, as binge-exposed adolescents have reduced dopamine release in adulthood [57]. These neuroadaptations likely underlie alterations in ethanol preference, as rats that were exposed to ethanol during adolescence, but not adulthood, had greater ethanol intake in the future [58], which mirrors the increased rate of future alcohol dependence seen in human adolescents [17]. Overall, preclinical findings mirror the ethanol intake patterns of human adolescents and suggest that alcohol use during adolescence can yield persistent changes in brain and behavior despite long periods of abstinence.

Marijuana

Cannabis is one of the most commonly used illicit drugs among adolescents and adults. The use of marijuana has remained stable the last few years, with over 20 % of 12th grade students reporting use in the previous month [1]. However, attitudes of greater acceptance and less perceived risk are becoming more prevalent among teenagers. In fact, only 36.1 % of high school seniors believe regular use puts them at great risk [1]. While public acceptance increases and legalization of marijuana continues in the United States, it largely remains unclear how cannabis may cause potential alterations in neuromaturational processes during adolescence.

Chronic marijuana use in early adolescence is associated with deficits in cognitive function in humans due to structural changes and decreased connectivity in brain regions important to learning and memory [59]. In fact, short-term memory impairments persist after 6 weeks of abstinence in cannabis-dependent adolescents [60]. Additionally, adolescent marijuana users perform worse on tests of executive functioning, correlating with the number of days of cannabis use in the past 30 days [61]. Although some studies suggest differences in learning and memory can recover to baseline levels following abstinence, attention deficits seem to be persistent [62].

Compelling evidence also suggests adolescent cannabis use is associated with the development of psychosis in adulthood. One prospective study showed an increased risk of psychotic disorders at age 26 associated with cannabis use in adolescence between ages 15–18 [63]. Other studies report early use of cannabis predicts a significant younger age of onset of psychosis and poorer treatment prognoses. Overall, the role of genetics and brain white matter maturation have been hypothesized to contribute to determining whether cannabis use may influence the development of adult psychosis in predisposed individuals.

Functional imaging studies report significant differences in brain activation patterns between adolescent marijuana users and nonusers. Marijuana users show more activation in areas of the brain associated with executive control during an inhibitory processing task, suggesting additional recruitment may be needed to maintain inhibition in adolescents with a history of marijuana use [64]. Additionally, initiation of cannabis use before age 16 is associated with increased brain activation during working memory tasks [65]. A recent longitudinal study found adolescents that reported weekly cannabis use prior to the age of 18 showed greater neuropsychological decline into adulthood, even following prolonged abstinence [66].

The major psychoactive component of cannabis smoke is Δ9-tetrahydrocannabinol (THC) and exerts its effects through agonism of cannabinoid-1 receptors (CB1Rs). Cannabinoid receptors are expressed throughout the brain, increasing during adolescence and are thought to influence gene expression critical for neural development [67]. Therefore, modulation of the endocannabinoid system during adolescence is likely to produce persistent neurological changes. Preclinical studies reveal baseline age-dependent differences in CB1R function that results in differential effects of THC at the CB1Rs. Adolescent CB1Rs are less sensitive to THC-induced desensitization, which corresponds with a lack of tolerance to the memory-impairing effects of THC [68]. Adults also develop tolerance to THC-induced memory impairments, indicating that adolescents may have greater memory impairments due to altered THC-induced neuroadaptations. Indeed, adolescent rats are more sensitive than adults to chronic THC-induced spatial memory impairments, especially at high doses [69, 70]. These spatial learning deficits in THC-treated adolescents can be attributed to an impaired ability to organize working memory [71] and may arise from THC-suppressing transcription of learning-induced neuroplasticity in the adolescent hippocampus [72].

THC exposure during adolescence has long-term consequences as well. Chronic exposure to THC during adolescence produces residual impairments in spatial working memory, changes in hippocampal morphology, and reduced markers of neuroplasticity that extend into adulthood even after 30 days of abstinence [73]. Additionally, adolescent females appear to be particularly vulnerable to both the short- and long-term consequences of THC exposure, as they are more sensitive to immediate memory disruptions [69] and exhibit depressive symptomology during adulthood [74]. These effects are associated with persistent sex-specific cognitive impairment and neuroplastic alterations of the prefrontal cortex [75, 76] and are mediated by ovarian hormones [77].

Adolescent THC exposure can also change responsiveness to future illicit drug intake. Subchronic cannabinoid treatment in adolescents and adults suppressed dopamine neuron firing; however, cross-tolerance to cocaine, amphetamine, and morphine was observed for only the adolescent rats exposed to cannabinoids [16]. Furthermore, THC enhances the effects of cocaine in adolescent, but not adult, rats [78]. There is some evidence that THC exposure during adolescence increases responding for heroin in adulthood [79] and subsequently increases heroin relapse rates [80]. This mirrors illicit drug use in surveys of human behavior: compared to adults who initiated marijuana use after 18 years of age, adults who began marijuana use before age 14 are 4.5 times more likely to be dependent on any illicit drug [2].

Together, human and preclinical research suggests marijuana use in adolescence can significantly impact both short- and long-term cognitive performance despite periods of abstinence. Additionally, adolescent marijuana use is associated with altered responses to other drugs of abuse, which likely contribute to the increased rates of illicit drug dependence in adults who began using marijuana during adolescence [2].

Conclusion

Adolescent drug experimentation is rather common [1], and after reviewing the effects of the three most commonly used drugs during adolescence [81], it is clear that this experimentation is not benign. Drug use during this time period is associated with excessive intake patterns [8–11], increased rates of future dependence [17, 18], and altered cognitive outcomes [44, 59, 60, 69, 70] compared to drug use during adulthood. While not all adolescents that experiment with drugs become dependent, adolescence represents a unique time period where the vulnerability to addiction is increased [12]. Adolescent drug use permanently changes future responses to substance use even after a period of abstinence, making drug use more likely to progress [13–16, 28, 31, 32].

Adolescents have a unique neurobiological composition, partly due to age-related changes in brain structure, function, and neurochemistry. It is likely that because of these innate differences, the effects of drug use during adolescence are different when compared to adulthood. While this has been appreciated in terms of research efforts for several years, it is also necessary to begin to alter therapy and/or treatment options to reflect the inherent differences that exist between adolescents and adults.

Initial onset of drug use during this developmental period is influenced by several factors, including changes in personality, mental health, parental supervision, autonomy, and impulsivity. Maturational changes are rampant during adolescence, with hormonal changes playing a primary role in development. For example, pubertal onset, especially early puberty in males, is associated with increases in substance use [82]. Indeed, the emergence of hormones can produce sex-dependent patterns of intake and escalation of drug use (for an excellent review, see [83]). For instance, unlike the majority of illicit drug use among teens [2], slightly more than half (52 %) of all adolescent prescription drug exposures requiring medical treatment involved females [84]. It is also worthwhile to mention that a significant proportion (38 %) of these prescription drug exposures were suspected suicide attempts [84], perhaps indicative of motivational differences in prescription drug use as compared to other drugs among a specific subset of youth.

Briefly, it is important to consider that other substances like anabolic androgenic steroids (AAS) may also be used during adolescence and emerging adulthood. Preclinical models of AAS use indicate that AAS administration during adolescence produces increased aggression, whereas no such change is observed in adulthood [85]. In humans, AAS use is associated with impaired attention and impulsivity in both ages, with adolescent-onset users displaying a greater sensitivity to these impairments [86]. Further, AAS use is associated with prescription drug misuse and illicit drug use [87]. This substance is relatively new compared to other drugs of abuse, so population usage data are scarce and its abuse potential has yet to be fully recognized at both the research and clinician levels [88].

Importantly, single substance use is hardly ever found in those who struggle with addiction. The vast majority of the current work, including the much of the current work reviewed here, does not consider the effects of polydrug use. This void of understanding needs to be addressed for research to more accurately address the needs of society.

In conclusion, substance use during adolescence continues to be a societal concern. While decreasing usage rates and further understanding of the neurobiological impact is in progress, additional resources, efforts, and new questions need to be acknowledged to better address the issue. Only through the continued collaboration between research and practitioners will the impact of drug use during adolescence be understood.

References

1. Johnston LD, O'Malley PM, Miech RA, Bachman JG, Schulenberg JE. Monitoring the future national survey results on drug use, 1975–2014: overview, key findings on adolescent drug use. Ann Arbor: Institute for Social Research, The University of Michigan; 2015.
2. Substance Abuse and Mental Health Services Administration. Results from the 2013 National Survey on Drug Use and Health: summary of national findings, NSDUH series H-48, HHS publication no. (SMA) 14–4863. Rockville: Substance Abuse and Mental Health Services Administration; 2014.
3. Grant BF. The impact of a family history of alcoholism on the relationship between age at onset of alcohol use and DSM-IV alcohol dependence: results from the National Longitudinal Alcohol Epidemiologic Survey. Alcohol Health Res World. 1998;22(2):144–7.
4. Bidwell LC, Knopik VS, Audrain-McGovern J, Glynn TR, Spillane NS, Ray LA, et al. Novelty seeking as a phenotypic marker of adolescent substance use. Subst Abuse. 2015;9 Suppl 1:1–10.
5. Steinberg L, Albert D, Cauffman E, Banich M, Graham S, Woolard J. Age differences in sensation seeking and impulsivity as indexed by behavior and self-report: evidence for a dual systems model. Dev Psychol. 2008;44(6):1764–78.
6. Crone EA, Bullens L, van der Plas EA, Kijkuit EJ, Zelazo PD. Developmental changes and individual differences in risk and perspective taking in adolescence. Dev Psychopathol. 2008;20(4):1213–29.
7. Macrì S, Adriani W, Chiarotti F, Laviola G. Risk taking during exploration of a plus-maze is greater in adolescent than in juvenile or adult mice. Anim Behav. 2002;64(4):541–6.
8. Masten AS, Faden VB, Zucker RA, Spear LP. A developmental perspective on underage alcohol use. Alcohol Res Health. 2009;32(1):3–15.

9. Levin ED, Slade S, Wells C, Cauley M, Petro A, Vendittelli A, et al. Threshold of adulthood for the onset of nicotine self-administration in male and female rats. Behav Brain Res. 2011;225(2):473–81.
10. Natividad LA, Torres OV, Friedman TC, O'Dell LE. Adolescence is a period of development characterized by short- and long-term vulnerability to the rewarding effects of nicotine and reduced sensitivity to the anorectic effects of this drug. Behav Brain Res. 2013;257:275–85.
11. Doremus TL, Brunell SC, Rajendran P, Spear LP. Factors influencing elevated ethanol consumption in adolescent relative to adult rats. Alcohol Clin Exp Res. 2005;29(10):1796–808.
12. Schramm-Sapyta NL, Walker QD, Caster JM, Levin ED, Kuhn CM. Are adolescents more vulnerable to drug addiction than adults? Evidence from animal models. Psychopharmacology (Berl). 2009;206(1):1–21.
13. Adriani W, Deroche-Gamonet V, Le Moal M, Laviola G, Piazza PV. Preexposure during or following adolescence differently affects nicotine-rewarding properties in adult rats. Psychopharmacology (Berl). 2006;184(3–4):382–90.
14. de la Peña JB, Ahsan HM, Botanas CJ, Sohn A, Yu GY, Cheong JH. Adolescent nicotine or cigarette smoke exposure changes subsequent response to nicotine conditioned place preference and self-administration. Behav Brain Res. 2014;272:156–64.
15. de la Peña JB, Ahsan HM, Tampus R, Botanas CJ, dela Peña IJ, Kim HJ, et al. Cigarette smoke exposure during adolescence enhances sensitivity to the rewarding effects of nicotine in adulthood, even after a long period of abstinence. Neuropharmacology. 2015;99:9–14.
16. Pistis M, Perra S, Pillolla G, Melis M, Muntoni AL, Gessa GL. Adolescent exposure to cannabinoids induces long-lasting changes in the response to drugs of abuse of rat midbrain dopamine neurons. Biol Psychiatry. 2004;56(2):86–94.
17. Grant BF, Dawson DA. Age at onset of alcohol use and its association with DSM-IV alcohol abuse and dependence: results from the National Longitudinal Alcohol Epidemiologic Survey. J Subst Abuse. 1997;9:103–10.
18. Chen K, Kandel DB. The natural history of drug use from adolescence to the mid-thirties in a general population sample. Am J Public Health. 1995;85(1):41–7.
19. Braams BR, van Duijvenvoorde AC, Peper JS. Longitudinal changes in adolescent risk-taking: a comprehensive study of neural responses to rewards, pubertal development, and risk-taking behavior. J Neurosci. 2015;35(18):7226–38.
20. Mills KL, Goddings AL, Clasen LS, Giedd JN, Blakemore SJ. The developmental mismatch in structural brain maturation during adolescence. Dev Neurosci. 2014;36(3–4):147–60.
21. Riggs NR, Chou CP, Li C, Pentz MA. Adolescent to emerging adulthood smoking trajectories: when do smoking trajectories diverge, and do they predict early adulthood nicotine dependence? Nicotine Tob Res. 2007;9(11):1147–54.
22. Wang MQ, Fitzhugh EC, Green BL, Turner LW, Eddy JM, Westerfield RC. Prospective social-psychological factors of adolescent smoking progression. J Adolesc Health. 1999;24(1):2–9.
23. Radziszewska B, Richardson JL, Dent CW, Flay BR. Parenting style and adolescent depressive symptoms, smoking, and academic achievement: ethnic, gender, and SES differences. J Behav Med. 1996;19(3):289–305.
24. Kandel DB, Davies M. Adult sequelae of adolescent depressive symptoms. Arch Gen Psychiatry. 1986;43(3):255–62.
25. Eissenberg T, Balster RL. Initial tobacco use episodes in children and adolescents: current knowledge, future directions. Drug Alcohol Depend. 2000;59 Suppl 1:S41–60.
26. Smith AE, Cavallo DA, Dahl T, Wu R, George TP, Krishnan-Sarin S. Effects of acute tobacco abstinence in adolescent smokers compared with nonsmokers. J Adolesc Health. 2008;43(1):46–54.
27. US Department of Health and Human Services. Preventing tobacco use among youth and young adults: a report of the Surgeon General. Atlanta: US Department of Health and Human Services, Centers for Disease Control and Prevention, National Center for Chronic Disease Prevention and Health Promotion, Office on Smoking and Health; 2012.
28. McQuown SC, Belluzzi JD, Leslie FM. Low dose nicotine treatment during early adolescence increases subsequent cocaine reward. Neurotoxicol Teratol. 2007;29(1):66–73.

29. Craig EL, Zhao B, Cui JZ, Novalen M, Miksys S, Tyndale RF. Nicotine pharmacokinetics in rats is altered as a function of age, impacting the interpretation of animal model data. Drug Metab Dispos. 2014;42(9):1447–55.
30. Belluzzi JD, Lee AG, Oliff HS, Leslie FM. Age-dependent effects of nicotine on locomotor activity and conditioned place preference in rats. Psychopharmacology (Berl). 2004;174(3): 389–95.
31. Werling LL, Reed SC, Wade D, Izenwasser S. Chronic nicotine alters cannabinoid-mediated locomotor activity and receptor density in periadolescent but not adult male rats. Int J Dev Neurosci. 2009;27(3):263–9.
32. Burns BE, Proctor WR. Cigarette smoke exposure greatly increases alcohol consumption in adolescent C57BL/6 mice. Alcohol Clin Exp Res. 2013;37 Suppl 1:E364–72.
33. Lydon DM, Wilson SJ, Child A, Geier CF. Adolescent brain maturation and smoking: what we know and where we're headed. Neurosci Biobehav Rev. 2014;45:323–42.
34. Jasinska AJ, Zorick T, Brody AL, Stein EA. Dual role of nicotine in addiction and cognition: a review of neuroimaging studies in humans. Neuropharmacology. 2014;84:111–22.
35. Baker LK, Mao D, Chi H, Govind AP, Vallejo YF, Iacoviello M, et al. Intermittent nicotine exposure upregulates nAChRs in VTA dopamine neurons and sensitises locomotor responding to the drug. Eur J Neurosci. 2013;37(6):1004–11.
36. Wu J, Liu Q, Yu K, Hu J, Kuo YP, Segerberg M, et al. Roles of nicotinic acetylcholine receptor beta subunits in function of human alpha4-containing nicotinic receptors. J Physiol. 2006;576(Pt 1):103–18.
37. Walters CL, Brown S, Changeux JP, Martin B, Damaj MI. The beta2 but not alpha7 subunit of the nicotinic acetylcholine receptor is required for nicotine-conditioned place preference in mice. Psychopharmacology (Berl). 2006;184(3–4):339–44.
38. McKee SA, Weinberger AH. How can we use our knowledge of alcohol-tobacco interactions to reduce alcohol use? Annu Rev Clin Psychol. 2013;9:649–74.
39. Doura MB, Gold AB, Keller AB, Perry DC. Adult and periadolescent rats differ in expression of nicotinic cholinergic receptor subtypes and in the response of these subtypes to chronic nicotine exposure. Brain Res. 2008;1215:40–52.
40. Champtiaux N, Gotti C, Cordero-Erausquin M, David DJ, Przybylski C, Lena C, et al. Subunit composition of functional nicotinic receptors in dopaminergic neurons investigated with knock-out mice. J Neurosci. 2003;23(21):7820–9.
41. Stoker AK, Markou A. Unraveling the neurobiology of nicotine dependence using genetically engineered mice. Curr Opin Neurobiol. 2013;23(4):493–9.
42. Trauth JA, Seidler FJ, McCook EC, Slotkin TA. Adolescent nicotine exposure causes persistent upregulation of nicotinic cholinergic receptors in rat brain regions. Brain Res. 1999;851(1–2):9–19.
43. Grant BF, Dawson DA, Stinson FS, Chou SP, Dufour MC, Pickering RP. The 12-month prevalence and trends in DSM-IV alcohol abuse and dependence: United States, 1991–1992 and 2001–2002. Drug Alcohol Depend. 2004;74(3):223–34.
44. Jacobus J, Tapert SF. Neurotoxic effects of alcohol in adolescence. Annu Rev Clin Psychol. 2013;9:703–21.
45. Tapert SF, Schweinsburg AD, Barlett VC, Brown SA, Frank LR, Brown GG, et al. Blood oxygen level dependent response and spatial working memory in adolescents with alcohol use disorders. Alcohol Clin Exp Res. 2004;28(10):1577–86.
46. Hommer D, Momenan R, Kaiser E, Rawlings R. Evidence for a gender-related effect of alcoholism on brain volumes. Am J Psychiatry. 2001;158(2):198–204.
47. Pfefferbaum A, Rosenbloom M, Deshmukh A, Sullivan E. Sex differences in the effects of alcohol on brain structure. Am J Psychiatry. 2001;158(2):188–97.
48. Squeglia LM, Boissoneault J, Van Skike CE, Nixon SJ, Matthews DB. Age-related effects of alcohol from adolescent, adult, and aged populations using human and animal models. Alcohol Clin Exp Res. 2014;38(10):2509–16.
49. Spear LP. Adolescent alcohol exposure: are there separable vulnerable periods within adolescence? Physiol Behav. 2015;148:122–30.

50. Van Skike CE, Botta P, Chin VS, Tokunaga S, McDaniel JM, Venard J, et al. Behavioral effects of ethanol in cerebellum are age dependent: potential system and molecular mechanisms. Alcohol Clin Exp Res. 2010;34(12):2070–80.
51. Spear LP, Varlinskaya EI. Adolescence. Alcohol sensitivity, tolerance, and intake. Recent Dev Alcohol. 2005;17:143–59.
52. Ehlers CL, Desikan A, Wills DN. Developmental differences in EEG and sleep responses to acute ethanol administration and its withdrawal (hangover) in adolescent and adult Wistar rats. Alcohol. 2013;47(8):601–10.
53. Lacaille H, Duterte-Boucher D, Liot D, Vaudry H, Naassila M, Vaudry D. Comparison of the deleterious effects of binge drinking-like alcohol exposure in adolescent and adult mice. J Neurochem. 2015;132(6):629–41.
54. Ehlers CL, Oguz I, Budin F, Wills DN, Crews FT. Peri-adolescent ethanol vapor exposure produces reductions in hippocampal volume that are correlated with deficits in prepulse inhibition of the startle. Alcohol Clin Exp Res. 2013;37(9):1466–75.
55. Ehlers CL, Liu W, Wills DN, Crews FT. Periadolescent ethanol vapor exposure persistently reduces measures of hippocampal neurogenesis that are associated with behavioral outcomes in adulthood. Neuroscience. 2013;244:1–15.
56. Schindler AG, Tsutsui KT, Clark JJ. Chronic alcohol intake during adolescence, but not adulthood, promotes persistent deficits in risk-based decision making. Alcohol Clin Exp Res. 2014;38(6):1622–9.
57. Zandy SL, Matthews DB, Tokunaga S, Miller AD, Blaha CD, Mittleman G. Reduced dopamine release in the nucleus accumbens core of adult rats following adolescent binge alcohol exposure: age and dose-dependent analysis. Psychopharmacology (Berl). 2015;232(4):777–84.
58. Fabio MC, Nizhnikov ME, Spear NE, Pautassi RM. Binge ethanol intoxication heightens subsequent ethanol intake in adolescent, but not adult, rats. Dev Psychobiol. 2014;56(3):574–83.
59. Renard J, Krebs MO, Le Pen G, Jay TM. Long-term consequences of adolescent cannabinoid exposure in adult psychopathology. Front Neurosci. 2014;8:361.
60. Schwartz RH, Gruenewald PJ, Klitzner M, Fedio P. Short-term memory impairment in cannabis-dependent adolescents. Am J Dis Child. 1989;143(10):1214–9.
61. Harvey MA, Sellman JD, Porter RJ, Frampton CM. The relationship between non-acute adolescent cannabis use and cognition. Drug Alcohol Rev. 2007;26(3):309–19.
62. Hanson KL, Winward JL, Schweinsburg AD, Medina KL, Brown SA, Tapert SF. Longitudinal study of cognition among adolescent marijuana users over three weeks of abstinence. Addict Behav. 2010;35(11):970–6.
63. Arseneault L, Cannon M, Poulton R, Murray R, Caspi A, Moffitt TE. Cannabis use in adolescence and risk for adult psychosis: longitudinal prospective study. BMJ. 2002;325(7374):1212–3.
64. Tapert SF, Schweinsburg AD, Drummond SP, Paulus MP, Brown SA, Yang TT, et al. Functional MRI of inhibitory processing in abstinent adolescent marijuana users. Psychopharmacology (Berl). 2007;194(2):173–83.
65. Becker B, Wagner D, Gouzoulis-Mayfrank E, Spuentrup E, Daumann J. The impact of early-onset cannabis use on functional brain correlates of working memory. Prog Neuropsychopharmacol Biol Psychiatry. 2010;34(6):837–45.
66. Meier MH, Caspi A, Ambler A, Harrington H, Houts R, Keefe RS, et al. Persistent cannabis users show neuropsychological decline from childhood to midlife. Proc Natl Acad Sci U S A. 2012;109(40):E2657–64.
67. Rubino T, Parolaro D. Long lasting consequences of cannabis exposure in adolescence. Mol Cell Endocrinol. 2008;286(1–2 Suppl 1):S108–13.
68. Moore NL, Greenleaf AL, Acheson SK, Wilson WA, Swartzwelder HS, Kuhn CM. Role of cannabinoid receptor type 1 desensitization in greater tetrahydrocannabinol impairment of memory in adolescent rats. J Pharmacol Exp Ther. 2010;335(2):294–301.
69. Cha YM, Jones KH, Kuhn CM, Wilson WA, Swartzwelder HS. Sex differences in the effects of delta9-tetrahydrocannabinol on spatial learning in adolescent and adult rats. Behav Pharmacol. 2007;18(5–6):563–9.

70. Cha YM, White AM, Kuhn CM, Wilson WA, Swartzwelder HS. Differential effects of delta9-THC on learning in adolescent and adult rats. Pharmacol Biochem Behav. 2006;83(3):448–55.
71. Steel RW, Miller JH, Sim DA, Day DJ. Learning impairment by Δ(9)-tetrahydrocannabinol in adolescence is attributable to deficits in chunking. Behav Pharmacol. 2011;22(8):837–46.
72. Steel RW, Miller JH, Sim DA, Day DJ. Delta-9-tetrahydrocannabinol disrupts hippocampal neuroplasticity and neurogenesis in trained, but not untrained adolescent Sprague–Dawley rats. Brain Res. 2014;1548:12–9.
73. Rubino T, Realini N, Braida D, Guidi S, Capurro V, Vigano D, et al. Changes in hippocampal morphology and neuroplasticity induced by adolescent THC treatment are associated with cognitive impairment in adulthood. Hippocampus. 2009;19(8):763–72.
74. Rubino T, Vigano D, Realini N, Guidali C, Braida D, Capurro V, et al. Chronic delta 9-tetrahydrocannabinol during adolescence provokes sex-dependent changes in the emotional profile in adult rats: behavioral and biochemical correlates. Neuropsychopharmacology. 2008;33(11):2760–71.
75. Rubino T, Prini P, Piscitelli F, Zamberletti E, Trusel M, Melis M, et al. Adolescent exposure to THC in female rats disrupts developmental changes in the prefrontal cortex. Neurobiol Dis. 2015;73:60–9.
76. Rubino T, Realini N, Braida D, Alberio T, Capurro V, Vigano D, et al. The depressive phenotype induced in adult female rats by adolescent exposure to THC is associated with cognitive impairment and altered neuroplasticity in the prefrontal cortex. Neurotox Res. 2009;15(4):291–302.
77. Winsauer PJ, Daniel JM, Filipeanu CM, Leonard ST, Hulst JL, Rodgers SP, et al. Long-term behavioral and pharmacodynamic effects of delta-9-tetrahydrocannabinol in female rats depend on ovarian hormone status. Addict Biol. 2011;16(1):64–81.
78. Dow-Edwards D, Izenwasser S. Pretreatment with Δ9-tetrahydrocannabinol (THC) increases cocaine-stimulated activity in adolescent but not adult male rats. Pharmacol Biochem Behav. 2012;100(3):587–91.
79. Ellgren M, Spano SM, Hurd YL. Adolescent cannabis exposure alters opiate intake and opioid limbic neuronal populations in adult rats. Neuropsychopharmacology. 2007;32(3):607–15.
80. Stopponi S, Soverchia L, Ubaldi M, Cippitelli A, Serpelloni G, Ciccocioppo R. Chronic THC during adolescence increases the vulnerability to stress-induced relapse to heroin seeking in adult rats. Eur Neuropsychopharmacol. 2014;24(7):1037–45.
81. Johnston LD, Miech RA, O'Malley PM, Bachman JG, Schulenberg JE. Use of alcohol, cigarettes, and number of illicit drugs declines among U.S. teens. Ann Arbor: University of Michigan News Service; 2014. http://www.monitoringthefuture.org. Retrieved 03 Aug 2015.
82. Kaltiala-Heino R, Koivisto AM, Marttunen M, Frojd S. Pubertal timing and substance use in middle adolescence: a 2-year follow-up study. J Youth Adolesc. 2011;40:1288–301.
83. Kuhn C. Emergence of sex differences in the development of substance use and abuse during adolescence. Pharmacol Ther. 2015;153:55–78.
84. Zosel A, Bartelson BB, Bailey E, Lowenstein S, Dart R. Characterization of adolescent prescription drug abuse and misuse using the Research Abuse Diversion and Addiction-related Surveillance (RADARS(®)) System. J Am Acad Child Adolesc Psychiatry. 2013;52:196–204.e2.
85. Morrison TR, Ricci LA, Melloni Jr RH. Anabolic/androgenic steroid administration during adolescence and adulthood differentially modulates aggression and anxiety. Horm Behav. 2015;69:132–8.
86. Hildebrandt T, Langenbucher JW, Flores A, Harty S, Berlin HA. The influence of age of onset and acute anabolic steroid exposure on cognitive performance, impulsivity, and aggression in men. Psychol Addict Behav. 2014;28:1096–104.
87. Hakansson A, Mickelsson K, Wallin C, Berglund M. Anabolic androgenic steroids in the general population: user characteristics and associations with substance use. Eur Addict Res. 2012;18:83–90.
88. Pope Jr HG, Kanayama G, Athey A, Ryan E, Hudson JI, Baggish A. The lifetime prevalence of anabolic-androgenic steroid use and dependence in Americans: current best estimates. Am J Addict. 2014;23:371–7.

Index

A
Adenosine triphosphate (ATP), 216
Adiponectin, 88
Adolescence
  alcohol consumption, 277
  cannabis, 278
  drug experimentation, 273
  in humans and rodents, 273
  inhibitory control, 277
  maturational changes, 280
  neuromaturational processes, 278
  nicotine, 276
  nicotine naïve, 276
  risk, 274
  smoking, 274
  THC exposure, 279
Adolescent development
  early adolescence, 264
  late adolescence, 265
  middle adolescence, 264
  normal and abnormal, 270
Adolescent growth (AG), 72
Adolescent stage, 65
Adolescent varicocele
  clinical examination, 216
  epidemiology, 212
  etiology, 212–214
  history, 211–212
  management, 218–220
  nitrous oxide, 215
  pathophysiologic mechanisms, 214
  sperm parameters, 218
  surgical approaches, 220–221
  testicular volume and consistency, 216
Adolescents
  vs. adults, regulations, 276
  alcohol dependence, 277
  cannabis, 278
  CB1Rs, 279
  chronic alcohol exposure, 278
  chronic THC-induced spatial memory impairments, 279
  drugs of abuse, 274
  e-cigarettes, 275
  fertility hormones, 257
  human, 278
  IGF-I, 253
  marijuana, 279
  neurobiology, 274
  nicotine use, 275
  smoking initiation, 275
  steroids, 253
Adoptees, 70
Adrenal reflux, 214
Adrenarche
  adrenal androgens, 40
  gonadal development, 40
  traditional understanding, 40
Age at menarche (AAM), 129–130
Age at peak height velocity (APHV), 69, 72
Age at take-off (ATO), 65, 72
Alcohol, 190
  drug by adolescents, 276
  induced neurotoxicity, 277
American Acne and Rosacea Society, 201–203, 206
Anabolic androgenic steroids (AAS), 281
Androgens, 24, 186, 199, 204, 205
Angiographic embolization, 223
Anosmin-1, 172
Anti-Müllerian hormone (AMH), 24, 238
Aromatase, 185, 187, 189, 190, 192

P. Kumanov, A. Agarwal (eds.), *Puberty*, DOI 10.1007/978-3-319-32122-6

Aromatase inhibitor testolacton, 194
Aromatase inhibitors, 165, 194
Axillarche, 40, 46, 53
Azoospermia, 50

B
Bisphenol A (BPA), 110
Body mass index (BMI), 95
Body weight
  anorexia nervosa, 95
  BMI, 95
  boys, 97–99
  breast tissue, 96
  girls, 96–97
  mean testicular volume (ml), 98, 99
  overweight and obesity, 95
  pubertal development, 105
  pubertal maturation, 96
  underweight, 95
Bone age (BA), 88–89
Bone development
  aromatase gene, 87
  calcium, 77
  correlation coefficients, 85
  hormonal group, 87
  mechanical barrier, 77
  meta-analysis, 85, 87
  microarchitectural parameters, 88
  normal-weight controls, 84
  nutrition, 86
  physical activity, 85
  pre- and midpuberty, 84
  prepubertal females, 87
  puberty, 86
  weight and height, 84
Bone mineral accretion, 81–84
Bone mineral content (BMC), 81
Bone mineral density (BMD), 81, 158
Bone morphogenetic proteins (BMPs), 78
Bone remodeling unit (BMU), 81
Breast development, 41, 42

C
Canadian Laboratory Initiative on Pediatric Reference Interval Database, 252
Cannabinoid-1 receptors (CB1Rs), 279
Caucasian, 155
Central precocious puberty
  causal lesions, 150
  GnRH agonists, 148–150
  retrospective analyses, 150
Central precocious puberty (CPP), 126, 138, 173
Cephalocaudal (head-to-tail) gradient of growth, 70
Cerebellar electrophysiology, 277
Chemiluminescent, 248
Children
  fertility hormones, 257
  GHD, 250, 252
  steroids, 253
Chronic marijuana, 278
Chronic renal failure, 190
Comedones, 199, 200, 203, 207
Conditional target height SDS (cTHSDS), 66
Constitutional delay of growth and puberty (CDGP), 157, 160
Constitutional delay of puberty (CDP), 156, 175
Conventional varicocelectomy, 221
Cooperation on Science and Technology organisation, 180
Cortisol-binding globulin (CBG), 254
Cosmetic Measures, 241
CpG islands (CGIs), 111
Cushing's syndrome, 205, 254
Cystic fibrosis (CF), 70

D
Dehydroepiandrosterone (DHEA), 40, 253
Dehydroepiandrosterone sulfate (DHEAS), 40, 99, 189
Delayed puberty, 156–158
Deviations from normal adolescent development, 263
DHEA-sulfate (DHEAS), 253
Dibromochloropropane (DBCP), 110
Dichlorodiethyl dichloroethane (DDE), 126
Dichlorodiphenyltrichloroethane (DDT), 110
Dihydrotestosterone (DHT), 165, 198
Distance curve, 65
DNA methylation, 111
DNA methyltransferases (DNMTs), 111
DXA-derived FN, 82

E
Electrochemiluminescent, 248
Endocrine disorder, 233
Endocrine disruptors/endocrine-disrupting chemicals (EDCs)
  anthropometric and pubertal measures, 126
  BPA, 126
  CNS regulation, 125

CPP, 126
DDE, 127
DDT, 126
estrogenic activity, 125
industry, 125
mimic/block hormone signaling, 125
pesticides, 126
phthalate diesters, 126
phytoestrogens, 125
pregnancy, 126
Endocrine imbalance, 214
Endocrine-disrupting chemicals (EDC), 110
Estradiol, 46, 185
Estradiol/testosterone ratio, 190
Estradiol–testosterone, 186
Estrogen, 29
Ethanol, 276–278
External genitalia, 47

F
Facial hair growth, 53–54
Familial short stature (FSS), 160
Female reproductive axis
birth and infancy, 29–30
childhood, 30–31
fetal life, 29
hormone levels, 29, 30
menstrual cycle, 32
puberty, 31
Fibroblast growth factor 8 (FGF8), 172
First conscious ejaculation (FCE), 50
Flutamide, 241
Follicle-stimulating hormone (FSH), 1, 49, 97, 111, 169
Follicle-stimulating hormone receptor (FSHR), 123

G
Galanin like peptide (GALP), 102
Gametogenesis
DNA methylation, 111
EDC, 110
environmental chemicals, 110
environmental factors, 109, 110
histone modifications, 112–113
imprinted genes, 112
miRNAs, 114–116
non-imprinted genes, 111–112
parabens and phthalates, 110
PCB, 110
protamination, 113
puberty, 109
urinary metabolite levels, 110
Gas chromatography–mass spectrometry (GC–MS), 256
Gaussian distribution of puberty, 160
Genome Wide Association Studies (GWAS), 122
GH and IGF-I assays
clinical significance, 251–253
GHRH, 247
IGFBP-3, 247, 250–251
IGF-I and IGFBP-3 immunoassays, 249–250
immunoassays, 248–249
steroid assays, 253–259
GH deficiency (GHD), 250
GH receptor (GHR), 248
GH stimulation testing, 165
GH therapy, 165
GH-binding protein (GHBP), 248
Glucose transporter type 4 (GLUT-4), 233
GnRH agonists
bone mineral density, 149
breast/testicular development, 149
long-term outcomes, 149
pituitary gonadotrophs, 148
tolerance, 149, 150
GnRH pulsatility
bioinformatic platforms, 180
constitutional pubertal delay, 179
functional categorization, 170, 171
KS/nIHH, 173
LH and FSH, 169
mini-puberty, 169–170
mouse hypogonadal (hpg) model, 173
neuroendocrine process, 169
neuron development, 172
pubertal prognosis, 179–180
puberty, 170
upstream inhibition, 170–172
GnRH signalling, 173
GnRH Stimulation Test, 219
GnRH/Gonadotropin-Releasing System
cues relieving prepubertal restraint, 6–7
estrogen-dependent and estrogen-independent prepubertal restraint, 4–6
KNDy neurons, 2–4
MUA volleys, 2
pubertal restraint, 4, 5
sexual maturation, 2
tonic and surge-mode, 2
Gonadal androgen secretion, 198

Gonadarche, 51–52
HPG reactivation, 40
pubertal key step, 40
somatotrophic axis, 40
Gonadotropin secretion, 156, 190
Gonadotropin-releasing hormone (GnRH), 13, 40, 97, 109, 159, 233
Gonadotropin-releasing hormone receptor (GNRHR) gene, 159
Gonadotropins, 24, 32, 165
GPR54 gene, 3
Grade III varicocele, 217
Growth factors, 87
Growth hormone (GH), 41, 67, 184, 199
Growth hormone (GH)/insulin-like growth factor (IGF) axis, 33
Growth in childhood
assortative mating, 66
centile, 65
distance curves, 65
dynamic process, 66
home-made measurements, 67
human development, 65
juvenile stage, 65
saltation and stasis, 67
short-term growth, 67
skeletal robustness, 71
Growth plate, 77–80

H
Height at take-off (HTO), 72
Hereditary predisposition, 237
High-risk behavior
adolescence, 267
alcohol and peers, 269
Hirsutism, 230, 240, 241
Hispanics, 155
Histone demethylases (HDM), 113
Histone methyltransferases (HTM), 113
Historia animalium, 127
Home-made measurements, 67
Hormonal changes
adrenal axis, 33
growth axis, 33–34
insulin and carbohydrate metabolism, 34–35
Hormonal imbalance, 229
Hormone-binding protein, 48
Human chorionic gonadotropin (hCG), 188
Human maturation
industrial revolution, 127
menarche, 127
metabolic syndrome, 121
physicians, 127
Hyperandrogenemia, 234–235
Hyperinsulinemia, 235
Hyperthyroidism, 189
Hypogonadotropic hypogonadism, 3
Hypothalamic amenorrhoea (HA), 171, 175
Hypothalamic regulation, gonadal axis
GnRH, 1
gonadotropins, 1
novel neuropeptide signaling, 2
Hypothalamic-pituitary-gonadal (HPG) axis, 23, 39, 96, 109, 121, 157, 170
Hypothalamic-pituitary-gonadal function, 164

I
Idiopathic hypogonadotropic hypogonadism (IHH), 159
Immunoassays (IAs)
IGF-I and IGFBP-3, 249–250
Immunoglobulin superfamily member 1 (IGSF1), 159
Infertility, 211, 212, 218–220
Inhibin B, 163
Insulin resistance, 233
Insulin sensitivity, 34
Insulin-like factor 3 (INSL3), 24
Insulin-like growth factor (IGF), 103
Insulin-like growth factor-1 (IGF1), 41
Internal genitalia, 46
Intrauterine growth retardation (IUGR), 174

J
Juvenile period, 6

K
Kallmann syndrome (KS), 172, 175
Kisspeptin, 3
Kisspeptin 1 (KISS-1), 102
Klinefelter syndrome, 187, 191
KNDy neurons, 2–4

L
Laparoscopic Varicocelectomy, 222
Leptin (LEP), 88, 176
Luteinizing hormone (LH), 1, 97, 169, 188
Lymphadenopathy, 193

M
Macrogynecomastia, 192
Macrophage colony-stimulating factor (M-CSF), 80

Magnetic resonance imaging (MRI), 146
Male reproductive axis
  AMH and inhibin B, 24
  birth and infancy, 24–26
  childhood, 26–27
  fetal life, 24
  hormone levels, 24, 25
  ontogeny, 24, 26
  puberty, 27–28
Mammography, 193
Marijuana, 278–280
Mass spectrometry (MS)
  GH, IGF-I and IGFBP-3, 250–251
  ID-MS-based assay, 252
  LC–MS/MS, 253–259
  steroid analysis, 256–257, (*see also* Steroid hormones)
McCune–Albright syndrome, 151
Medial preoptic area (mPOA), 5
Medical therapy, 194
Menarche, 46–47
Menstrual irregularities, 235–242
Metastin, 2
Metformin, 239–240
MicroRNAs (miRNAs)
  Dicer1 gene, 114
  Drosha knockouts, 114
  endo-siRNAs, 116
  environmental pollution, 115
  fertility biomarkers, 115
  meiotic and mitotic phases, 115
  next-generation sequencing analysis, 114
  spermatogenesis, 114, 115
Microsurgical varicocelectomy, 222
Migrants, 70
Mini-puberty, 169–170
Multiple unit neuronal activity (MUA), 2

N
nAChR expression, 276
Nasal embryonic LHRH factor (*NELF*), 172
National Center for Health Statistics, 124
National Health and Nutrition Examination Survey (NHANES), 98
National Institute of Biological Standards and Control (NIBSC), 249
Neuroadaptations, 278
Neurobiology, 274, 276, 277, 280
Neurokinin B (NKB), 3
Neuropeptide Y/agouti-related protein (NPY/AgRP)-expressing neurons, 101
Nicotine, 274–276
Nicotine pharmacokinetics, 275
Nicotine-induced upregulation, 276
Nicotinic acetylcholine receptor (nAChR) expression, 276
Normosmic idiopathic hypogonadotropic hypogonadism (nIHH), 170, 175

O
Obesity, 187, 235
Old World Europeans, 74
Oligomenorrhea, 229, 230, 232, 235
Oligo-ovulation, 234
Onset of puberty, 121, 124, 125, 127–131
  boys
    genital area, 130
    genital stage 2 (G2), 130
    pubertal maturation, 130
    pubic hair development and longitudinal, 130
    spermarche (ejacularche), 131
    testicular growth and pubic hair development, 131
    TV, 131
  environmental factors
    childhood, 125
    chronic illnesses, 125
    health hazard, 124
    parental education, 125
    pubertal timing, 125
    sexual maturation, 125
  ethnic/racial influences, 124
  factors, 122, 123
  genetic and epigenetic, 122–123
  girls
    AAM, 129–130
    BMI, 128
    breast and pubic hair development, 128
    cross-sectional and longitudinal, 128
    maturational tempo and age, menarche, 130
    PH2, 128
    PROS, 128
    socioeconomic conditions and the hygiene, 127
    transitional society, 128
  HPG, 121
Onset of pubic hair development (PH2), 128
Osteoblastogenesis, 80–81
Osteoclastogenesis, 80–81
Ovarian dysfunction, 236
Overweight and obesity
  adipocytes and hormone leptin, 103, 104
  childhood, 100
  critical body weight, 100
  dual-energy X-ray absorptiometry, 100
  endocrine organ, 101

Overweight and obesity (*cont.*)
fat mass, 102
GALP, 102
gonadal steroids, 100
gonadotropins, 100
hypothalamic nucleus arcuatus, 101
hypothalamic pulse generator, 100
insulin, 102
insulin resistance, 103
kisspeptin, 102
leptin, 101
milk feeding, 103
neurotransmitter and neuromodulatory systems, 100
puberty, 100
testosterone, 101

P
Paracrine Regulation, 215
Parathyroid hormone-related peptide (PTHrp), 79, 184
Peak bone mass (PBM), 84
Peak height velocity (PHV), 43, 48, 66–68
Pediatric Research in Office Settings (PROS), 128
Penile growth, 54–55
Peripheral precocious puberty
causal lesions, 150
medications, 151
Persistent organic pollutants (POP), 110
Peutz–Jeghers syndrome, 189
Polychlorinated biphenyls (PCBs), 110
Polycomb group proteins, 123
Polycystic ovarian syndrome (PCOS), 149
AMH levels, 239
clinical features, 230–231
definition, 229
diagnosis, 231, 238
endocrine disorder, 233
epidemiology, 230
GnRH, 234
insulin resistance, 233
lifestyle modification, 239
management, 239
prevalence, 230
valproic acid, 236
Postmenarcheal age, 47
Preadolescent period (Stage B1), 41
Precocious puberty (PP)
breast development, 141
central/peripheral mechanisms, 137
definition, 137
GnRH stimulation tests, 138
growth velocity, 141
identification, 137
neuroimaging, 146
pelvic ultrasound scans, 145
precocious puberty *vs.* slowly progressive forms, 146
premature sexual maturation, 137
puberty timing, 142
sexual abuse, 142
Premature pubarche, 148
Premature sexual development
clinical diagnosis, 142–144
CPP, 138, 139
etiologies and mechanisms, 138–139
gonadotropin determinations, 145
isolated premature breast development/ premature thelarche, 147
peripheral precocious puberty, 138, 140–141
precocious puberty, 143–147
psychosocial aspects, 148
pubic hair/premature pubarche, 148
sex steroid determinations, 144–145
slow progression, 148
Premature thelarche, 147
Pri-miRNAs, 114
Primordial germ cells (PGCs), 111
Progestogens, 241
Prolactin receptors, 189
Proopiomelanocortin/cocaine- and amphetamine-regulated transcript (POMC/CART)-expressing neurons, 101
Proportional age, 71
Psychosocial development, 264, 265
adolescence, 263
adolescents, 269–270
brain, 269
eating behaviors, 266
environment and family, 268
individual, 267–268
neuropsychological changes, 263
normal development
early adolescence, 264
late adolescence, 265
middle adolescence, 264
peers, 268–269
pubertal, 269
sexual activity, 266
substance use, 266
suicide, 265
violence, 266
YRBSS, 265
Pubarche, 40, 44–46, 53

Pubertal acne
adrenal androgens, 205
clinical features, 199
epidemiology and demographic profile, 197
etiopathogenesis, 198
GH, 199
microcomedone, 200
microcomedone formation, 206
pathogenesis, 200
prognosis, 207
pubertal and prepubertal, 205
Quality of Life, 207
sebum production, 197
Pubertal delay
adult-onset idiopathic hypogonadotropic hypogonadism, 175
CDP, 175
DAX1, 177
FGFR1, 178
genetic testing, 176
GnRH deficiency, 176, 177
HA, 175
micropenis/cryptorchidism, 175
monogenicity *vs.* oligogenicity, 178–179
nonreproductive features, 175
phenotypic clues, 176–178
PROK2, 178
skeletal defects, 175
SOX10, 178
Pubertal gonadotropin stimulation, 156
Pubertal gynecomastia
breast development, 184–185
estrogen and progesterone, 185
estrogen receptor, 184
etiology and pathogenesis, 185–191
mammary glandular tissues, 183
mammography, 193
prevalence, 185, 189
steroids, 183
treatment, 193–194
Pubertal height spurt, 47–48, 55
Pubertal maturation, 204
Pubertal timing
environmental factors, 174
genetics, 173
Pubertal weight, 48, 55
Puberty, 155–156
adolescence, 13
classical diagrams, 57
definition, 13
delayed, 156–158
environmental influences, 19
factors, 14
functional pubertal delay, 157
Gaussian distribution, 160
genes, 16, 17
genetic factors, 15–17
GnRH, 13
gonadal failure, 157
gonadotropins, 39
hypothalamic-pituitary dysfunction, 157
laboratory assessment, 162–164
mechanisms, 14
metabolic control, 17–19
neuropeptide regulation, 14–15
physical changes, 264
physical observations, 162
psychosocial challenges, 266–267
pubertal development, 269
secondary sex characteristics, 39
steroid levels, 56
Tanner stage, 155
timing and tempo, 155
transcriptional regulation, 17, 18
Pubic hair (PH), 44
development stages, 45
growth, 155

Q

Quality control (QC) materials, 249

R

RNA-induced silencing complex (RISC), 114
Rochester orchidometer, 217
Rostral periventricular area of the third ventricle (RP3V), 169

S

Saliva steroid, 254
Semen analysis, 218, 220, 223
Sertoli cell dysfunction, 215
Sertoli cells, 111
Sex hormone-binding globulin (SHBG), 101, 185, 236, 254
Sex steroids, 79
Sex-corrected midparental, 165
Sperm chromatin packaging, 113
Spermarche, 50, 53
Spironolactone, 241
Split hand/foot malformation (SHFM), 178
Standard deviation or Z-scores (SDS), 68
Standard deviation scores (SDS), 66
Stein–Leventhal syndrome, 229

Steroid hormones
adrenal gland, 253
analytical methods, 253
by mass spectrometry, 256–257
estradiol, 253
free *vs.* total steroid measurement, 254–255
immunochemical assays, 255–256
results and reference intervals, 257–259
synthesis, 253
Subinguinal approach, 221
Substance use
AAS, 281
adolescence, 273
adolescence permanently changes, 274
adolescent neurobiology, 274
adolescents, 280
developmental period, 280
environmental and psychosocial factors, 273
ethanol, 276–278
in mind, 274
marijuana, 278–280
nicotine, 274–276
preclinical research, 274
prefrontal cortex, 274
progression, 274
societal concern, 281

T
"T"-zone, 204
Tanner stage 4, 86
Tanner stages, 41, 53, 155
Tanner–Whitehouse method, 68
Target height (TH), 66
Target-seeking process, 66
Tempo
acceleration, 68
and amplitude, 72
biological age, 68
catch-up growth, 70
growth as a target-seeking process, 74
pubertal maturity, 68
skeletal maturity, 68
Testicular development, 48–50
Testicular neoplasms, 188
Testicular volume (TV), 55, 121, 213, 215, 216, 218, 219
Testosterone response to hCG, 163
Testosterone therapy, 165
THC-induced memory, 279
The Avon Longitudinal Study, 44
The US Centers for Disease Control (CDC), 265
Thyreostimulating hormone (TSH), 192
Thyroid transcription factor 1 (TTF1), 17
Transition proteins (TPs), 113
Transvaginal or transrectal ultrasound, 238
Tubular duct system, 184

U
Ultrasonography (US), 122, 192
Underweight, 103–105
3′ untranslated region (3′UTR), 114

V
Valproic acid, 236–237
Varicocele, 188
Vascular endothelial growth factor (VEGF), 79
Velocity curve, 65
Voice break, 54

W
Waardenburg syndrome (WS), 178

Y
Youth Risk Behavior Surveillance System (YRBSS), 265

Printed by Printforce, the Netherlands